The Cranial Nerves in Neurology

Wolfgang Grisold · Walter Struhal
Anna Grisold

The Cranial Nerves in Neurology

A comprehensive and systematic evaluation of cranial nerves, pathology and specific conditions

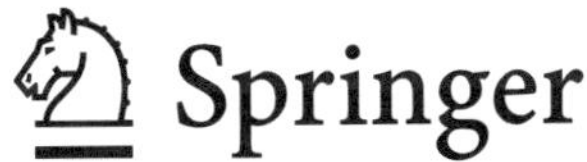 Springer

Wolfgang Grisold
Ludwig Boltzmann Institute for
Experimental und Clinical Traumatology
Vienna, Austria

Anna Grisold
Department of Neurology
Medical University of Vienna
Vienna, Austria

Walter Struhal
Karl Landsteiner University of Health
Sciences, Division of Neurology
University Clinic Tulln
Tulln, Austria

ISBN 978-3-031-43083-1   ISBN 978-3-031-43081-7 (eBook)
https://doi.org/10.1007/978-3-031-43081-7

This Springer imprint is published by the registered company Springer Nature Switzerland AG
The registered company address is: Gewerbestrasse 11, 6330 Cham, Switzerland

Paper in this product is recyclable.

Acknowledgment

The editors thank all contributors of this book, which has been stimulated by the Atlas of Neuromuscular Disease (now in its third edition). The Atlas has an important and useful chapter on CNs that was used as the basis for Part II of this book and has been completely updated. The co-editors of the Atlas III Eva Feldman, James Russell, Wolfgang Löscher, and Stefan Meng, as well as Udo Zifko for the first edition, need acknowledgment, as do several authors of specific chapters who stimulated the previous chapter on CNs.

This book is also a multi-author book, mainly but not exclusively from neurologists, and we want to thank our coauthors. This collection of authors also shows how important interdisciplinary work is, and particularly in the field of CNs there is a strong interdependency of various medical and surgical fields.

In each book, there is also a longer history, and I want to acknowledge my clinical teacher and mentor Kurt Jellinger, who stimulated neurology from the classical view of neuropathology and localization and inspired me to engage in neurophysiology and the use of imaging.

My other clinical teacher, Prof. Stacher, a hematologist-oncologist, stimulated my scientific career and taught me humanities in regard to patients and their caregivers.

My co-editors, Walter Struhal and my daughter Anna Grisold, are two further generations of neurology whom I have had the pleasure to work with in many neurological aspects, and I want to thank them for their vigor and contributions.

Stacey Sakowski has also edited the book with us, and we thank her for her excellent and diligent work.

Contents

Part III   The Cranial Nerves in Specific Conditions (Diseases)

Contributors

Naela Alhani Karl Landsteiner University of Health Sciences, University Clinic of Neurology, University Hospital Tulln, Tulln, Austria

Vera Bril Division of Neurology, Ellen and Martin Prosserman Centre for Neuromuscular Disorders, University Health Network, University of Toronto, Toronto, ON, Canada

Silvia Casagrande Neurology Unit, Azienda Provinciale per i Servizi Sanitari (APSS), Trento, Italy

Kristl G. Claeys Department of Neurology, University Hospitals Leuven, Leuven, Belgium

Laboratory for Muscle Diseases and Neuropathies, Department of Neurosciences, KU Leuven, Leuven, Belgium

Yosef Ellenbogen Division of Neurosurgery, University of Toronto, Toronto, ON, Canada

Bruno Giometto Neurology Unit, Azienda Provinciale per i Servizi Sanitari (APSS), Trento, Italy

University of Trento, Trento, Italy

Anna Grisold Department of Neurology, Medical University of Vienna, Vienna, Austria

Simon Grisold Psychiatry, ESRA, Psychosoziales Zentrum, Vienna, Austria

Wolfgang Grisold Ludwig Boltzmann Institute for Experimental und Clinical Traumatology, Vienna, Austria

Carrie Katherine Grouse Department of Neurology, and Ambulatory Informatics, UCSF Health, University of California San Francisco, San Francisco, CA, USA

A. Hainfellner Division of Anatomy and Medical Imaging Cluster, Medical University of Vienna, Vienna, Austria

Johannes Herta Department of Neurosurgery, General Hospital Vienna, Medical University of Vienna, Vienna, Austria

Barbara Horvath-Mechtler Department of Radiology, Favoriten Clinic, Vienna, Austria

Diagnostic Center 22, Vienna, Austria

Satish V. Khadilkar Department of Neurology, Bombay Hospital Institute of Medical Sciences, Mumbai, India

Matthew C. Kiernan Neurology, Brain and Mind Centre, University of Sydney, Sydney, NSW, Australia
Neurology, Royal Prince Alfred Hospital, Camperdown, NSW, Australia

Martin Krenn Department of Neurology, Medical University of Vienna, Vienna, Austria

Helmar Lehmann Department of Neurology, Medical Faculty University Hospital Cologne, Köln, Germany

Stefan Leis Department of Neurology, Christian Doppler Klinik, University Hospital Salzburg, Paracelsus Medical University Salzburg, Salzburg, Austria

Steven L. Lewis World Federation of Neurology, London, UK
Neurology, Lehigh Valley Fleming Neuroscience Institute, Lehigh Valley Health Network, Allentown, PA, USA

Wolfgang N. Löscher Department of Neurology, Medical University Innsbruck, Innsbruck, Tyrol, Austria

Doriana Lupescu Department of Anaesthesia and Intensive Care, Buftea Obstetrics and Gynaecology Hospital, Buftea, Ilfov County, Romania

Tudor Lupescu Department of Neurology, "Prof. Dr. Agrippa Ionescu" Emergency Clinical Hospital, Bucharest, Romania

Stefan Meng Division of Anatomy and Medical Imaging Cluster, Medical University of Vienna, Vienna, Austria
Department of Radiology, Hanusch Hospital, Vienna, Austria

Deepak Menon Ellen and Martin Prosserman Centre for Neuromuscular Disorders, University Health Network, University of Toronto, Toronto, ON, Canada

Susanna B. Park Faculty of Medicine and Health, Brain and Mind Centre, University of Sydney, Camperdown, NSW, Australia

Riddhi Patel Department of Neurology, Bombay Hospital Institute of Medical Sciences, Mumbai, India

Franz Riederer Department of Neurology, Clinic Hietzing, Vienna, Austria
Faculty of Medicine, University of Zurich, Zürich, Switzerland

Karl Roessler Department of Neurosurgery, Medical University of Vienna, Vienna, Austria

Stacey A. Sakowski Department of Neurology, University of Michigan, Ann Arbor, MI, USA

Robert Schmidhammer Millesi Center for Surgery of Peripheral Nerves, Vienna Private Clinic, Vienna, Austria

Walter Struhal Karl Landsteiner University of Health Sciences, Division of Neurology, University Clinic Tulln, Tulln, Austria

Suganth Suppiah Division of Neurosurgery, University of Toronto, Toronto, ON, Canada

Savas Tsolakidis Millesi Center for Surgery of Peripheral Nerves, Vienna Private Clinic, Vienna, Austria

W. J. Weninger Division of Anatomy and Medical Imaging Cluster, Medical University of Vienna, Vienna, Austria

Fabian Winter Department of Neurosurgery, Medical University of Vienna, Vienna, Austria

Gelareh Zadeh Division of Neurosurgery, University of Toronto, Toronto, ON, Canada

Udo A. Zifko Department of Neurology, Evangelisches Krankenhaus, Vienna, Austria

CNs are the most important connections of the brain, with motor, sensory, autonomic, and sense functions, and they are also essential for our communication with the environment. Part II of this book discusses all CNs and has an additional chapter on functions that involve several CNs at the same time. These chapters are based on the anatomic details and the possibilities of imaging and electrophysiology from Part I.

Conventionally, we distinguish 12 pairs of CNs, which all have their nuclei in the brainstem except for CNs I and II. Historically, several other classifications were used, but modern neurology uses this present classification successfully. The course of each CN is described in regard to intracranial and extracranial locations, as well as the site of the exit of the skull. The extracavitary route of the CNs can be short (e.g., ending in the orbit), or long (e.g., vagal nerve). After the CNs leave the skull, the CNs (except CN I and II) are considered peripheral nerves, are dependent on local changes, and need blood supply from extracranial arteries. CNs are connected by several anastomosis, particularly of autonomic fibers. In the cervical region, anastomoses with the cervical plexus is also of importance.

These features of anatomy are more complex, with the CNs bearing special senses, such as vision, smell, taste, hearing, and balance. Electrophysiological properties allow testing of function, and recent imaging progress has allowed an even closer look at their anatomy and structure.

CNs can be restricted or damaged in their function within the CNS, resulting in impairment of complex tasks (optomotor system, facial expression, deglutition, and swallowing), or as a focal lesion, usually in the brainstem, or in the intracranial course. All CNs have defined and marked points of transition through the skull, and specific syndromes are described according to the site of the lesion. These lesions of the exit of CNs are usually characterized by characteristic syndromes defined by the vicinity of several structures, such as vessels and lymph nodes.

Part II of the book is a classical account of the descriptions and functions of CNs I–XII, which is based on symptoms, signs, localization of lesions, and causes. Chapter 18 summarizes functions that cannot be attributed to a single CN but are always executed in synergy. Examples are the pupil, the eyelid function, and others.

Complex optomotor functions, such as gaze paralysis, nystagmus, internuclear ophthalmoplegia, saccadic eye movements, are briefly discussed in Chap. 19, and the reader is referred to textbooks on optomotor function.

Part III of this book describes specific situations and diseases and related CN functions and might help to identify CN lesions in trauma, diabetes, inflammatory disease, and toxic causes, among others. Also, a summary of phenomena in psychiatric disorders is presented, as it is helpful to consider these rare phenomena.

A book on CNs can never be complete since different accents and deeper and more detailed associations can be found from the point of other specialty fields, such as ophthalmology, ENT, and neurosurgery. This summary aims to be comprehensive and useful for neurologists and is based on anatomy, imaging, electrophysiology, and clinical neurological investigations. It acknowledges the need to consult with other specialties in many cases.

Anatomy of the Cranial Nerves: Novel Concepts and Traditional Descriptions

1

Bullet Points

- This chapter describes and richly illustrates the anatomy of the cranial nerves and the visceral (vegetative) nervous pathways in the head.
- It pragmatically relies on traditional systematics; however, it discusses inadequacies in terminology and acknowledges the direction of action potential conduction for describing course and branching.

Introduction

Cranial nerves (CNs) are defined as bundles of nerve fibers, which leave or enter the brain. Hence, they are the white matter of the peripheral nervous system, with all its consequences (*e.g.,* regeneration after injury).

Reflecting the body symmetry, cranial nerves are always paired. The perikarya of the neurons are either located in motor or parasympathetic brain nuclei (multipolar neurons of efferent fibers) or in bipolar or pseudounipolar ganglia along their course (pseudounipolar or bipolar neurons of afferent fibers). The central axons emerging from the pseudounipolar or bipolar ganglion cells then synapse with multipolar neurons in sensory nuclei.

When leaving or entering the brain, the nerves may comprise fibers of all qualities, except for sympathetic. Yet, especially when derived from perikarya located in the superior cervical ganglion, postganglionic sympathetic fibers often join branches of cranial nerves. They use them to travel to blood vessels, brain structures, and glands, particularly salivary and sweat glands in the skin. On their way, they often do not stick to one nerve but "hop" from nerve to nerve or branch to branch until they enter their targets.

Traditionally, some nerves are described as purely sensory (afferent) or purely motor (efferent). However, in most cases, this is a simplification. At least some segments of almost all nerves comprise afferent and efferent fibers. As an example, motor nerves innervate muscle fibers. However, afferent fibers derived from proprioceptors travel as part of the terminal branches.

In the head, a noteworthy general phenomenon is that cranial nerves extensively feature "fiber exchange." This, as in modern literature, is better described as "fiber hopping." Nerve fibers often consecutively join and leave several nerves until they reach their targets. Hence, several cranial nerves and sympathetic fibers resemble a large nerve plexus rather than a system of distinct nerves. The branches of CN V especially "hop on" and "hop off" of nerve fibers. For example, the lingual nerve, a branch of the mandibular nerve, is considered to be composed of general

---

Authors of this chapter: Weninger W. J. and Hainfellner A.

© The Author(s), under exclusive license to Springer Nature Switzerland AG 2023
W. Grisold et al., *The Cranial Nerves in Neurology*, https://doi.org/10.1007/978-3-031-43081-7_1

somatic afferent (GSA) fibers. However, certain peripheral segments also comprise pre- and post-ganglionic parasympathetic, sympathetic, and special visceral afferent (SVA) fibers in various combinations (see sections "CN V" and "parasympathetic Ganglia"). To overcome the problem of the changing fiber compositions in the description of the "fiber quality" of cranial nerves along their way from the periphery to the brain or vice versa, the following chapters primarily consider the composition of nerves at their exit/entrance from/into the brain or their most central portion when defining general fiber quality.

Systematics

Classic textbooks (*e.g.,* Gray's Anatomy [1]) distinguish twelve pairs of cranial nerves. They are referred to as left and right CN I to CN XII. The sequence reflects the position at which the nerves leave the brain and at which they perforate the dura mater encephali (Fig. 1.1).

However, this traditional classification is highly insufficient and confusing. It essentially ignores many facts learned in the last centuries. Most prominently, it ignores the existence of the terminal nerve (CN 0 or CN XIII) and the true nature of CN II as white matter of the central nervous system. It also considers the motor portion of CN V as part of CN V at large, summarizes the intermediate and facial nerves as CN VII, considers CN XI as a nerve formed by a cranial and a spinal root, and ignores phylogenetic considerations regarding CN XI and CN XII. These weaknesses of traditional nomenclature have triggered a large number of alternative classifications [2–9], and each one makes fair points. Yet, until now, none of the alternatives was successful in replacing the traditional nomenclature.

This chapter will therefore pragmatically rely on the traditional terminology. However, it will group the pairs of cranial nerves relying on obvious similarities and refer to the most prominent of the countless inconsistencies when describing the single "nerves" (Table 1.1).

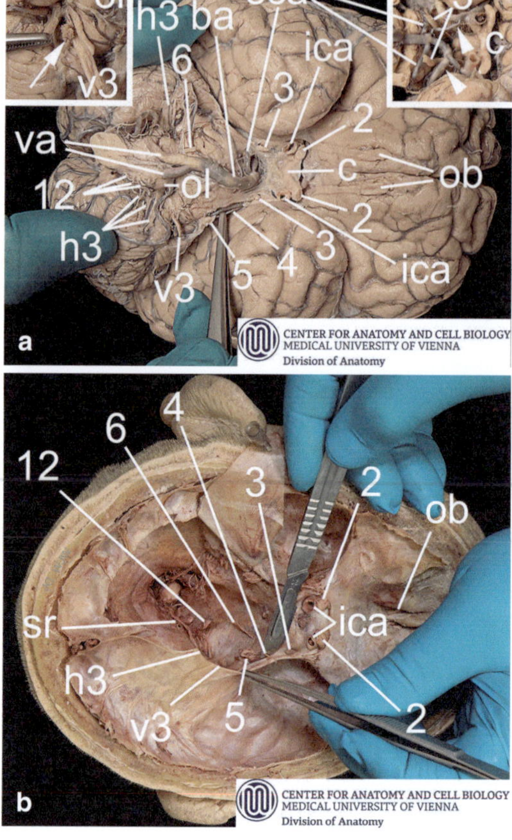

Fig. 1.1 Sequence of cranial nerves (CN) according to conventional nomenclature. Frontal to the right. Note the sequential brain and dura exit/entrance of the cranial nerves. Numbers refer to respective CNs. (**a**) Base of the brain. Except for the pontal cistern, the arachnoid mater forming the basal cisterns is largely preserved. The arachnoid mater covering the ambient cistern is opened, and CN IV [4] is lifted with a forceps. Left-sided inlay highlights the relationship of the nerves of the cerebellopontine angle (v3), Bochdalek's flower basket (arrow), and CN IX (held in forceps) as the most rostral nerve of those, exiting at the anterolateral sulcus (h3). Right-sided inlay magnifies the relationship of CN III [3] with the superior cerebellar (sca) and posterior cerebral arteries (arrowhead). Arachnoid mater of the basal cisterns is removed. The brain displayed in the inlay is different from the brain displayed in the main panel. Note the dimension of the left-sided posterior cerebral artery. (**b**) Skull base with cranial nerves, cut near their penetration through the dura mater. Stumps of right-sided cranial nerves are labeled with numbers. 2, CN II; 3, CN III; 4, CN IV; 5, CN V; 6, CN VI; 12, CN XII; ob, olfactory bulb; ica, internal carotid artery; ba, basilar artery; va, vertebral artery; ol, oliva; c, optic chiasm; sr, sinus rectus

Table 1.1 Traditional systematics of cranial nerves

Cranial nerve	Brain nuclei	Gross position of nuclei in CNS	Skull transition	Inconsistencies with official nomenclature
CN I	Olfactory bulb	Telencephalon	Cribriform plate	Definition of terminal nerve (CN 0, CN XIII)
CN II		Diencephalon	Optic canal	Definition of "nerve" (PNS) versus "tract" (CNS)
CN III	Oculomotor nucleus Accessory oculomotor nucleus	Mesencephalon	Superior orbital fissure	
CN IV	Trochlear nucleus	Mesencephalon	Superior orbital fissure	
CN V	Motor nucleus Mesencephalic nucleus Principal sensory nucleus Spinal trigeminal nucleus	Mesencephalon, Rhombencephalon, Spinal cord	Superior orbital fissure Foramen rotundum Foramen ovale	2 nerves (independent motor and sensory portion)
CN VI	Abducens nucleus	Rhombencephalon	Superior orbital fissure	
CN VII	Motor nucleus Lacrimal nucleus Salivatory nucleus Solitary nucleus	Rhombencephalon	Internal acoustic meatus	2 nerves (N. intermedius and N. facialis)
CN VIII	4 vestibular nuclei (Bechterew, Schwalbe, Roller, Deiters) 2 cochlear nuclei (dorsal, ventral)	Rhombencephalon	Internal acoustic meatus	2 nerves instead of 2 portions of 1 nerve
CN IX	Sensory nucleus Nucleus ambiguous Spinal trigeminal nucleus Solitary nucleus Inferior salivatory nucleus	Rhombencephalon	Nervous part of jugular foramen	
CN X	Dorsal nucleus Nucleus ambiguous Solitary nucleus Spinal trigeminal nucleus	Rhombencephalon	Nervous part of jugular foramen	
CN XI	Nucleus ambiguous Spinal nucleus	Rhombencephalon Spinal cord	Nervous part of jugular foramen	Cranial radix is part of CN X
CN XII	Hypoglossal nucleus	Rhombencephalon	Hypoglossal canal	United segmental nerves

CN cranial nerve, *PNS* peripheral nervous system, *CNS* central nervous system

Thematically, the chapter does not aim to describe every single detail of cranial nerve systematics and topology but merely intends to provide a comprehensive overview. Furthermore, in contrast to traditional textbooks, the descriptions will follow the direction of action potentials whenever possible. This means that afferent (*e.g.,* sensory) nerves are described from the periphery to the central nervous system and efferent (*e.g.,* motor, parasympathetic) nerves from the central nervous system to the periphery. Finally, relationships of cranial nerves and the visceral (autonomic) nervous system will be described in Chap. 27, following the systematic descriptions of the cranial nerves.

Cranial Nerves

Olfactory Nerve (CN I)

CN I is a sensory nerve communicating olfactory information via SVA fibers. The fibers emanate from neurons, which are located in the mucosa overlying the upper nasal concha and septum nasi and ascend toward the cribriform plate. They form bundles, called fila olfactoria. The sum of the fila olfactory is referred to as CN I (Fig. 1.2).

The fila pass separately through the foramina of the cribriform plate and perforate the overlying dura and arachnoid mater. They then immediately enter the olfactory bulb and synapse with its multipolar neurons. Axons of the neurons of the

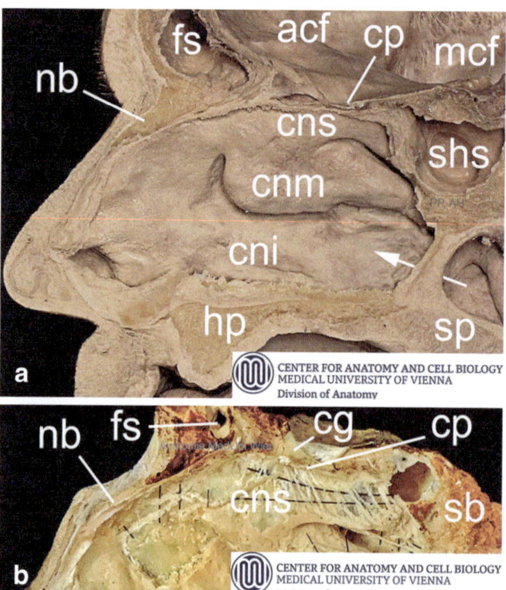

Fig. 1.2 Cranial nerve (CN) I. Lateral wall of left-sided nasal cavities. Frontal to the left. (**a**) Undissected specimen, showing the mucosa covering the concha nasalis superior (cns), concha nasalis medialis (cnm), concha nasalis inferior (cni), and the rest of the lateral nasal cavity. Note the thinness of the cribriform plate (cp), which borders anterior cranial fossa (acf) and nasal cavity. (**b**) Specimen from the historical collection of the Division of Anatomy of the Medical University of Vienna. The mucosa is removed from the cns and the fila olfactoria are displayed. Mcf, medial cranial fossa; cg, crista galli; hp., hard palate; sp., soft palate; sb, sphenoid bone; shs, sphenoid sinus; fs, frontal sinus; nb, nasal bone; arrow points through right choana

olfactory bulb converge and form the olfactory tract, which travels occipitally, toward the trigonum nuclei and the telencephalic cortex. Although the olfactory bulb and tract are distinct structures, located beneath and isolated from the frontal lobe of the telencephalon (Figs. 1.1 and 1.3), they are the central nervous system.

Terminal Nerve (CN 0, CN XIII)

SVA fibers, connected to pheromone receptors in the mucosa of the anterior septum, are often considered to be part of CN I. However, their course substantially differs from the course of the fibers forming the fila olfactoria.

In the mucosa, these fibers have a close relationship to the branches of the trigeminal nerve. However, they soon leave them and ascend towards the cribriform plate. They perforate this plate, but, contrary to fibers of CN I, they do not penetrate the dura and arachnoidea mater encephali and do not enter the gray matter of the olfactory bulb. Instead, they stay extradural and form an elongated plexus, which extends medially and in parallel to the olfactory tract toward the jugum sphenoidale. Only here do the fibers perforate both the dura and arachnoid mater to continue their occipital course in the subarachnoid space. Finally, the fibers reach and enter the forebrain at the terminal lamina, where they synapse with central neurons.

Considering the course of the fibers of the terminal nerve, their bypassing of the olfactory bulb and the arrangement that permits instant transfer of information to a telencephalic cortical region implies that these fibers have to be considered as a distinct nerve. Since the nerve enters at the terminal lamina, the name "terminal nerve" was suggested, although CN 0 or CN XIII are also in use [5–8].

Optic "Nerve" (CN II)

The optic "nerve" is a component of the visual system (Fig. 1.3). It is traditionally referred to as a nerve, comprising special somatic (SSA) fibers.

Fig. 1.3 Cranial nerve (CN) II [2], according to conventional terminology. (**a**) Topology of CN II in the orbit. Silicon preserved coronal section through a human head. Specimen from the Anatomy Teaching Unit of the Medical University of Vienna. Dorsal view. Inlay magnifies CN II in the right orbit. It is surrounded by meninges and subarachnoid space (as). In its center travels the central retinal artery (cra). Main panel shows the relationship of CN II and the inferior (irm), lateral (lrm), superior (srm), and medial (mrm) rectus muscles. Small branches of CN III and CN V are discernable near them. The supraorbital nerve (son) is visible beneath the orbital roof and the infraorbital nerve (ion) in a groove at the orbit floor. Also, note the transition zone between the olfactory bulb and tract (ot). (**b**) Three-dimensional (3D) computer model of the forming brain of an early mouse embryo (left view). Optic stalk (os), which remodels to CN II, and optic cup (arrows) are lateral extensions of the gray and white matter of the diencephalon (di). Inlay shows these structures from the anterior. to, tongue; m, mandible; slg, sublingual gland; tel, telencephalon; osm, oblique superior muscle; mes, mesencephalon; c, anlage of cerebellum; po, pons; my, myelencephalon; sc, spinal cord

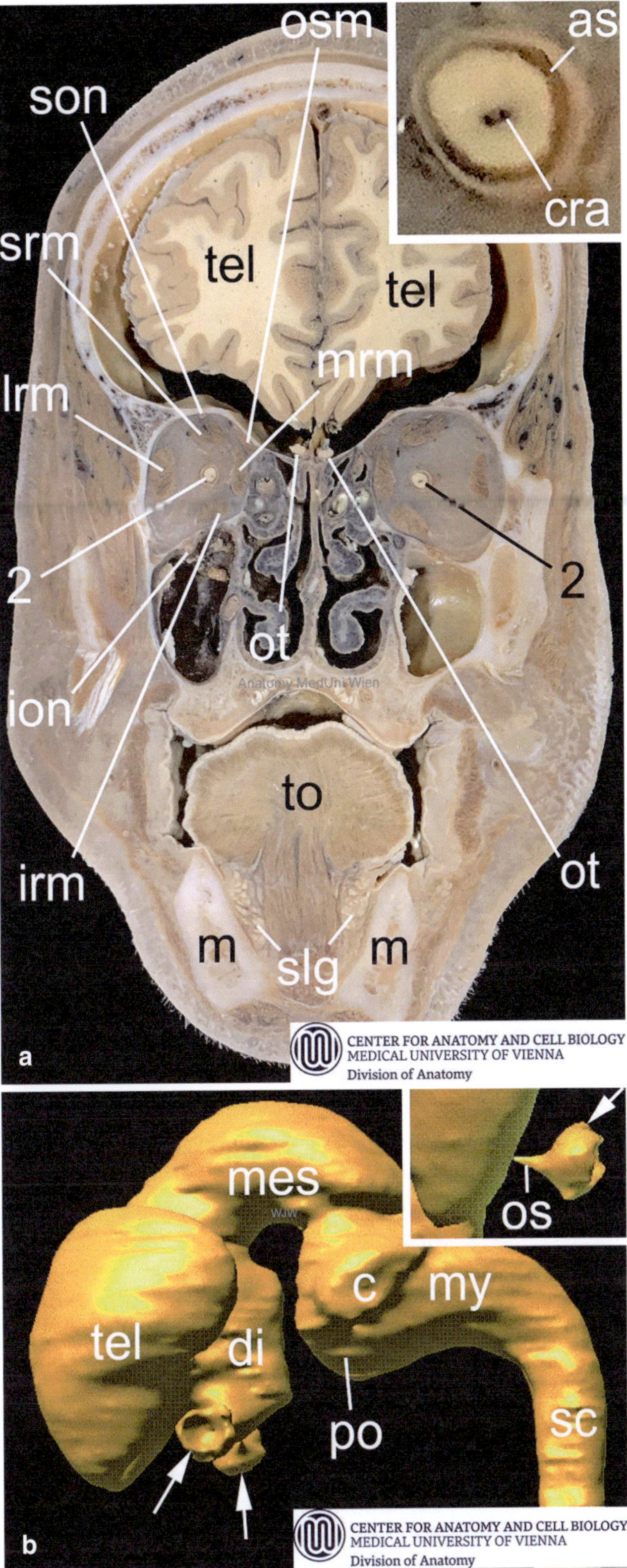

Yet, the fiber bundle named as CN II is not a nerve, but the white matter of the diencephalon. Per definition, a nerve is a component of the peripheral nervous system, whereas the "optic nerve" and the retina are integral parts of the central nervous system, as clearly visible in early embryos (Fig. 1.3b). The consequences include meningeal cover of the nerve and suppression of regeneration of injured optic nerve fibers, etc.

Ignoring the true nature of the fibers, textbooks usually describe the fiber bundle between the eyeball and optic chiasm as optic nerve. The fibers emerge from the third of the three neurons, which are consecutively arranged in the retina. The first are the sensors, the second are bipolar interneurons connecting the first and third neurons, and the third are the axons, which leave the retina at the optic disc to continue as optic nerve.

Per definition, the optic nerve ends at the optic chiasm. However, this structure does not hold perikaryal, and no fibers terminate or synapse in this structure. There is merely a crossing of fibers derived from neurons located in the nasal segments of the retina. Together with fibers emerging from neurons of the temporal segments of the retina of the ipsilateral eye (which do not cross in the chiasm), they continue as optic tract and finally terminate in the lateral geniculate nucleus of the thalamus. Hence, the axons of the third retinal neurons leaving the retina in the optic disc are the first part of the so-called optic nerve, then of the optic chiasm, and finally of the optic tract, before they synapse with neurons forming the lateral geniculate body (nucleus) of the thalamus.

The optic nerve passes the skull through the optic canal. This canal is also used by the ophthalmic artery, which is the first branch of the subarachnoid segment of the internal carotid artery. The artery transits the canal running below CN II. Once in the orbit, it splits and its terminal branch, the central retinal artery, pierces into the nerve. Surrounded by the nerve fibers, it enters the retina and ramifies in its inner layers.

Inside the optic canal and the orbit, both the artery and the nerve are surrounded by extensions of the dura and arachnoid mater and, consequently, are bathed in cerebrospinal fluid (Fig. 1.3a, inlay).

Nerves Associated with the Parasellar (Cavernous Sinus) Region: CN III to CN VI

CN III–CN VI are in close relationship with the parasellar region (PSR). Hence, the systematic description of CNs III to VI will start with a brief description of the PSR's composition and topology.

Since the PSR is also an important crossroad for sympathetic fibers emerging from the superior cervical ganglion [10], the following passage will also provide a brief description of the pathways of these nerves.

Composition of the parasellar (cavernous sinus) region: The region lateral to the sella turcica is traditionally termed as cavernous sinus due to its resemblance to the corpus cavernosum penis in histologic sections. However, in the last century, it became evident that the extradural space lateral to the sella turcica is not a spongiform sinus formed by interconnected cavernous spaces. The space rather holds a plexus of differently sized veins. To acknowledge this clinically important fact and to acknowledge the composition of its anterior section, this chapter will use PSR instead of cavernous sinus [11].

Detailed analysis revealed that the PSR consists of three compartments, which are separated by connective tissue [11–14]. Two of them, the orbital and pterygopalatine compartments, represent extensions of the extracranial tissue spaces of the orbit and the pterygopalatine fossa. They protrude into the cranial cavity through the superior orbital fissure and are named the orbital and pterygopalatine compartment of the PSR [10, 11]. They have their greatest relative extension in the fetus and infant [12]. The third and largest compartment of the PSR is the lateral sellar compartment, which holds the parasellar venous plexus. Between its venous channel, numerous arteries and nerves make their way toward intra- and extracranial targets (see below).

The parasellar venous plexus receives the superior ophthalmic vein, which drains blood from the orbit and enters through the superior orbital fissure. It also receives the sphenoparietal sinus and, sometimes, superficial cerebral veins.

Occipitally, the veins of the plexus drain into the superior and inferior petrous sinus and the basilar plexus, which in turn connects to the internal vertebral venous plexus. Laterally, the veins of the plexus connect to the veins of the infratemporal region and pterygopalatine fossa through the foramen ovale, spinosum, and rotundum. Finally, the left and right-sided parasellar venous plexus are connected via the midline through highly variable vascular channels, forming the so-called intercavernous sinus. Thus, functionally, the parasellar plexus is part of an extradural venous pathway, connecting the internal vertebral venous plexus and the orbit [15].

Surrounded by the veins of the parasellar plexus, the internal carotid artery takes its course from the internal ostium of the eponymous canal toward the anterior clinoid process. In fetuses and infants, the artery runs rather straight, while in adults it forms the characteristic spiraled siphon [12, 13, 16]. It gives rise to two large trunks, the meningohypophyseal and lateral trunk [17, 18], and to several small vessels. Lateral to the artery, and also embedded in the venous plexus, CN VI makes its way from Dorello's canal toward the superior orbital fissure. In the tissues of the lateral wall, which borders the PSR and middle cerebral fossa, CN III, CN IV, and CN V₁ are arranged to form Parkinson's triangle (Fig. 1.4), with CN IV showing a high variability in course [12, 13, 19].

Parasellar sympathetic pathways: Several sympathetic fiber bundles, which originate in the superior cervical ganglion, transit the carotid canal and enter the PSR together with the internal carotid artery. At least in infants, the bundles enter frontally and occipitally to the artery, and most of the bundles join to form a parasellar sympathetic trunk below the internal carotid artery and medially to CN VI. Often, one of the bundles entering occipitally directly joins CN VI.

The sympathetic parasellar trunk first splits into a large fiber bundle, which joins CN VI. Second, several fiber bundles travel back to the carotid artery. Third, a very small fiber bundle enters the pterygopalatine compartment to connect to the ganglion resting in this compartment [10]. The sympathetic fibers that joined CN VI soon leave it to become integrated in CN V₁. Inside the orbit, some of these fibers form the "sympathetic root" of the ciliary ganglion (see below). The rest use the cutaneous branches of CN V₁ to reach their targets in the skin innervated by CN V₁.

Oculomotor Nerve (CN III)

CN III comprises motor and preganglionic parasympathetic fibers. The motor fibers target the rectus superior, inferior, and medial, and inferior oblique muscles of the eyeball. The parasympathetic fibers synapse in the ciliary ganglion to trigger activation of the sphincter pupillae and ciliary muscle and body.

CN III leaves the mesencephalon at the interpeduncular fossa and enters the interpeduncular cistern. Passing between the superior cerebellar and posterior cerebral artery, it travels toward the PSR and dives into the dura mater forming its roof (Fig. 1.1b and 1.5). It then shifts laterally and descends in the layers of the lateral wall of the PSR to reach the superior orbital fissure (Fig. 1.4b). Here, it usually splits into a superior and inferior branch, which both enter the orbit running inside the annular tendon of Zinn.

The superior branch sends fibers to innervate the levator palpebrae superioris and superior rectus muscles. The inferior branch sends preganglionic parasympathetic fibers to the ciliary ganglion (see section "Parasympathetic Ganglia") and motor fibers towards the medial and inferior rectus and the inferior oblique muscles of the eyeball.

Trochlear Nerve (CN IV)

CN IV leaves the caudal mesencephalon lateral to the frenulum veli medullaris superioris. It comprises motor fibers, which innervate the superior oblique muscle of the eyeball.

CN IV is the only cranial nerve leaving the brain dorsally. Consequently, it passes the ipsilateral pedunculus cerebri to reach the skull base with its foramina. On its way, it travels inside the

Fig. 1.4 Parasellar region (PSR) and sinus cavernosus, respectively. Frontal to the right. Numbers refer to respective cranial nerves (CNs). (**a**) Adult skull base from superior for orientation. Relevant, right-sided osseous structures related to sella turcica and PSR are labeled. Note this specimen's bilaterally fused anterior (ac) and middle (mcp) clinoid processes. (**b**) Lateral wall of an infant's PSR. Dura mater removed. CN III, CN IV, and CN V_1 are arranged in Parkinson's triangle (asterisk) and head for the superior orbital fissure (sof). The sensory ophthalmic (5_1), maxillary (5_2), and mandibular (5_3) nerves join to form the semilunar trigeminal ganglion (^). The central processes of the pseudounipolar ganglion cells run as sensory portion of CN V (s5) toward the brain. The superior recess of Meckel's cave (arrow) is visible. Proximal to the foramen ovale (fo), CN V_3 is joined by the motor portion of CN V (m5). Note the connective tissue sheath covering the adipose tissue of the pterygopalatine compartment (+). (**c**) Sympathetic pathways in the PSR of an infant. The connective tissue of the lateral wall but also the venous parasellar plexus, s5, m5, semilunar ganglion, and V_3 are removed. V_1 is cut near the ganglion, and V_2 is shifted anterolaterally. Postganglionic sympathetic fibers (sf) enter the PSR through the internal aperture of the carotid canal (ioa), running frontal and occipital to the internal carotid artery (ica). The occipital fibers join the CN VI. The frontal fibers, together with fibers entering the frontomedial, form a parasellar trunk (hidden by CN VI). From here fibers join CN VI and others run back to the ica (arrowheads). Note that fibers connecting CN VI and CN V_1 are covered by the stump of CN V_1. acf, anterior cranial fossa; mcf, middle cranial fossa; pcf, posterior cranial fossa; cl, clivus; fs, foramen spinosum; fro, foramen rotundum; oca, entrance into optic canal, mcp, middle clinoid process; hf, hypophysial fossa; gws, greater wing of sphenoid bone; pc, posterior clinoid process

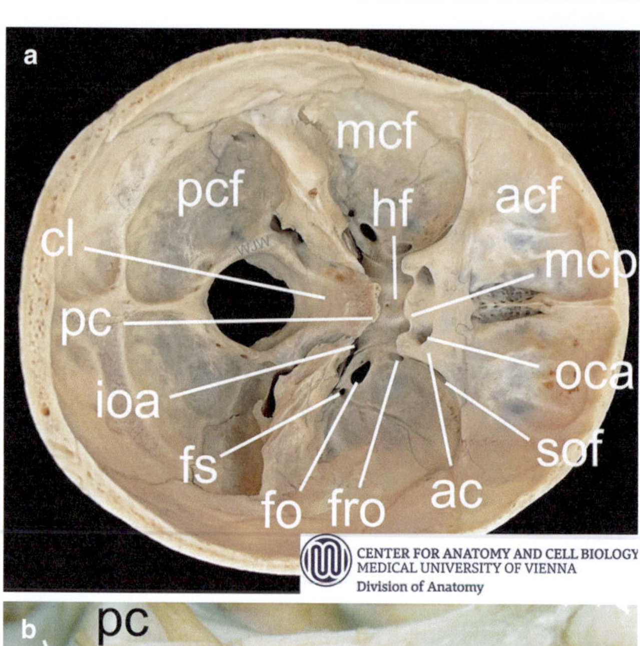

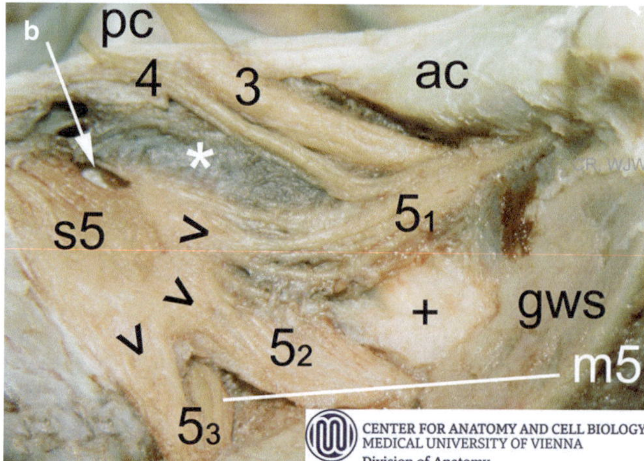

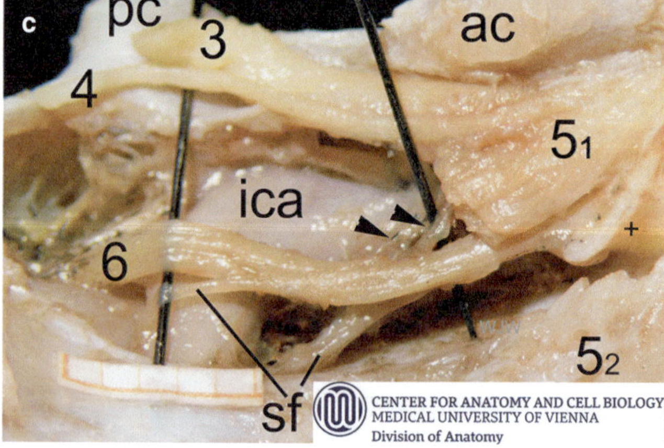

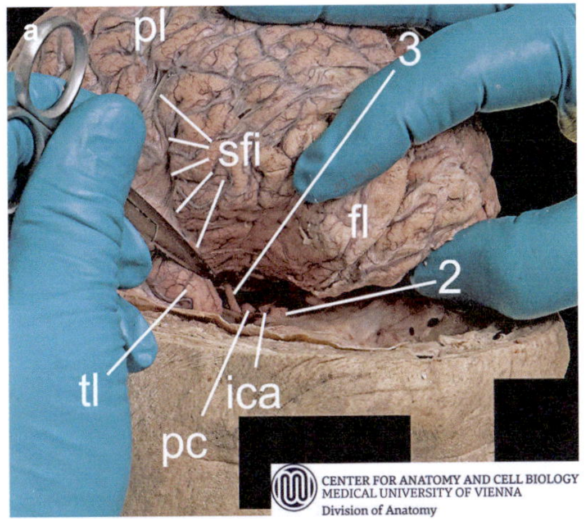

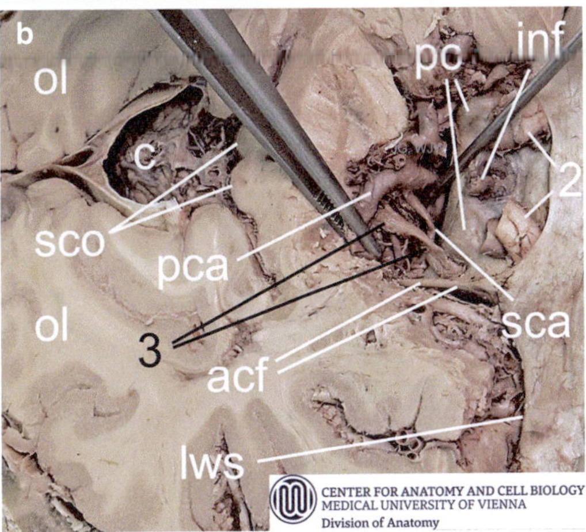

Fig. 1.5 Subarachnoid course of cranial nerve (CN) III. Frontal to the right. Numbers represent respective CNs. Compare with Fig. 1.4. (**a**) Descent to roof of the parasellar region (PSR). Right, frontolateral view of a head after removal of the calvaria with dura mater. Frontal lobe (fl) of telencephalon is lifted and temporal lobe (tl), pressed occipitally by scissor. (**b**) Topology of CN III in the interpeduncular fossa and perforation of the roof of the PSR, near the posterior clinoid process (pc). Superior view at a dissected brain resting in the skull base. Note the relationship of CN III to the posterior cerebral (pca) and superior cerebellar (sca) arteries. pl, parietal lobe, ol, occipital lobe; ica, internal carotid artery; 2, optic nerve; sfi, Sylvian fissure (lateral sulcus); inf, infundibulum of pituitary gland; c, cerebellum; lws, lesser wing of sphenoid bone; acf, anterior petroclinoid fold, forming the edge between roof and lateral wall of PSR; sco, superior colliculi of lamina tecti

ambient cistern near the basal vein of Rosenthal and the posterior cerebral artery. As soon as it arrives at the anterior petroclinoid fold, it enters it to run along the edge between roof and lateral wall of the PSR (Fig. 1.6). However, it soon descends between the layers of the PSR's lateral wall (Fig. 1.4b) and passes into the orbit superolateral to the annular tendon of Zinn. Once inside the orbit, it penetrates the superior oblique muscle from above.

Trigeminal Nerve (CN V)

CN V comprises a sensory and a motor portion and forms three divisions, traditionally termed as "nerves" (CN V_1, CN V_2, CN V_3). It innervates the skin of the face and most of the mucosa of the nasal and oral cavity and the paranasal sinuses, as well as the tensor tympani, the masticatory muscles, and muscles of the diaphragma oris.

Sensory portion of CN V: The perikarya of the pseudounipolar neurons of the sensory portion are located in the trigeminal (semilunar) ganglion of Gasser (Fig. 1.4). The latter is positioned anterior to Meckel's cave, a recess of the subarachnoid space in the occipital part of the PSR's lateral wall (Figs. 1.6 and 1.7). The central processes of the axons of the pseudounipolar neurons travel to the brain and enter it laterally to the pons. The peripheral processes form the ophthalmic, maxillary, and mandibular nerves (Fig. 1.4).

The fibers of CN V, which innervate the skin of the face, are specially arranged. All thicker bundles run between periosteum and mimic muscles, forcing the nerve fibers which start in the skin to perforate the muscles. On their passage, some are joined by fibers innervating the proprioceptors located between the muscle fibers of the mimic muscles.

In general, similar connections exist with many other motor nerves. Therefore, proprioceptive fibers of the muscles of the head largely use CN V to enter the brain.

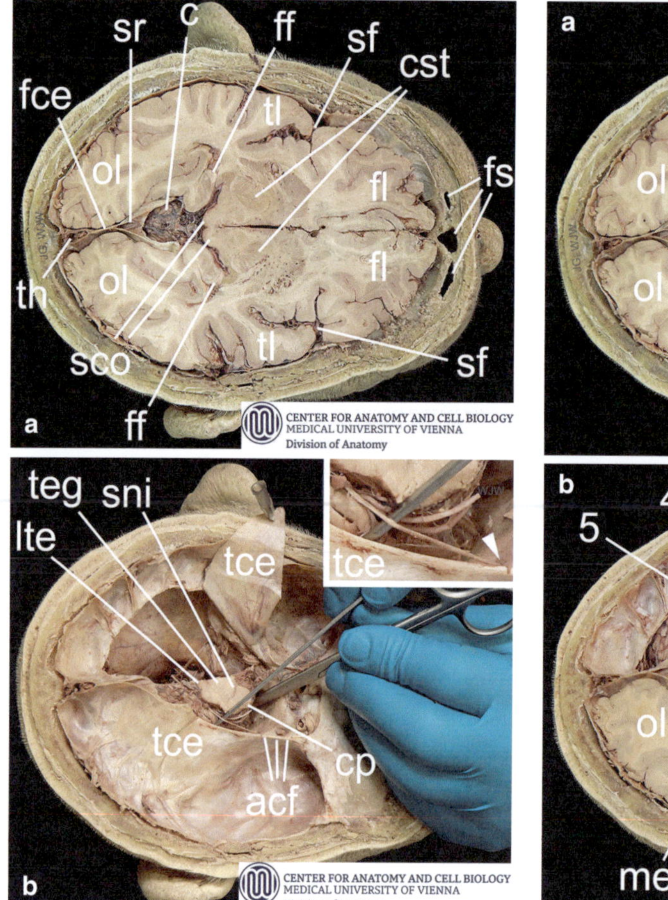

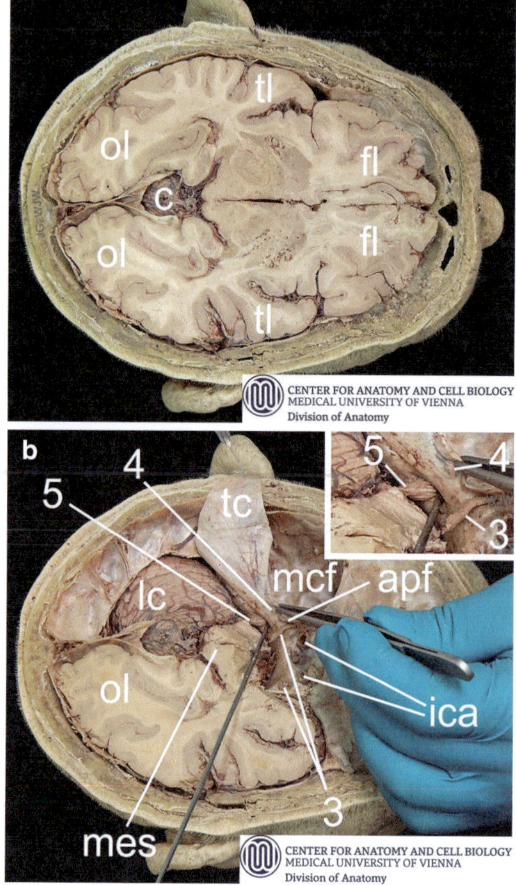

Fig. 1.6 Subarachnoid segment of cranial nerve (CN) IV. Numbers represent respective CNs. Axially cut head from superior. Frontal to the right. Calvaria and upper parts of the brain removed. (**a**) Topology of brain structures in relation to skull base and meninges for orientation. (**b**) Topology of CN IV. Left-sided telencephalon and entire diencephalon are removed. The left-sided tentorium cerebelli (tce) is cut along the transverse sinus and hinged superiorly along the superior petrosal sinus. The brain stem is cut at the level of the caudal mesencephalon and in the midline. Brain material on the left is removed. The right-sided ambient cistern is open. CN IV is exposed and lifted by a probe. Passing the cerebral peduncle (cp) laterally, it runs straight toward the lateral PSR. Inlay magnifies the entrance of CN IV into the anterior petroclinoid fold (acf, arrowhead). Note the superior cerebellar vessels below the probe. fs, frontal sinus; ol, occipital lobe; tl, temporal lobe; fl, frontal lobe; sf, Sylvian fissure; c, cerebellum; fce, falx cerebri; sr, sinus rectus; th, torcular Herophili (confluens of sinuses); ff, fimbria of fornix (hippocampus) emerging from hippocampus formation; sco, right-sided superior colliculus of lamina tecti (lte); cst, corticospinal tract later forming the center of cp; teg, tegmentum; sni, substantia nigra

Fig. 1.7 Subarachnoid segment of cranial nerve (CN) V. Numbers refer to respective CNs. Axially cut head from superior. Frontal to the right. Calvaria and upper parts of the brain removed. (**a**) Topology of brain structures in relation to skull base and meninges for orientation. Compare to Fig. 1.6. (**b**) Topology of nerve. Left-sided telencephalon, entire diencephalon, and entire right-sided telencephalon are removed. The left-sided tentorium cerebelli (tce) is cut along the transverse sinus and hinged superiorly along the superior petrosal sinus. The brain stem is cut at the level of the caudal mesencephalon (mes). The tip of a probe is inserted in Meckel's cave. Inlay shows the relation of CN V and Meckel's cave. Ol, occipital lobe; tl, temporal lobe; fl, frontal lobe; c, cerebellum; lc, left cerebellar hemisphere; mcf; middle cranial fossa; ica; anterior petroclinoid fold; internal carotid artery; apf, anterior petoclinoid fold; 3, CN III; 4, CN IV; 5, CN V

Ophthalmic nerve (CN V₁): CN V_1 is composed of GSA fibers, which innervate the tentorium cerebelli, forehead, upper orbit, superior nasal cavity, nasal ridge, and the mucosa of the frontal sinus, sphenoid sinus, and ethmoidal cells. The nerve is formed inside the skull, near the superior orbital fissure, by fusion of three main nerve bundles, named lacrimal, frontal, and nasociliary nerve. Inside the skull, it passes in the layers of the lateral wall of the PSR and receives a meningeal branch, which chiefly innervates the tentorium cerebelli. Postganglionic sympathetic fibers from the superior cervical ganglion traveling via the internal carotid nerve, the parasellar trunk, and CN VI join it (see above).

- *Lacrimal nerve*: The nerve comprises fibers which innervate the lacrimal gland and the nearby tissues, including the conjunctiva. In the upper orbit, it is joined by postganglionic sympathetic and parasympathetic fibers (Fig. 1.8) that had used the zygomatic nerve to enter the orbit via the inferior orbital fissure (see section "Parasympathetic Ganglia"). Finally, the nerve enters the skull via the superior orbital fissure, running inside the annular tendon of Zinn.

- *Frontal nerve*: The nerve is formed by unification of the supratrochlear and supraorbital nerves [20]. The supratrochlear nerve comprises fibers innervating the skin of the medial forehead, while the supraorbital nerve fibers innervate the skin of the lateral forehead (Fig. 1.3a). Both turn around the superior rim of the orbit, with the supraorbital nerve using the foramen/incisura supraorbitalis (Fig. 1.8b). Once in the orbit, the nerves pass between the periosteum of the roof of the orbit and the levator palpebrae superioris muscle and unite. The resulting frontal nerve enters the skull through the superior orbital fissure, above Zinn's tendon.

- *Nasociliary nerve*: The nasociliary nerve is formed in the orbit by unification of the anterior and posterior ethmoidal nerves. The anterior ethmoidal nerve starts as the external nasal nerve in the skin overlying the nasal ridge. It enters the nasal cavity between nasal bone and cartilage. Inside the cavity, it ascends along the nasal bone toward the cribriform plate and is constantly joined by fibers coming from the local mucosa. It then changes name

to anterior ethmoidal nerve and enters the skull through the anterior part of the cribriform plate. Staying beneath the dura mater, it runs for a few millimeters occipitally and then dives into the ethmoid cells. Here, it again receives fibers innervating the local mucosa before it enters the orbit through the anterior ethmoidal foramen. Inside the orbit, the nerve is joined by the posterior ethmoidal nerve, which comprises fibers innervating the mucosa of the posterior ethmoidal cells and sphenoid sinus.

- The nasociliary nerve connects with the ciliary ganglion. The connecting fibers had started in the cornea, ciliary body, and iris and reached the ganglion as part of the long ciliary nerves (compare to section "Parasympathetic Ganglia"). After this, the nerve also receives the infratrochlear nerve, which is formed by fibers innervating the skin of the medial canthus, skin and conjunctiva of the medial eyelids, and the tissues of and near the lacrimal sac.

- After having received all these nerve bundles, the nasociliary nerve transits the superior orbital fissure inside the tendinous annulus of Zinn and joins the lacrimal and frontal nerves inside the skull.

Maxillary nerve (CN V_2): CN V_2 comprises GSA fibers from the lower nasal cavity, soft palate and the teeth, mucosa, gingiva, and skin associated with the maxilla, palatine, and zygomatic bone.

The nerve is formed in the pterygopalatine fossa by unification of the infraorbital and zygomatic nerve and a small branch communicating with the pterygopalatine ganglion (Fig. 1.8). It enters the skull through the foramen rotundum and continues in the lateral wall of the parasellar region (Fig. 1.4b). Here, it is joined by a meningeal nerve, which innervates significant parts of the dura of the middle cranial fossa.

- *Infraorbital nerve*: Three main branches form the infraorbital nerve. The external nasal branches start in the skin of the lateral nose; the inferior palpebral branches in the skin of

Fig. 1.8 Peripheral branches of cranial nerve (CN) V. Numbers refer to respective CNs. (**a**) Head specimen from the historical collection of the Division of Anatomy of the Medical University of Vienna. Parasellar region, lateral orbit, and the neurovascular bundle (nvb) of the lateropharyngeal region are exposed by removing soft tissues and bones. The main stem of CN V and the trigeminal ganglion are resected. The intracranial segment of CN V_1 is hinged laterally, and the venous plexus of the PSR is removed to expose CN VI [6] and the internal carotid artery (ica), forming the carotid siphon. In the orbit, the ciliary ganglion (cg) with branches and the inferior branch of CN III (ib3) are visible. The lacrimal nerve (ln) receives postganglionic parasympathetic fiber (arrow) from the pterygopalatine ganglion via the zygomaticotemporal (ztn) and the zygomatic nerve (compare section "Parasympathetic Ganglia"). The bones shielding the upper lateral parts of the pterygopalatine fossa and the lateral foramen rotundum are removed. The infraorbital (ion) nerve and the posterior superior alveolar branches (psab) are discernable. Likewise, the lateral border of the foramen ovale is cleared away, and the sensory nerves of CN V_3, such as the buccal (bn), lingual (lin), inferior alveolar (ian), and auriculotemporal (atn) nerves, are exposed. The two latter are cut, since the mandible (m) is split and the two processes are removed. (**b**) Skull from ventral, showing the osseous structures, where the mental, infraorbital, and frontal nerves transit. p, pterygopalatine process; max, maxilla; e, auricle; 5_2, maxillary nerve; mf, mental foramen; iof, infraorbital foramen; sof, supraorbital foramen

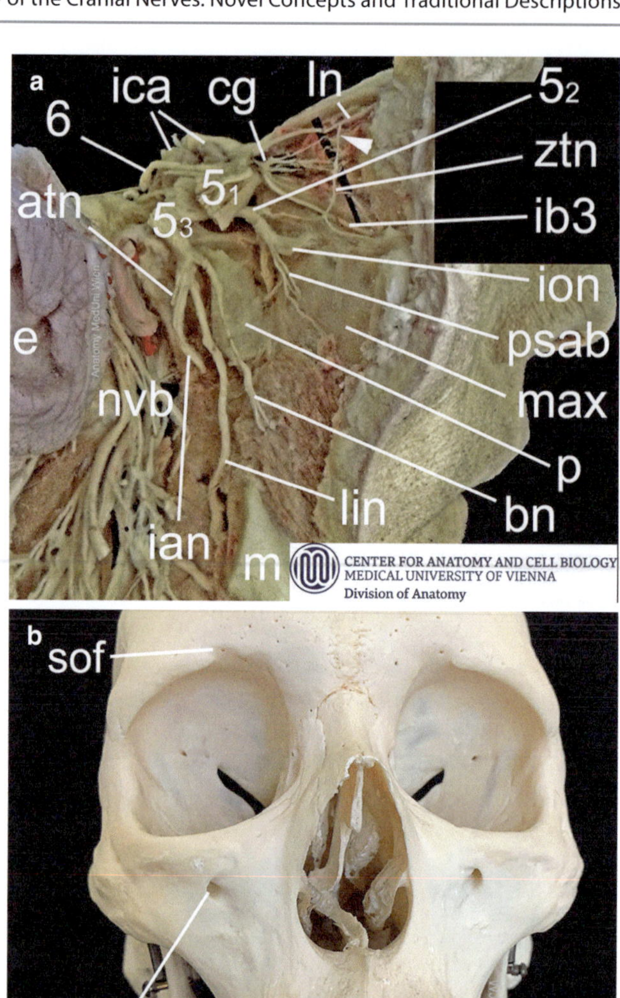

the lower lid; and the superior labial branches in the skin of the upper lip. They converge near the infraorbital foramen and the resulting infraorbital nerve immediately enters the infraorbital foramen (Fig. 1.8b). It continues inside a canal or semicanal at the bottom of the orbit (Fig. 1.3a), which almost extends toward the inferior orbital fissure at the apex of the orbit. Inside the canal, the nerve receives branches from teeth and associated structures (*i.e.*, anterior and middle superior alveolar nerves) and from the mucosa covering the maxillary sinus. Transiting the inferior orbital fissure, the nerve dives into the pterygopalatine fossa and receives posterior superior alveolar branches from the posterior teeth and associated structures (Fig. 1.8).

- *Zygomatic nerve*: The zygomatic nerve is formed in the lateral orbit by union of the zygomaticofacial and zygomaticotemporal nerves. It enters the pterygopalatine fossa through the inferior orbital fissure. The zygomaticofacial nerve collects fibers from the skin of the upper cheek and the zygomaticotemporal nerve fibers from the skin of the temple. Both nerves enter the orbit through eponymous foramina (also compare Figs. 1.14 and 1.15). Inside the orbit, the zygomaticotemporal nerve connects with the lacrimal nerve and exchanges fibers with the lacrimal nerve (Fig. 1.8; also compare section "Parasympathetic Ganglia").

Mandibular nerve (CN V₃): CN V_3 is the division of CN V which is composed of GSA fibers but also joined by motor fibers. The latter run medially to the sensory part of CN V and meet the sensory fibers near the oval foramen (Fig. 1.4b). Together, the motor and sensory fibers transit the oval foramen and enter the infratemporal fossa.

Sensory portion: The sensory portion of the mandibular nerve is formed near the oval foramen by unification of the sensory fibers traveling with the inferior alveolar, lingual, buccal, and auriculotemporal nerve.

- *Inferior alveolar nerve*: This nerve starts as the so-called mental nerve, which enters the mandibular canal through the mental foramen after having collected cutaneous branches from the lower lip and anterior lower jaw (Fig. 1.8b). Inside the canal, it changes its name to inferior alveolar nerve, which runs close to the inferior alveolar vessels. On its way it continuously thickens by receiving fibers from the teeth and associated apparatuses. Finally, the nerve leaves the canal through the mandibular foramen and ascends between the medial and lateral pterygoid muscles. From the mandibular to the oval foramen, the nerve runs close to, but independent

from, the lingual nerve, although they often exchange fibers. Motor fibers ultimately forming the mylohyoid nerve accompany this segment.

- *Lingual nerve*: This nerve has GSA and SVA fibers. The GSA fibers innervate tactile receptors of the anterior 2/3 of the tongue (anterior to the terminal sulcus), the mucosa of the floor of the mouth, and parts of the gingiva of the lower yaw. Its stem runs between the tongue and mandible and then between the medial and lateral pterygoid muscles toward the oval foramen.
- Near the tongue, the nerve also receives SVA fibers from the taste buds of the anterior 2/3 of the tongue. They travel as part of the nerve until the nerve has reached the level of the pterygoid muscles. Here, these fibers leave the lingual nerve and form the chorda tympani—a nerve fiber bundle comprised of SVA and preganglionic parasympathetic fibers, which finally enter the brain as part of Wrisberg's nerve (see CN VII). The preganglionic parasympathetic fibers entering the lingual nerve via the chorda tympani use the nerve to travel toward the submandibular region, where they leave the nerve to synapse at perikarya of the submandibular ganglion (see section "Parasympathetic Ganglia").
- *Buccal nerve*: The buccal nerve starts in the mucosa and skin of the cheek and squeezes between the venters of the lateral pterygoid muscle to join CN V_3 below the oval foramen (Fig. 1.8).
- *Auriculotemporal nerve*: The auriculotemporal nerve starts in the skin of the temple, external acoustic meatus, tympanic membrane, tragus, and a small region immediately anterior to the ear. In the temple, it runs together with the superficial temporal artery. The nerve enters the tissues of the parotid gland anterior to the tragus and then passes medially to the temporomandibular joint to join CN V_3 below the oval foramen (Fig. 1.8). When passing below the foramen spinosum, the nerve is joined by a meningeal branch. It innervates the dura mater of the middle cranial fossa and leaves the skull through the foramen.

- Occipital to the foramen spinosum, the auriculotemporal nerve is joined by postganglionic parasympathetic fibers arising from the otic ganglion and sympathetic fibers, leaving the plexus surrounding the middle meningeal artery. They accompany the nerve toward the parotid gland, where they leave it to join CN VII (see section "Parasympathetic Ganglia").

Motor portion of CN V and CN V_3: The perikarya of the motor portion are located in the motor (masticator) nucleus. They leave the brain lateral to the pons. Running below and often separated from the sensory fibers, they head for the oval foramen, where they join CN V_3 medially (Fig. 1.4b). As soon as CN V_3 has passed the foramen, most of the motor fibers split off to innervate the masticatory, tensor tympani, and tensor veli palatini muscles. Merely a few motor fibers continue as part of the inferior alveolar nerve and soon leave it as the mylohyoid nerve. Hence, the motor fibers of CN V are only integrated for an astonishingly short distance in the main stem of CN V_3 and one of its branches.

- *Branches to muscles of mastication*: Once the motor portion has entered the infratemporal fossa as part of CN V_3, the fibers spread for the masticatory muscles. Thus, they form a masseteric nerve, which passes through the incisura mandibulae; a medial pterygoid nerve, which enters the medial pterygoid muscle; a lateral pterygoid nerve, which innervates the lateral pterygoid muscle; and several deep temporal nerves, which ascend toward the temporal muscle. Quite frequently, the fibers of the lateral pterygoid nerve stay as part of the buccal nerve until it squeezes between the bellies of the lateral pterygoid muscle.
- *Branches to muscles of the skull base and auditory system*: Immediately below the foramen ovale, CN V_3 also gives rise to fibers, which head for the tensor tympani and tensor veli palatini muscles.
- *Mylohyoid nerve*: A larger bundle of motor fibers stays with the inferior alveolar nerve. Before it enters the mandibular foramen and the mandibular canal, this bundle leaves the

nerve as mylohyoid nerve. This descends toward the diaphragma oris to innervate the mylohyoid and anterior belly of digastric muscle.

CN V—peculiarities: The motor portion of CN V can be considered as more or less entirely separated from the sensory portion. It often exits the brain independent from the sensory portion and merely joins the sensory CN V_3 near the oval foramen to immediately split into motor nerves outside the skull. The only exceptions are the mylohyoid nerve, which travels for a short distance as part of the inferior alveolar nerve, and in some variation the lateral pterygoid nerve, which may travel for a short distance with the very proximal portion of the buccal nerve. Consequently, it seems to be much more correct to consider CN V as two separate nerves: a sensory CN V and a motor CN V.

Many branches of CN V are joined by visceral (autonomous) nerve fibers. Their precise cranial course and connections are described in the section "Parasympathetic Ganglia".

Abducens Nerve (CN VI)

CN VI leaves the brain near the caudal rim of the pons. It comprises motor fibers, which innervate the lateral rectus muscle of the eyeball.

From its exit, CN VI ascends and perforates the dura mater covering the clivus. Amidst the veins of the basilar plexus, it continues its ascend and enters the PSR through the canal of Dorello. Inside the PSR, it runs lateral to the internal carotid artery, surrounded by the veins of the parasellar venous plexus (Fig. 1.4c).

The parasellar segment of CN VI is joined by postganglionic sympathetic nerve fibers, which instantly leave it for CN V_1 (compare section "Parasellar Sympathetic Pathways"). CN VI finally leaves the PSR through the superior orbital fissure, running inside the annulus tendon of Zinn. In the orbit, it heads for the lateral rectus muscle and innervates it. Quite frequently it transits the PSR as two roundish bundles [21].

Nerves of the Cerebellopontine Angle (CN VII and CN VIII)

The fibers of CN VII and CN VIII leave/enter the brain in close vicinity at the site where the pons, medulla oblongata, and cerebellum, respectively, its inferior peduncle, come together (cerebellopontine angle). Running in the cerebellopontine cisterna, they head for the internal acoustic meatus and leave/enter it together with the labyrinthine artery (Fig. 1.9).

(Intermedio) Facial Nerve (CN VII)

CN VII is composed of two bundles. One is the "proper" facial nerve consisting of motor fibers. The second is the nervus intermedius (intermediate nerve of Wrisberg) comprising preganglionic parasympathetic, GSA, and SVA fibers. Quite frequently, the motor fibers and the intermediate nerve leave the brain separately and join near the internal acoustic porus. Together, they pass through the meatus and enter the facial (Fallopian) canal, which branches off from the internal acoustic meatus in a frontolateral direction.

The canal changes its direction twice and consequently has three segments. The first (labyrinthine) segment continues the frontolateral direction of the internal acoustic meatus. After a knee-like bend, the second (tympanic) segment heads occipitolaterally. Then, the canal curves downwards, and the third (mastoid) segment descends and terminates at the stylomastoid foramen. Consequently, the intrapetrous portion of CN VII features three eponymous segments and two curves. The first curve, between the labyrinthine and tympanic segments, is termed as the external knee of the facial nerve. It is formed by all fibers of CN VII. The internal knee of the facial nerve is formed inside the brain and only by motor fibers, which round the abducens nucleus and curl up the facial colliculus of the rhomboid fossa.

Intermediate nerve: Wrisberg's nerve holds efferent (preganglionic parasympathetic) and afferent (GSA and SVA) fibers. It innervates the lacrimal, submandibular, sublingual, and small

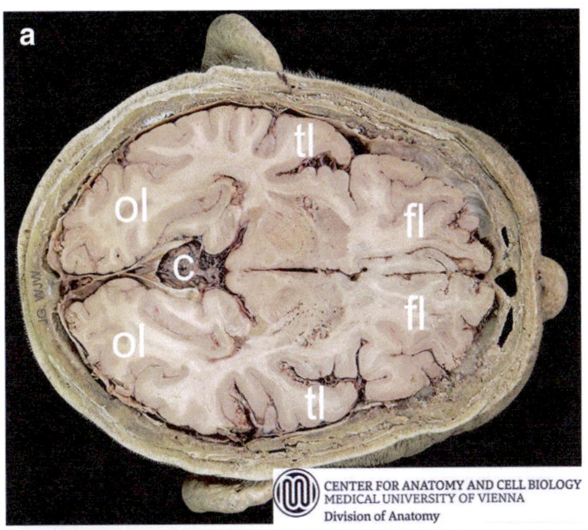

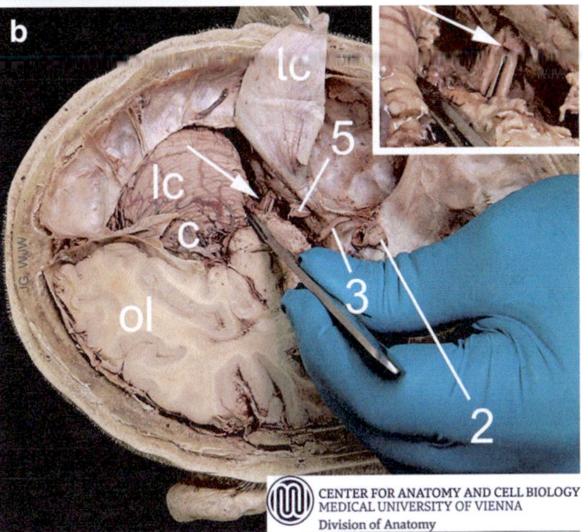

Fig. 1.9 Subarachnoid course of the nerves of the cerebellopontine angel (v3)—*i.e.,* cranial nerve (CN) VII and CN VIII. Numbers refer to respective CNs. Axially cut head from superior. Frontal to the right. Calvaria and upper parts of the brain removed. (**a**) Topology of brain structures in relation to skull base and meninges for orientation. Compare to Fig. 1.6. (**b**) v3 and labyrinthine artery (arrow). The left-sided telencephalon and the entire diencephalon are removed. The left-sided tentorium cerebelli (tc) is cut along the transverse sinus and hinged superiorly along the superior petrosal sinus. The brain stem is cut at the level of the caudal mesencephalon and in the midline. Brain stem material on the left is removed. Inlay magnifies the situation at the internal acoustic porus, the opening leading into the internal acoustic meatus. ol, occipital lobe; tl, temporal lobe; fl, frontal lobe; c, cerebellum; lc, left cerebellar hemisphere; tc, hinged left tentorium cerebelli; 2, cranial nerve (CN) II; 3, CN III; 5, CN V

salivatory glands, taste buds at the anterior 2/3 of the tongue and in the palatal mucosa, and a small skin area at the outer ear. The perikarya of the afferent neurons form the geniculate ganglion, a ganglion located at the apogee of the external knee of CN VII.

The nerve splits into two large nerve bundles, the greater petrosal nerve and the chorda tympani. In addition, a small connection exists between CN X and the mastoid segment of CN VII, which transfers GSA fibers innervating the skin of the external acoustic meatus, mastoid, and pinna. All bundles that leave the intracanalicular segment of CN VII travel in osseous canals (see section "Parasympathetic Ganglia").

- *Greater petrosal nerve*: It comprises SVA fibers and preganglionic parasympathetic fibers and joins CN VII at its external knee. The SVA fibers start at the taste buds of the palatal mucosa. The parasympathetic fibers travel quite complexly to the pterygopalatine ganglion (see section "Parasympathetic Ganglia").
- *Chorda tympani*: The chorda tympani connects the mastoid segment of CN VII and the lingual nerve at its transition between the medial and lateral pterygoid muscles. It comprises SVA fibers and preganglionic parasympathetic fibers. The SVA fibers start from taste buds at the anterior 2/3 of the tongue (anterior to the terminal sulcus) and accompany the lingual nerve all the way from the tongue to the connection with the chorda tympani. The preganglionic parasympathetic fibers join the lingual nerve as part of the chorda tympani and leave the nerve proximal to the submandibular fossa to enter the submandibular ganglion (see section "Parasympathetic Ganglia").

Motor fibers/nerves of CN VII: The motor fibers of CN VII innervate the stapedius, mimic, some auricular, and the posterior suprahyoid muscles.

The first motor nerve arising from CN VII is the stapedial nerve. It splits from its mastoid segment proximal to the chorda tympani and runs in an osseous canal toward the eponymous muscle.

Immediately after passing through the stylomastoid foramen, three branches split from CN VII. First is the posterior auricular nerve, which ascends occipital to the pinna to innervate the occipital belly of the occipitofrontalis muscle. It also forms small branches to innervate the rudimentary posterior auricular and upper intrinsic muscles of the auricle. Second is the stylohyoid nerve, which leaves for the stylohyoid muscle. Third is the digastric nerve, which heads for the posterior belly of the digastric muscle.

The main stem of the facial nerve then dives into the parotid gland and usually splits into two main trunci, named cervicofacial and temporofacial division, although there is a broad variability. The branches of the trunci form a plexus between the superficial and profound portion of the parotid gland (Fig. 1.10). From this plexus, a highly variable number of fiber bundles are formed, which emerge from the anteroinferior borders of the parotid gland (Fig. 1.10a). According to their targets, five main groups are usually distinguished. They are termed as temporal, zygomatic, buccal, marginal mandibular, and cervical branches and spread toward the mimic muscles located in the respective areas [22, 23].

Vestibulocochlear Nerve (CN VIII)

CN VIII is composed of a cochlear and vestibular portion. It comprises sensory and motor fibers and is involved in hearing and balance.

Sensory fibers: CN VIII mainly comprises SSA fibers stemming from bipolar neurons in the modiolus of the cochlea (spiral ganglion) and the internal acoustic meatus (vestibular ganglion of Scarpa).

The central (efferent) axons of both ganglia join and straightly run toward the cerebellopontine angle. The cochlear portion synapses in the ventral and dorsal cochlear nucleus; the vestibular portion in the medial (Schwalbe), lateral (Deiters), superior (Bechterew), and inferior (Roller) vestibular nucleus. All these nuclei are located ventral to the rhomboid fossa.

The peripheral (afferent) axons of the spiral ganglion connect with inner and outer hair cells of Corti's organ. The peripheral (afferent) axons of the vestibular ganglion reach the ganglion as two fiber bundles. The inferior bundle starts at sensory cells of the anterior and lateral semicir-

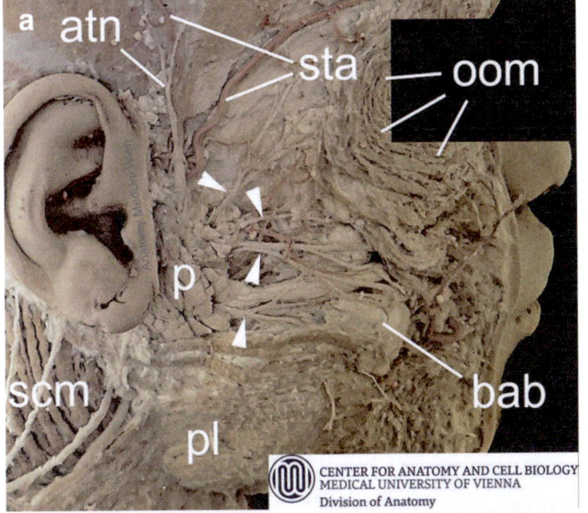

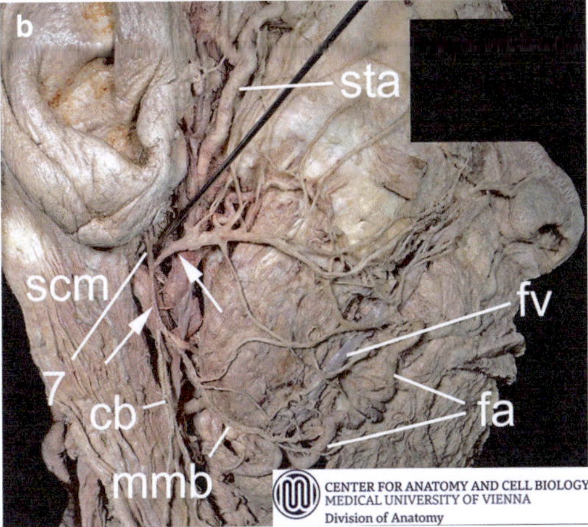

Fig. 1.10 Extracranial branches of cranial nerve (CN) VII. Numbers refer to respective CNs. Head specimen from right. Skin and subcutis are removed. Frontal to the right. (**a**) Specimen from the historical collection of the Division of Anatomy of the Medical University of Vienna. Major terminal motor branches of CN VII (arrowheads) leave the parotid gland (p) at its borders. The inferior branches are covered by the platysma (pl). Note the relationship between auriculotemporal nerve (atn), a branch of CN V₃ and the branches of the superficial temporal artery (sta). (**b**) Specimen, in which platysma and parotid gland are removed. CN VII splits into a superior and inferior trunk (arrows). The cervical branch (cb) and the marginalis mandibulae branch (mmb), both formed by the inferior trunk, are now visible. Note that branching of CN VII is highly variable, and this is only one of many normal variations. oom, orbicularis oculi muscle; scm, sternocleidomastoid muscle; fv, facial vein; fa, facial artery; bab, buccal adipose body (Bichat's fat pad)

cular canals and the utriculus. The superior bundle starts at sensory cells of the posterior semicircular canal and the sacculus.

Motor fibers: In addition to SSA fibers, both the cochlear and vestibular portion hold motor fibers, which emerge from the superior olivary complex and the ventral rhombencephalon, respectively [24, 25]. They terminate at sensory cells and are considered to modulate their responsiveness [26].

Nerves Exiting from the Anterolateral Sulcus (CN IX–CN XI)

A large number of nerve fiber bundles exit the brain at the posterolateral (dorsolateral) sulcus (retroolivary groove) of the medulla oblongata, ventral to the oliva, and caudal to Bochdalek's flower basket (Fig. 1.1). They head for the nervous part of the jugular foramen (Fig. 1.11). On their way, the three to four most rostral bundles join to form CN IX, the next eight to ten form CN X, and the most caudal ones form the cranial root of CN XI. Inside the jugular foramen, the nerves are ensheathed by a recess formed by dura and arachnoid mater. A connective tissue septum divides the recess in two compartments. One contains CN X and CN XI; the other contains CN IX.

CN IX and CN X comprise both efferent and afferent fibers. Hence, each of the two nerves has two pseudounipolar ganglia; one inside and a second just below the jugular foramen. At the level of its superior ganglion, the vagus nerve is joined by a large nerve fiber bundle, the "internal ramus" of CN XI (see below).

Glossopharyngeal Nerve (CN IX)

CN IX innervates parts of the tympanic cavity, pharynx, pharyngeal isthmus, parotid gland, and both the taste buds and sensory receptors of the posterior 1/3 of the tongue (posterior to the terminal sulcus). It comprises GSA, SVA, and preganglionic parasympathetic and motor fibers, which contribute to various plexus and some small nerves.

Tympanic plexus: The first branch of CN IX is the tympanic (Jacobson's) nerve. It comprises most of the preganglionic parasympathetic fibers

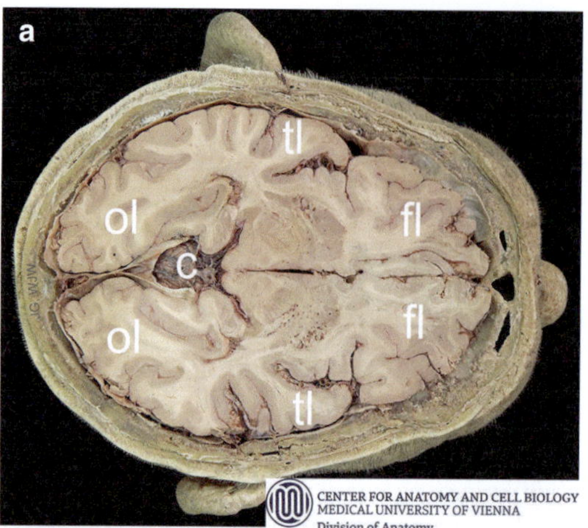

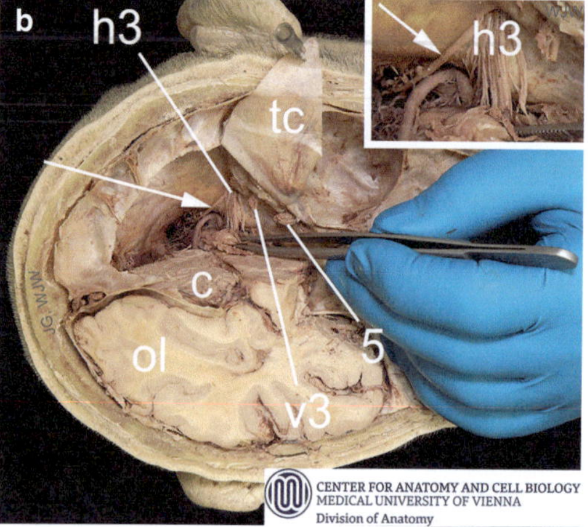

Fig. 1.11 Subarachnoid course of the nerves exiting from the anterolateral sulcus (h3), *i.e.,* cranial nerve (CN) IX, CN X, and CN XI. Numbers refer to respective CNs. Axially cut head from superior. Frontal to the right. Calvaria and upper parts of the brain removed. (**a**) Topology of brain structures in relation to skull base and meninges for orientation. Compare to Fig. 1.6. (**b**) Topology of h3 at the entrance into the pars nervosa of the jugular foramen. Left-sided telencephalon and entire diencephalon are removed. The left-sided tentorium cerebelli (tc) is cut along the transverse sinus and hinged superiorly along the superior petrosal sinus. The brain stem is cut at the level of the caudal mesencephalon and in the midline. Brain stem material on the left is removed. Note the plethora of rootlets and the spinal root of CN XI (arrow). Inlay magnifies the situation. ol, occipital lobe; tl, temporal lobe; fl, frontal lobe; c, cerebellum; tc, hinged left tentorium cerebelli; v3, nerves of the cerebellopontine angle; 5, trigeminal nerve

of CN IX and a small number of sensory fibers. The nerve leaves CN IX near its inferior ganglion, ascends, and enters the tympanic cavity through the tympanic canaliculus (compare Fig. 1.14). Inside the tympanic cavity, it splits into a plexus (tympanic plexus), innervates the local mucosa and the mucosa of the mastoid cells and tuba Eustachii, and connects with the greater petrosal nerve. Finally, some plexus fibers converge again and form a small nerve bundle, the lesser petrosal nerve. This nerve comprises the preganglionic parasympathetic fibers, which head for the otic ganglion (see section "Parasympathetic Ganglia").

Pharyngeal plexus: After exiting from the nervous part of the jugular foramen, the main stem of CN IX accompanies the levator pharyngis muscle toward the pharynx (Fig. 1.12). Here, its fibers become part of the pharyngeal plexus. This plexus innervates the mucosa and the muscles of the pharynx and is described to be built up by both CN IX and CN X; the fibers of CN IX chiefly contribute to the cranial part of the plexus and consequently innervate the proximal segments of the pharynx.

Tonsillar plexus: Together with the middle and posterior palatine nerves (see below), fibers of CN IX form a tonsillar plexus, which innervates the mucosa and intrinsic muscles of the soft palate, the levator veli palatini, the pharyngeal isthmus, and the tonsils.

Lingual branches: CN IX receives sensory fibers from the tongue. These lingual branches comprise GSA and SVA fibers and innervate both the mucosa and taste bodies of the tongue posterior to the terminal sulcus.

Carotid sinus nerve: Finally, a small bundle of nerve fibers connects CN IX with sensors located in the glomus body and the wall of the carotid sinus near the carotid bifurcation.

Vagus Nerve (CN X)

CN X innervates targets not only in the head and neck region but also in the thorax and abdomen. It comprises GSA, SVA, preganglionic parasympathetic, and motor fibers.

The nerve leaves the skull through the jugular foramen and descends in the parapharyngeal space, running inside the carotid sheath, sand-

Fig. 1.12 Cranial nerves (CN) IX, CN X, CN XI, and CN XII in the neck. Numbers refer to respective CNs. (**a**) Specimen from the historical collection of the Division of Anatomy of the Medical University of Vienna. Dorsal wall of pharynx and the parapharyngeal neurovascular bundles are exposed. Dorsal view. Branches of CN IX run along the stylopharyngeus muscle (spm) toward the constrictor pharyngis muscles (cpm). Arrowheads indicate branches of CN IX and CN X that form the pharyngeal plexus. Note the spiral course of CN XII [12] and the external ramus of CN XI (e11). (**b**) Left-sided parapharyngeal nerves and vessels from anterolateral. Skin, subcutis, superficial, and middle cervical fasciae, and vagina carotica are removed. Platysma (pl) with innervating cervical branch of CN VII (cb7) and sternocleidomastoid (scm) muscle are hinged superolaterally. The omohyoid muscle is cut, and its cranially shifted venter superior (soh) is positioned between the superficial and deep veins of the neck. CN X, descending between common carotid artery (cca) and internal jugular vein (ijv), is held and lifted by a forceps. ob, occipital bone; cmh, dorsal tip of larger horn of hyoid bone; scg, superior cervical ganglion (of sympathicus); ms, manubrium of sternum; lcl, left clavicle; smg, submandibular gland; shm, sternohyoid muscle

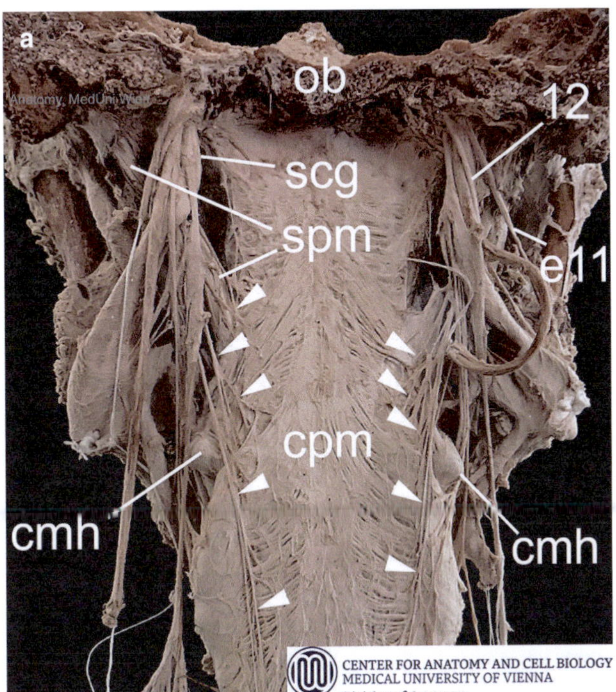

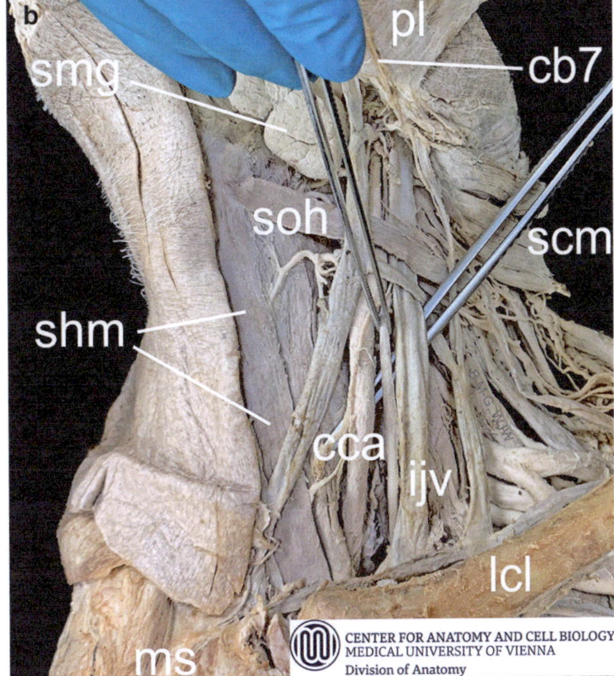

wiched between internal carotid artery and jugular vein (Fig. 1.12b). It enters the thorax and passes dorsal to the hilum of the lung to join the esophagus. In the caudal mediastinum, the left CN X shifts anterior and, together with a few fibers of the right, forms the anterior vagal trunk, which passes the esophageal hiatus of the diaphragm anterior to the esophagus. On the contralateral side, the majority of the fibers of the right CN X shift posteriorly and form the posterior vagal trunk. This passes the diaphragm also through the esophageal hiatus but posterior to the esophagus. In the abdomen, the trunks spread to form a plexus anteriorly and posteriorly to the stomach. The shift of the majority of the left CN X to the anterior and the right CN X to the posterior wall of the stomach has its reason in the leftward rotation of the stomach's greater curvature in early embryogenesis.

Segment of CN X inside the jugular foramen: Inside the jugular foramen, at the level of its superior ganglion, the nerve is joined by a meningeal branch and an auricular branch (Arnold's nerve). The first innervates the dura mater of the posterior cranial fossa, the second the skin of the inner parts of the concha, the posterior wall, and floor of the external acoustic meatus and adjacent parts of the tympanic membrane. It enters the jugular foramen through the mastoid canaliculus and connects to CN VII.

Head and neck segment of CN X: In the neck, CN X occasionally receives fibers of the cervical spinal nerves via the ansa cervicalis [27]. It gives rise to GSA and motor fibers, which contribute to the pharyngeal plexus and innervate the caudal parts of the pharynx (Fig. 1.12b). Small bundles of GSA and SVA fibers run toward and innervate the mucosa and extralingual taste buds located at and near the epiglottis [28].

Preganglionic parasympathetic fibers of the neck segment also form superior cardiac branches. Independently from the main stem of the nerve, they descend to ganglia near the heart. This reflects the early innervation of the heart during embryogenesis, which starts prior to the relative "descensus" of the heart into the thorax.

Finally, the neck segment forms the superior laryngeal nerve, which splits into an external and internal laryngeal nerve. The external innervates the cricothyroid muscle, the internal the mucosa of the cranial larynx.

Thoracic segment of CN X: Inside the chest, CN X gives rise to the recurrent laryngeal nerve.

It comprises GSA, preganglionic parasympathetic, and motor fibers. On the left side, the nerve slings around the aortic arch segment between the origin of the left common carotid and left subclavian artery and then ascends between esophagus and trachea toward the laryngopharynx. On the right side, it slings around the proximal segment of the right subclavian artery and then takes a comparable course—the rounded aortic arch and right subclavian artery segments are both derivatives of the fourth pair of pharyngeal (aortic) arch arteries [29].

The nerve enters the pharynx and continues climbing cranially by running below the mucosa covering the piriform recess and the posterior cricoarytenoid muscle. It changes name to the inferior laryngeal nerve and connects to the superior laryngeal nerve, thereby forming the ansa galeni. The branches of the inferior laryngeal nerve innervate the local pharynx mucosa, the larynx mucosa caudal to the vocal fold, and the inner muscles of the larynx.

The recurrent nerve gives rise to the inferior cardiac branch. This comprises preganglionic parasympathetic fibers, which chiefly synapse in Wrisberg's ganglion, near the heart.

In addition to the recurrent laryngeal nerve, the thoracic portion also forms a pulmonary plexus dorsal to the lung hilum. Fibers of this plexus enter the ipsilateral lung to innervate bronchial glands and muscles.

Abdominal segment of CN X: The abdominal segment is responsible for the parasympathetic innervation of the components of the gastrointestinal tract, from esophagus to Cannon's point (see "Parasympathetic Ganglia" section). Fibers of the vagal trunks become integrated into the celiac and superior mesenteric plexus. These plexuses form around the eponymous arteries and are also named as solar plexus. They contain preganglionic parasympathetic (fibers of CN X), postganglionic sympathetic, and GVA fibers.

The fibers of the vagus nerves finally synapse at intramural ganglion cells of the organs orally to Cannon's point (compare to "Parasympathetic Ganglia" section).

Accessory Nerve (CN XI)

CN XI is traditionally considered as a motor nerve with a cranial and spinal root. Each root has several rootlets. The cranial rootlets leave the posterolateral (dorsolateral) sulcus of the medulla oblongata caudal to the rootlets of CN X. The spinal rootlets leave the segments C1–C5 of the spinal cord, between the ventral and dorsal roots of the cervical spinal nerves. The rootlets of the spinal root ascend and consecutively unify, wherefore a single spinal root then transits the foramen magnum and runs toward the nervous portion of the jugular foramen (Figs. 1.1 and 1.11). Here, it meets the cranial root to form CN XI.

Transiting the foramen in the same compartment of the dura and arachnoid recesses that holds CN X, CN XI splits into an external and internal ramus. The internal becomes integrated in CN X. The external—essentially the fibers of the spinal root—exits the jugular foramen separately and runs to the dorsal aspect of the sternocleidomastoid muscle (Fig. 1.12). Then, it crosses the posterior triangle of the neck in a characteristic meandering course and enters the trapezius muscle [30]. It innervates these muscles together with branches directly emerging from the cervical plexus (sternocleidomastoid and trapezius branch).

Even traditional textbooks (*e.g.,* [1]) emphasize that the concept of a two-rooted CN XI is unsatisfactory. Considering the cranial radix as part of CN X and the spinal radix as CN XI would be more appropriate, since the fibers forming the external ramus essentially emerge from segments of the cervical spine. Hence, both, the sternocleidomastoid and trapezius muscle, are innervated by neurons of the perikarya, which are located in the anterior cornua of segments of the cervical spinal cord.

Hypoglossal Nerve (CN XII)

CN XII is composed of motor fibers innervating the intrinsic and extrinsic muscles of the tongue. It leaves the anterolateral (ventrolateral) sulcus of the medulla spinalis in several rootlets. They pass the vertebral artery (Fig. 1.13) and unify into 1–3 (but in principle up to four) bundles, which head for the hypoglossal canal. The canal is usually composed of 1–2 tunnels, with up to four being possible. Inside the canal, each nerve bundle is surrounded by an extension of dura and arachnoid mater.

After leaving its canal, CN XII is situated dorsal to the vein and nerves transiting the jugular foramen. It starts descending and spirals these nerves and vessels (Fig. 1.12). Then, it curves and crosses the parapharyngeal bundle anteriorly to enter the gap between the mylohyoid and hyoglossus muscles. The curved segment is crossed by the stylomastoid artery on its way from the external carotid artery to the eponymous muscle. Finally, CN XII splits and terminates inside the muscles of the tongue.

The nerve innervates all ipsilateral intrinsic tongue muscles (transversal, vertical, and longitudinal muscle fiber bundles) as well as all muscles connecting the tongue to skeletal elements (genioglossus, hyoglossus, and styloglossus muscles).

Intracranially, CN XII is joined by a meningeal branch consisting of GSA fibers innervating the dura mater of the posterior cranial fossa. They are considered to merely join CN XII for the transit from intra- to extracranially. Extracranially, these fibers immediately leave CN XII to join CN X. Together with these fibers, postganglionic sympathetic fibers starting in the superior cervical ganglion are exchanged. They leave C12 with the meningeal branch and travel with it into the cranial cavity to innervate the arteries of the posterior cranial fossa.

In the neck, large fiber bundles from spinal nerves C1 and C2 join CN XII. These fibers accompany the nerve only for a few millimeters and leave it to form the upper root (superior radix) of the ansa cervicalis (profunda), which innervates the infrahyoid muscles.

The multi-sectioned canal and the existence of several nerve bundles reflect that CN XII is essentially formed by the fusion of the anterior roots of four spinal nerves, which emerge between the occipital somites and fail to form dorsal roots—occipital somites exist in the early embryo and contribute to the occipital bone. Hence, the status of CN XII as a "cranial nerve" is questionable from an anatomic perspective.

Parasympathetic Ganglia and Postganglionic Nerves in the Head and Neck

Four cranial nerves (CNs III, VII, IX, and X) comprise, among others, preganglionic parasympathetic fibers when exiting the brain. Those of CN III, VII, and IX head for four large multipolar or one of the several, very small scattered visceral ganglia located in the head. On the contrary, the parasympathetic fibers of CN X synapse at intramural ganglion cells of the intestine and ganglia scattered near the large organs of thorax and abdomen.

As all ganglion cells, those of the visceral ganglia are derived from neural crest cells, migrating into the body tissues during early embryogenesis. Usually, there is an amplification, with one preganglionic fiber on average synapsing with three postganglionic neurons.

The four main head ganglia are briefly characterized in Table 1.2. The ganglia only comprise multipolar perikarya of parasympathetic neurons. Yet, the ganglia also connect to postganglionic sympathetic and general somatic afferent (GSA) nerves. Therefore, nerves emerging from the ganglia, or at least the nerves joined by postganglionic parasympathetic fibers, hold postganglionic parasympathetic, postganglionic sympathetic, and GSA fibers.

Ciliary Ganglion

The ciliary ganglion rests in the orbit, temporal to the optic nerve and approximately halfway between the eyeball and the apex of the orbit (Fig. 1.8). Preganglionic parasympathetic fibers, derived from the accessory nucleus of the oculomotor nerve (Edinger Westphal), synapse. They reach the ganglion by traveling as part of CN III.

GSA fibers of CN V_1 and postganglionic sympathetic fibers traveling as part of the nasociliary nerve also enter the ganglion, with the latter having joined the parasellar segment of CN V_1. They do not synapse but merely pass through and become integrated in the nerves leaving the ganglion.

The ganglion gives rise to so-called short ciliary nerves, which hold GSA and postsynaptic sympathetic and parasympathetic fibers. These nerves enter the eyeball. The parasympathetic fibers innervate the ciliary body and muscle and sphincter pupillae. The sympathetic fibers innervate the dilatator pupillae and occasionally travel with the long ciliary nerves (direct branch of nasociliary nerve) instead of passing through the ganglion.

Pterygopalatine Ganglion

The pterygopalatine ganglion rests in the pterygopalatine fossa. It receives preganglionic parasympathetic fibers from the superior part of the salivatory nucleus (lacrimal nucleus) via the intermediate, greater petrosal, and Vidian nerve (nerve of the pterygoid canal).

Table 1.2 Cranial parasympathetic ganglia

	Position	Preganglionic neurons	Preganglionic fibers (CN)	Parasympathetic targets
Ciliary	Orbit	Nucleus of Edinger-Westphal (accessory nucleus)	CN III	Sphincter pupillae, ciliary muscle, and body
Pterygopalatine	Pterygopalatine fossa	Superior salivatory nucleus	CN VII (intermediate)	Lacrimal gland
Submandibular	Submandibular region	Superior salivatory nucleus	CN VII (intermediate)	Submandibular gland
Otic	Infratemporal fossa, near oval foramen	Inferior salivatory nucleus	CN IX	Parotid gland

The greater petrosal nerve splits off the intermediate nerve of Wrisberg at the level of the external knee of CN VII. It carries GSA and SVA fibers and passes in an osseous canal through the petrosal part of the temporal bone. After leaving the canal and entering the middle cranial fossa through a small hiatus (hiatus of greater petrosal nerve), it continues extradurally in a small osseous groove towards the foramen lacerum. After passing through this foramen, it joins the profound petrosal nerve. This is a bundle of postganglionic sympathetic fibers, which branches from the internal carotid nerve before it enters the carotid canal (compare Fig. 1.13).

The unified greater and profound petrosal nerves are named as nerve of the pterygoid canal (Vidian nerve). This passes through the eponymous canal at the base of the pterygoid process (Vidian canal) and reaches the pterygopalatine ganglion in the pterygopalatine fossa (Fig. 1.14).

The pterygopalatine ganglion is situated below the level of the foramen rotundum and is also entered by a big bundle of sensory fibers from CN V_2 (compare to CN V). The parasympathetic fibers synapse, while the sympathetic GSA and SVA fibers only pass through. Hence, the nerves arising from the ganglion are composed of postganglionic parasympathetic and sympathetic fibers, as well as two types of sensory fibers.

Most of the nerves arising from the ganglion descend to innervate the mucosa, taste buds, and minor salivary glands of the palate, nasopharynx, and posterior and lower nasal cavity. Two ascend through the inferior orbital fissure to reach targets in the orbit (Fig. 1.15).

Nasopharyngeal nerve: The nerve passes through the palatovaginal canal to reach the nasopharynx near the ostium of the auditory tube.

Greater palatine nerve: The nerve gives rise to lateral posterior inferior nasal branches and then transits the greater palatine foramen to innervate most of the hard palate (Fig. 1.15b).

Lesser palatine nerves: These are usually 2–3 nerves which pass through the lesser palatine canal and innervate the soft palate, uvula, and palatine tonsil.

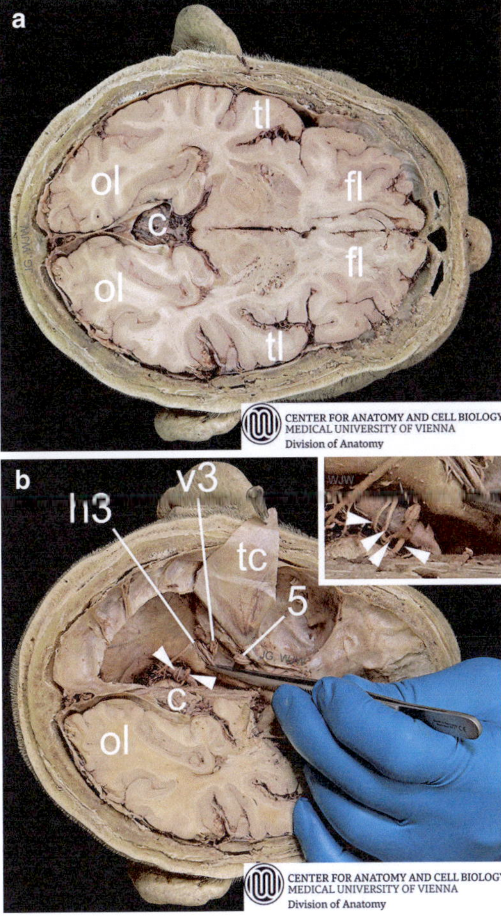

Fig. 1.13 Cranial nerve (CN) XII. Numbers refer to respective CNs. Axially cut head from superior. Frontal to the right. Calvaria and upper parts of the brain removed. (**a**) Topology of brain structures in relation to skull base and meninges for orientation. Compare to Fig. 1.6. (**b**) Intracranial course of CN XII. Left-sided telencephalon and entire diencephalon are removed. The left-sided tentorium cerebelli (tce) is cut along the transverse sinus and hinged superiorly along the superior petrosal sinus. The brain stem is cut at the level of the caudal mesencephalon and in the midline. Brain stem material on the left is removed. Inlay magnifies the situation near the hypoglossal canal. The rootlets of the nerves, which leave the brain at the anterior lateral sulcus (h3) are shifted frontally by a forceps to expose CN XII. Its rootlets (arrowheads) converge and enter a bipartite hypoglossal canal. Note their relationship to the vertebral artery. ol, occipital lobe; tl, temporal lobe; fl, frontal lobe; c, cerebellum; tc, hinged left tentorium cerebelli; v3, cranial nerves of the cerebellopontine angle

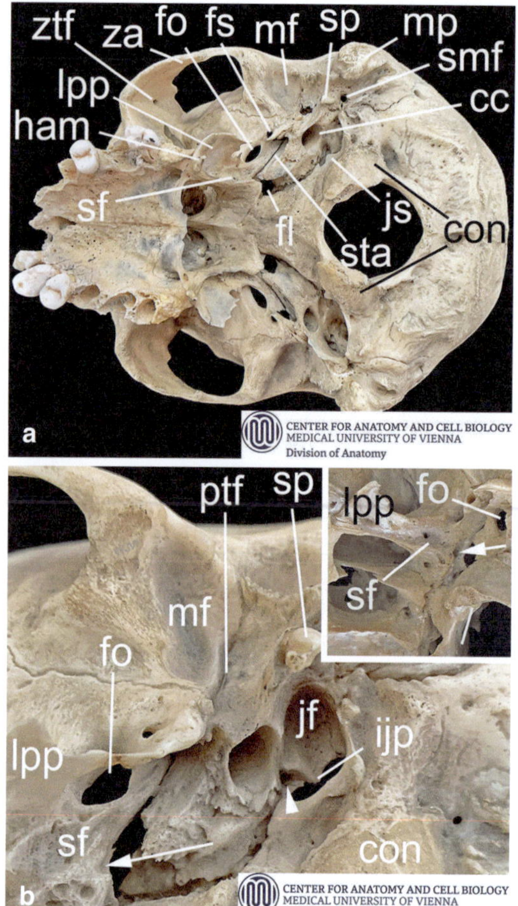

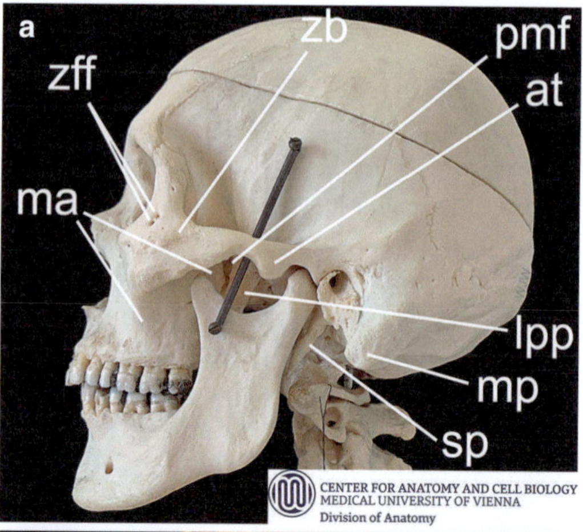

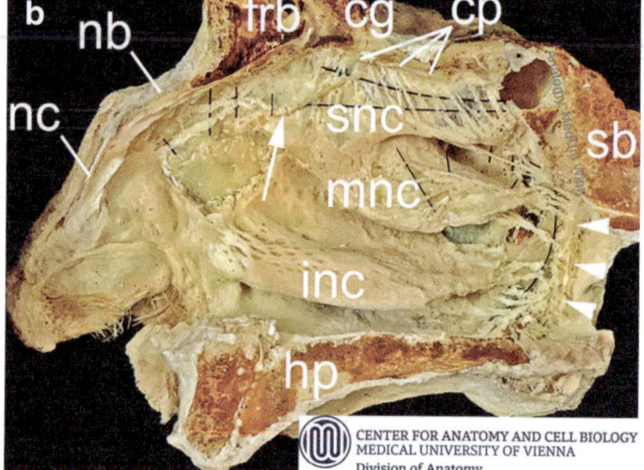

Fig. 1.14 Osseous pathways taken by postganglionic parasympathetic nerve fibers. Skull base from inferior. Frontal to the left. (**a**) Overview for orientation. (**b**) Magnification of A in a slightly oblique angle showing basal parts of the temporal and adjacent sphenoidal and occipital bones. The petrotympanic fissure (ptf), being the passage for the chorda tympani, and the tympanic canal (arrowhead), being the passage for the tympanic nerve, are clearly visible. The tympanic canal starts at the nervous portion of the jugular foramen, medial to the jugular spine (intrajugular process, ijp) of the temporal bone. Note the jugular fossa (jf) lateral to the spine. Inlay shows again a magnification of this specimen in again a slightly different angle. It highlights the entrance into the pterygoid (Vidian) canal (arrow) beneath the scaphoid fossa (sf), which is the passage of the Vidian nerve into the pterygopalatine fossa (compare Fig. 1.15). con, condyle; mp, mastoid process; smf, sp., styloid process; smf, stylomastoid foramen; cc, external ostium of carotid canal; js, jugular spine (intrajugular process of occipital bone; mf, mandibular fossa; lpp, lateral pterygoid plate; fo, foramen ovale; fs, foramen spinosum; sta, (semi-)canal for pharyngotympanic tube; fl, foramen lacerum; lpp, lateral pterygoid plate; ham, hamulus on medial pterygoid plate; za, zygomatic arch; ztf, zygomaticotemporal foramen

Fig. 1.15 Major nerves arising from the pterygopalatine ganglion to innervate the lateral wall of the nasal cavity. Frontal to the left. (**a**) Skull from left. Note the pterygomaxillary fissure (pmf) as entrance into the pterygopalatine fossa. (**b**) Lateral wall of a right nasal cavity. Specimen from the historical collection of the Division of Anatomy of the Medical University of Vienna. The mucosa is partly removed. The fila olfactoria emerging from the superior nasal concha (snc) are displayed (compare with Fig. 1.2). The bones parting nasal cavity and pterygopalatine fossa (arrowheads) are removed. The greater and palatine lesser nerves descend toward their eponymous foramina (arrowheads). The lateral posterior superior and lateral posterior inferior nasal nerves are exposed. Note the lateral internal nasal branch of the anterior ethmoidal nerve (arrow)—a branch forming CN V_1. mp, mastoid process; sp., styloid process; lpp, lateral pterygoid plate; at, articular tubercle; zb, zygomatic bone; zff, zygomaticofacial foramen; ma, maxilla; frb, frontal bone; nc, nasal cartilage; nb, nasal bone; sb, sphenoid bone; cg, crista galli; cp, cribriform plate; mnc, medial nasal concha; inc, inferior nasal concha; hp, hard palate

Sphenopalatine nerve: This represents a bundle of nerve fibers, which passes through the sphenopalatine foramen into the nasal cavity. In the majority of individuals, it splits into six lateral posterior superior nasal nerves, three medial posterior superior nasal nerves, and the nasopalatine nerve. The lateral posterior superior nasal nerves innervate the posterior parts of the middle and superior concha (Fig. 1.15b); the medial posterior superior nasal nerves are the septum nasi. The nasopalatine nerve runs anteriorly along the lower parts of the vomer and descends through the incisive (nasopalatine) foramen to the anterior section of the palate.

Nerve for orbital (Müller) muscle: The minority of fibers emerging from the pterygopalatine ganglion ascend toward the inferior orbital fissure. They form several bundles, composed of sympathetic and GSA fibers, which enter the orbital muscle of Müller and the local periosteum, a region which is also reached by fibers emerging from the ganglion located in the pterygopalatine compartment of the PSR [10].

Communicating branch with zygomatic nerve: A single bundle of postganglionic sympathetic and parasympathetic fibers ascends from the ganglion and joins the zygomatic nerve. When splitting into the zygomaticotemporal and zygomaticofrontal nerve, it stays with the zygomaticotemporal before it transits to the lacrimal nerve (Fig. 1.8) to reach and innervate both lobes of the lacrimal gland.

Submandibular Ganglion

The submandibular ganglion rests in the submandibular region, superior to the hilum of the submandibular gland. It is targeted by preganglionic parasympathetic fibers, which emerge from the superior salivatory nucleus. They leave the brain as part of Wrisberg's nerve and branch from the mastoid segment of CN VII as part of the chorda tympani. The chorda tympani also holds GSA and SVA fibers (see above).

As suggested by its name, the chorda tympani enters the tympanic cavity. Running near the tympanic membrane, it passes below the joint linking hamulus and incus in a highly variable distance and then leaves the cavity through the petrotympanic (glaserian) fissure (Fig. 1.14) to enter the infratemporal fossa. Here, it joins the lingual nerve (see CN V$_3$). The preganglionic parasympathetic fibers and a few GSA fibers leave the nerve near the submandibular fossa of the mandible and descend to the submandibular ganglion. This link between lingual nerve and ganglion is named the "posterior filament."

In addition to the preganglionic parasympathetic and the sensory fibers forming the posterior filament, postganglionic sympathetic fibers enter the submandibular ganglion. They emerge from perikarya located in the superior cervical ganglion and travel to the region as part of the visceral plexus surrounding the facial artery. While the parasympathetic fibers synapse, the sensory and sympathetic fibers merely pass through the ganglion. Five to six fiber bundles (filaments) holding postganglionic parasympathetic, sympathetic, and GSA fibers leave the ganglion to enter and innervate the submandibular gland. In addition, a single filament, the "anterior filament," arises from the ganglion. It holds postganglionic parasympathetic and sympathetic fibers and ascends to join the lingual nerve. Step by step, small fiber bundles leave the nerve to target minor salivary glands. The majority of the fibers however travels with the lingual nerve toward the sublingual fossa of the mandible, where they leave the nerve to innervate the sublingual gland.

Otic Ganglion

The otic ganglion is located in the infratemporal fossa, near the oval foramen. Here, preganglionic parasympathetic fibers stemming from perikarya in the inferior segments of the salivatory nucleus synapse. These fibers leave the brain together with CN IX. They branch off as part of the tympanic nerve and reach the tympanic cavity through the tympanic canal (Fig. 1.14). Inside the tympanic cavity, the tympanic nerve forms the tympanic plexus on the promontorium (cochlear promontorium), which also receives a small amount of fibers from the greater petrosal nerve. Out of this plexus, a portion of fibers converge and form a single nerve, the lesser petrosal nerve. This leaves the tympanic cavity through an osseous canal, which ends with a hiatus at the internal side of the petrous part of the temporal bone. In an eponymous groove, it then runs in middle cranial fossa in the direction of the oval foramen and passes through an osseous canal into the infratemporal fossa, where it terminates in the otic ganglion (see also CN IX).

The lesser petrosal nerve is the only nerve fiber bundle that joins the otic ganglion. Its fibers synapse and the postganglionic parasympathetic fibers pass posteriorly to the middle meningeal artery to join the sensory auriculotemporal nerve, which passes the meningeal artery anteriorly. While passing the artery, postganglionic sympathetic fibers arriving as part of the plexus surrounding the middle meningeal artery also join the auriculotemporal nerve. Hence, when entering the parotid gland, the auriculotemporal nerve carries GSA, postganglionic sympathetic, and postganglionic parasympathetic fibers. Once inside the parotid gland, these fibers leave the nerve and join CN VII. As part of the branches of CN VII, they spread through the parotid gland and innervate it.

References

1. Williams PL, Gray H. Gray's anatomy. 37th ed. Edinburgh: Churchill Livingstone; 1989.
2. Apaydin N, Kendir S, Karahan ST. The anatomical relationships of the ocular motor nerves with an emphasis on surgical anatomy of the orbit. Anat Rec (Hoboken). 2019;302(4):568–74.
3. Porras-Gallo MI, Pena-Meliaan A, Viejo F, Hernaandez T, Puelles E, Echevarria D, et al. Overview of the history of the cranial nerves: from galen to the 21st century. Anat Rec (Hoboken). 2019;302(3):381–93.
4. Martinez-Marcos A, Sanudo JR. Cranial nerves: phylogeny and ontogeny. Anat Rec (Hoboken). 2019;302(3):378–80.
5. Fuller GN, Burger PC. Nervus terminalis (cranial nerve zero) in the adult human. Clin Neuropathol. 1990;9(6):279–83.
6. Pineda AG, Leon-Sarmiento FE, Doty RL. Cranial nerve 13. Handb Clin Neurol. 2019;164:135–44.
7. Vilensky JA. The neglected cranial nerve: nervus terminalis (cranial nerve N). Clin Anat. 2014;27(1):46–53.
8. Pena-Melian A, Cabello-de la Rosa JP, Gallardo-Alcaniz MJ, Vaamonde-Gamo J, Relea-Calatayud F, Gonzalez-Lopez L, et al. Cranial pair 0: the nervus terminalis. Anat Rec (Hoboken). 2019;302(3):394–404.
9. Benninger B, McNeil J. Transitional nerve: a new and original classification of a peripheral nerve supported by the nature of the accessory nerve (CN XI). Neurol Res Int. 2010;2010:476018.
10. Weninger WJ, Müller GB. The sympathetic nerves of the parasellar region: pathways to the orbit and the brain. Acta Anat (Basel). 1997;160(4):254–60.
11. Weninger WJ, Streicher J, Müller GB. Anatomical compartments of the parasellar region: adipose tissue bodies represent intracranial continuations of extracranial spaces. J Anat. 1997;191(Pt 2):269–75.
12. Weninger WJ, Müller GB. The parasellar region of human infants: cavernous sinus topography and surgical approaches. J Neurosurg. 1999;90(3):484–90.
13. Weninger WJ, Pramhas D. Compartments of the adult parasellar region. J Anat. 2000;197(Pt 4):681–6.
14. Weninger WJ, Prokop M. In vivo 3D analysis of the adipose tissue in the orbital apex and the compartments of the parasellar region. Clin Anat. 2004;17(2):112–7.
15. Parkinson D. Lateral sellar compartment: history and anatomy. J Craniofac Surg. 1995;6(1):55–68.
16. Meng S, Geyer SH, Costa Lda F, Viana MP, Weninger WJ. Objective characterization of the course of the parasellar internal carotid artery using mathematical tools. Surg Radiol Anat. 2008;30(6):519–26.
17. Parkinson D. Collateral circulation of cavernous carotid artery: anatomy. Can J Surg. 1964;7:251–68.
18. Lasjaunias PL. Anatomy of the tentorial arteries. J Neurosurg. 1984;61(6):1159–60.
19. Parkinson D. A surgical approach to the cavernous portion of the carotid artery. Anatomical studies and case report. J Neurosurg. 1965;23(5):474–83.
20. Gyori E, Tzou CH, Weninger WJ, Reissig L, Schmidt-Erfurth U, Radtke C, et al. Axon numbers and landmarks of trigeminal donor nerves for corneal neurotization. PLoS One. 2018;13(10):e0206642.
21. Tv L, Wachsmuth W. Praktische anatomie. Erster Band, erster Teil: Kopf. Berlin: Springer Verlag; 1985.
22. Heber UM, Weninger WJ. In: Tzou CJ, Rodriguez-Lorenzo A, editors. Anatomy of the facial nerve. Facial palsy: Springer Cham; 2021. p. 71–8.

23. Jensson D, Weninger WJ, Schmid M, Meng S, Jonsson L, Tzou CJ, et al. Oculo-zygomatic nerve transfer for facial synkinesis: an anatomical feasibility study. Microsurgery. 2019;39(7):629–33.

24. Lopez-Poveda EA. Olivocochlear efferents in animals and humans: from anatomy to clinical relevance. Front Neurol. 2018;9:197.

25. Mathews MA, Camp AJ, Murray AJ. Reviewing the role of the efferent vestibular system in motor and vestibular circuits. Front Physiol. 2017;8:552.

26. Raghu V, Salvi R, Sadeghi SG. Efferent inputs are required for normal function of vestibular nerve afferents. J Neurosci. 2019;39(35):6922–35.

27. Banneheka S, Tokita K, Kumaki K. Nerve fiber analysis of ansa cervicalis-vagus communications. Anat Sci Int. 2008;83(3):145–51.

28. Rabl H. Notiz zur Morphologie der Geschmacksknospen auf der Epiglottis. Anat Anz. 1895;11:153–6.

29. Geyer SH, Weninger WJ. Some mice feature 5th pharyngeal arch arteries and double-lumen aortic arch malformations. Cells Tissues Organs. 2012;196(1):90–8.

30. Placheta E, Tinhofer I, Schmid M, Reissig LF, Pona I, Weninger W, et al. The spinal accessory nerve for functional muscle innervation in facial reanimation surgery: an anatomical and histomorphometric study. Ann Plast Surg. 2016;77(6):640–4.

Introduction

Magnetic resonance imaging (MRI) is the main imaging modality in the diagnostic workup of neurologic symptoms regarding cranial nerves. Superior soft tissue contrast and advanced MRI techniques allow a thorough assessment of the nervous system. With appropriate sequences, 3 T MRI systems offer a better signal-to-noise ratio and superior spatial resolution. Due to many medical and nonmedical reasons, MRI systems with 1.5 T are more common. In short, systems with 3 T are more cost-intensive as they are technically more demanding. For most anatomical regions, any MRI system requires a dedicated radiofrequency coil, which has to be changed if an examination exceeds the anatomical range of the specific coil. MRI is a safe examination technique. However, checking patient history for metal foreign objects or incompatible implants is time-consuming. Websites offer a thorough database free of charge, e.g., www.MRIsafety.com/list.html. For several examinations, intravenous contrast agents are not necessary. In some cases, the examination protocol must be adapted after evaluation of the first sequences, and application of a contrast agent may be necessary. Sedation with an appropriate monitoring can be helpful for patients with claustrophobia and infants but demands much organizational effort.

Direct visualization of nerves is possible. Due to the small size and complex surroundings, the depiction of most cranial nerves in the extracranial segments is difficult and strongly depends on the anatomical region. In all cases, MRI visualizes the presumed pathway of the nerve. With high sensitivity, MRI depicts denervation edema in muscles. The pattern of denervated muscles in turn may indicate the affected nerve. A reliable depiction of perineural spread of neoplastic processes is a unique and valuable feature of MRI and is essential in the staging of head and neck cancer.

The role of computed tomography (CT) in the diagnostic workup of cranial nerve pathologies is very limited. Processes in cranial nerve nuclei or tracts, *e.g.,* infarction or hemorrhages, are depicted identically to processes in other parts of the central nervous system, with commonly known weaknesses in comparison to

Authors of this chapter: Stefan Meng and Barbara Horvath-Mechtler.

© The Author(s), under exclusive license to Springer Nature Switzerland AG 2023

W. Grisold et al., *The Cranial Nerves in Neurology*, https://doi.org/10.1007/978-3-031-43081-7_2

MRI. Although the spatial resolution of standard CT systems is superior to standard MRI systems, the much lower soft tissue contrast limits CT to the visualization of osteolytic, osteoblastic, or traumatic processes of the skull base. A direct visualization of a cranial nerve either intra- or extracranially is not feasible.

Ultrasound is a cost-effective, high-resolution imaging modality. There are virtually no contraindications for diagnostic ultrasound. Natural limitations are the bone barrier, gas-filled spaces, and nerves lying deeply in the body. Thus, intracranial and intraosseous segments of cranial nerves cannot be examined in clinical routine. Just outside the skull base, some of the cranial nerves may be directly visualized by ultrasound. Deep lying nerves can be reached by ultrasound using low frequencies only, which in turn yield low resolution images [1]. While the course of the vagus nerve in the neck can be visualized easily by ultrasound, the branches in the abdomen cannot be routinely examined. In addition to bones, gas also represents an absolute barrier for ultrasound, so the course of the vagal branches in the thorax is invisible for ultrasound. Unfortunately, ultrasound of nerves has not been established as a standard tool in many clinical facilities. This might be due to the limitation that ultrasound is strongly dependent on the skills of the examiner.

In this chapter, we will provide a concise radiological overview of imaging for each cranial nerve. Imaging modalities will be discussed regarding the respective anatomical segment. For selected diseases, we also present imaging modality recommendations. Finally, special regions will be discussed.

Cranial Nerve I: Olfactory Nerve

Using MRI, depiction the olfactory mucosa of the nasal cavity is feasible, but the diagnostic value exceeding the possibilities of an endoscopy might depend on the individual case.

The osseous structure of the nasal cavity and the paranasal sinuses as well as the base of the anterior fossa – especially of the cribriform plate –are adequately examined by CT [2].

Although visualization of the fila olfactoria is technically feasible in experimental settings using high-resolution MRI systems, the detection of a traumatic rupture of these thin structures is not a routine examination [3].

The olfactory system, beginning at the bulb of the olfactory nerve, can be routinely visualized by MRI systems with a field strength of 1.5 and 3 T. Here, T2-weighted images show a strong contrast between the bright cerebrospinal fluid and the dark nervous structures. At the same time, there is poor contrast between the individual nervous structures of the olfactory system, the brain, and local bone structures [2].

Congenital anosmia: MRI is the imaging modality of choice for delineation of hypoplastic or even absent olfactory bulbs (Fig. 2.1).

Local tumor process: MRI and CT, both with contrast, are necessary to assess the intra- and extracranial tumor extent. MRI is necessary to evaluate the soft tissue and CT is necessary for detection of bone destruction (Fig. 2.2).

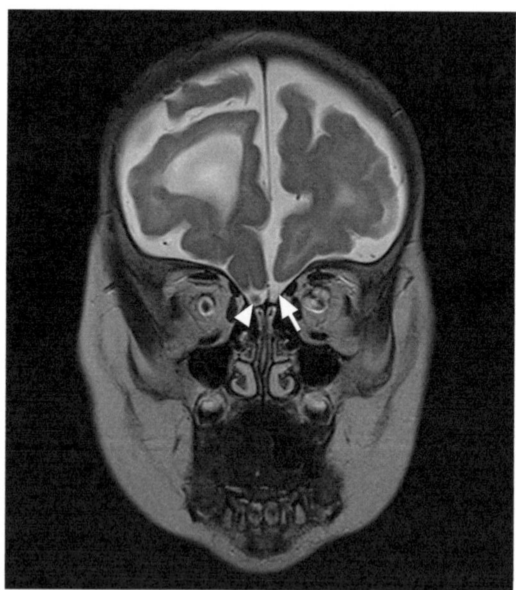

Fig. 2.1 Olfactory nerve aplasia. Coronal T2w MRI. Olfactory bulb aplasia on the patient's left side (arrow) and regular anatomical situation on the right side (arrowhead)

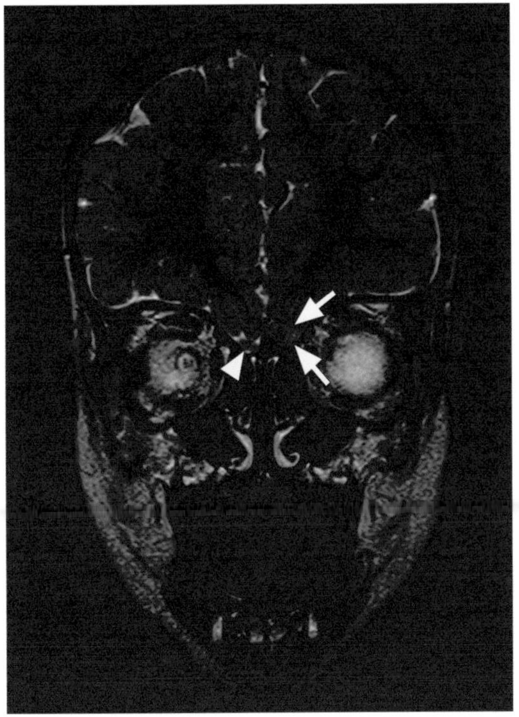

Fig. 2.2 Medulloblastoma. Coronal T2w MRI. Patient with an medulloblastoma which is extending into the olfactory nerve on the left side (arrows). Regular nerve on the right patient side (arrowhead)

Cranial Nerve II: Optic Nerve

Due to motion, ocular globes are difficult to scan with high resolution MRI. Technically, ophthalmic ultrasound can visualize the posterior segment of the eye, retina, and the macula as well as the beginning of the optic nerve. Optic nerve head drusen, detachments of the retina, and tumors can be detected. Furthermore, ultrasound is able to detect elevated intracranial pressure, which leads to a widening of the optic nerve sheath [4].

The method of choice for the intraorbital segment of the optic nerve and its surroundings is MRI. The use of contrast agent is advised in most cases as the optic nerve shows no enhancement; thus, enhancing pathological processes may support easier detection. The orbital wall and the optic canal are assessed best with CT and multiplanar reconstructions.

MRI is the best modality for the intracranial part of the optic nerve, the optic chiasm, and the optic tracts. High-resolution 3D T1- and T2-weighted sequences are recommended. 3D reformations simplify the assessment of the visual pathway [5]. Diffusion tensor imaging may depict the composition of the nerve fibers.

Idiopathic orbital inflammation: The recommended imaging modality is MRI with contrast, which shows inflammatory changes in the orbital soft tissue. Alternatively, CT with contrast may be used.

Optic neuritis: The best imaging modality is MRI with contrast. Alternatively, sequences without contrast (T2w with fat saturation) might be helpful. Considering possible underlying diseases, such as neuromyelitis optica or multiple sclerosis, extension of the field of view to the entire brain is recommended (Fig. 2.3)

Graves disease: For surgical planning, CT as well as MRI are indicated.

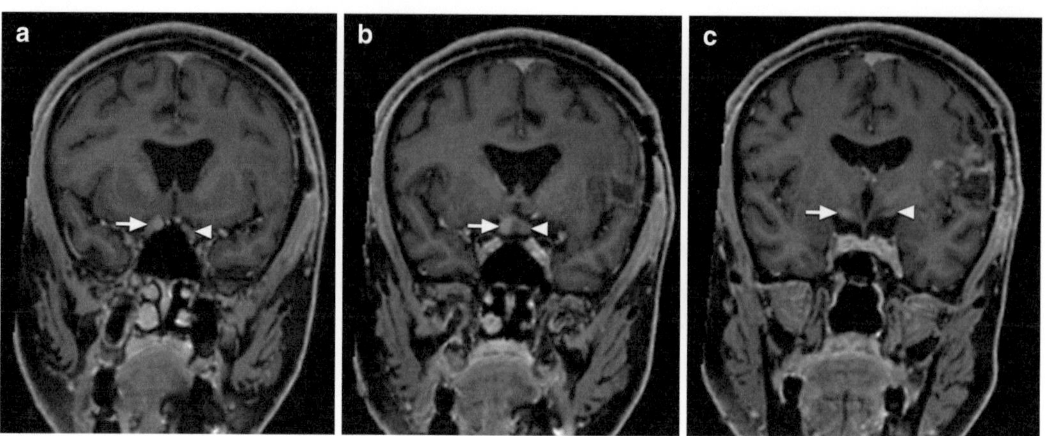

Fig. 2.3 Optic neuritis. Coronal T1w MRI with contrast. Marked enhancement of the right visual pathway (arrows) and regular depiction on the left side (arrowheads). (**a**) optic nerve; (**b**) optic chiasm; (**c**) optic tract

Cranial Nerve III: Oculomotor Nerve

The course of the oculomotor nerve can be divided into seven segments, which are the mesencephalon, interpeduncular cistern, petroclinoid segment, trigonal segment, cavernous segment, fissural segment, and orbit.

For the mesencephalic to the cavernous segment, MRI with high-resolution T2w sequences in axial and coronal planes are advised. In the cavernous segment, the nerve lies within the lateral wall of the cavernous sinus just below the anterior clinoid process (Fig. 2.4). Of all cranial nerves (oculomotor, trochlear, ophthalmic, and maxillary) in the lateral wall, the oculomotor nerve is the most superior [6].

The oculomotor nerve enters the orbit via the superior orbital fissure. Bony structures should be assessed by CT. Depiction of the oculomotor nerve divisions in the orbit may be difficult.

Aneurysms: Due to the close proximity of the oculomotor nerve to the posterior communicating artery, posterior cerebral artery, and the superior cerebellar artery, isolated symptoms of the oculomotor nerve indicate the search for an aneurysm of the arteries, preferably with MRI or alternatively with CT.

Uncal herniation: In cases of trauma to the head, an isolated lesion of the oculomotor nerve might result from a nerve entrapment by uncal herniation. MRI is the imaging modality to assess any brain parenchyma dislocation.

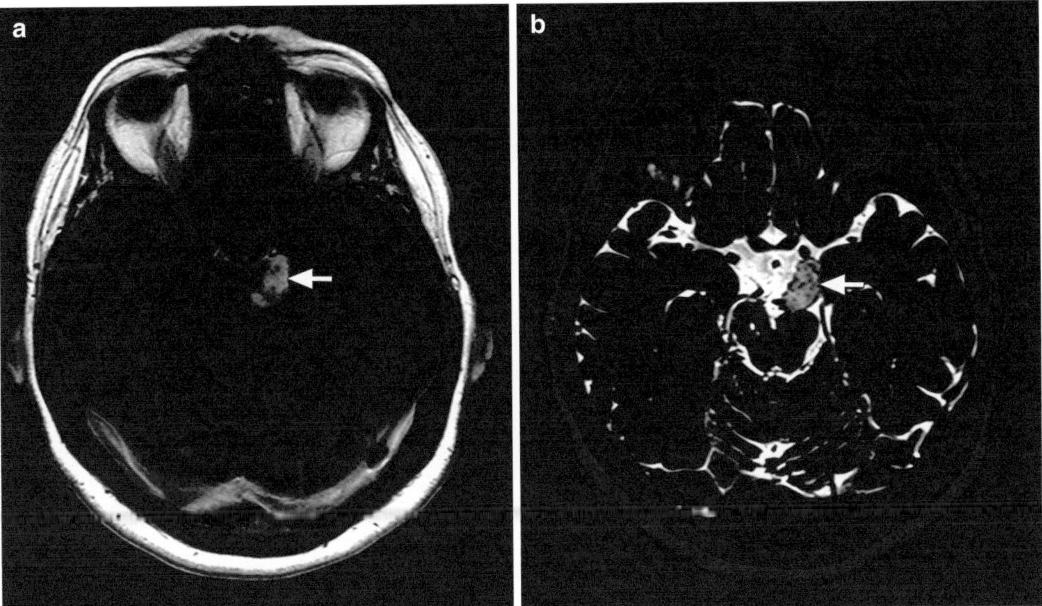

Fig. 2.4 Oculomotor nerve schwannoma. (**a**) Axial T1w contrast-enhanced MRI. (**b**) Axial space MRI. Bulky, enhancing oculomotor nerve schwannoma on the left side (arrow)

Cranial Nerve IV: Trochlear Nerve

The nuclei of each trochlear nerve lie contralateral to the side of the course and muscle of the nerve.

Inferior to the colliculus, the nerve leaves the brain stem as the only cranial nerve exiting from the brain stem dorsally. Through the quadrigeminal and ambient cistern, the nerve travels frontal between the posterior cerebral artery and the superior cerebellar artery (Fig. 2.5). From below the edge of the tentorium, the nerve enters the lateral wall of the cavernous sinus just below the course of the oculomotor nerve. Finally, the nerve enters the orbit via the superior orbital fissure above the annulus of Zinn. The course of the nerve from the nuclei to the superior orbital fissure can be visualized by MRI. Direct visualization of the nuclei is not possible. Due to the small size of the nerve, visualization of the nerve can be challenging. High-resolution sequences in coronal and axial planes are recommended. Bony structures are depicted best with CT.

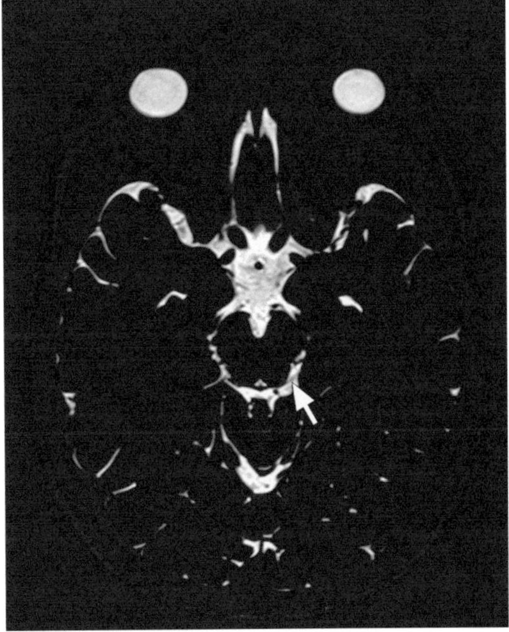

Fig. 2.5 Regular trochlear nerve depiction. Axial space MRI. Routine depiction of the trochlear nerve may be demanding as demonstrated here. The course of the nerve (arrow) is just visible

Isolated lesions of the nerve are based on trauma. Complex neuropathies with the association of other local cranial nerves occur due to tumors, stroke, and processes in the cavernous sinus or orbit [7].

Aneurysm: Isolated lesions of the trochlear nerve might result from an aneurysm of the superior cerebellar nerve. Here, MRI is the primary imaging modality, and the secondary modality is CT.

Trauma: Injuries of the trochlear nerve due to trauma may be assessed with MRI.

Cranial Nerve V: Trigeminal Nerve

The origin of the trigeminal nerve is in the mesencephalon, pons, and the medulla oblongata as well as the cervical spinal cord (Fig. 2.6). In the cisternal segment, the nerve lies in the prepontine cistern. Then, the trigeminal nerve lies as a trigeminal ganglion in a dural space called Meckel's cave. In the abovementioned segments, the trigeminal nerve can be examined with MRI.

At the trigeminal ganglion, the three branches of the trigeminal nerve separate and head to different directions:

1. The ophthalmic branch (V1) enters the lateral wall of the cavernous sinus just below the trochlear nerve and enters the orbit via the superior orbital fissure. For the cavernous sinus, MRI is the primary modality. In the orbit, direct visualization of the ophthalmic nerve branches is difficult. The tiny sensory terminal branches of the ophthalmic nerve, the supraorbital and supratrochlear branches, can be examined directly with high resolution ultrasound beginning at the superior rim of the orbit into the periphery.
2. The maxillary branch (V2) also enters the lateral wall of the cavernous sinus below the ophthalmic branch. Again, MRI is the modality of choice. The maxillary branch enters the foramen rotundum, passes the superior part of the pterygopalatine fossa, and enters the orbital region through the inferior orbital fissure. In the orbital floor, the nerve travels frontally in the infraorbital canal (Fig. 2.7)

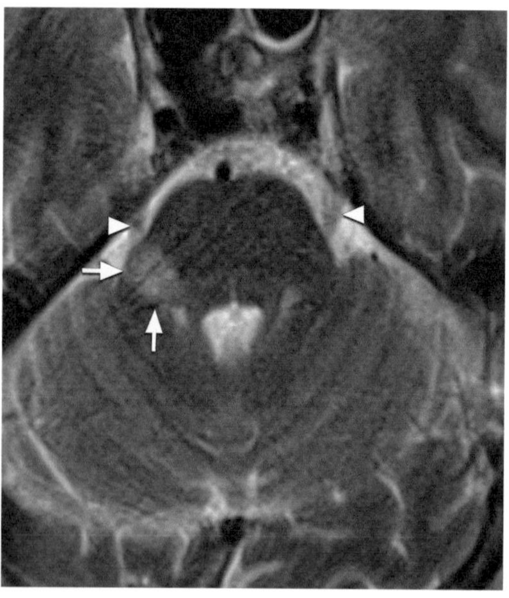

Fig. 2.6 Multiple sclerosis plaque in trigeminal nuclei. Axial T2w MRI. Multiple sclerosis plaque in the right intra-axial trigeminal nerve origin (arrows). Regular trigeminal nerve roots on both sides (arrowheads)

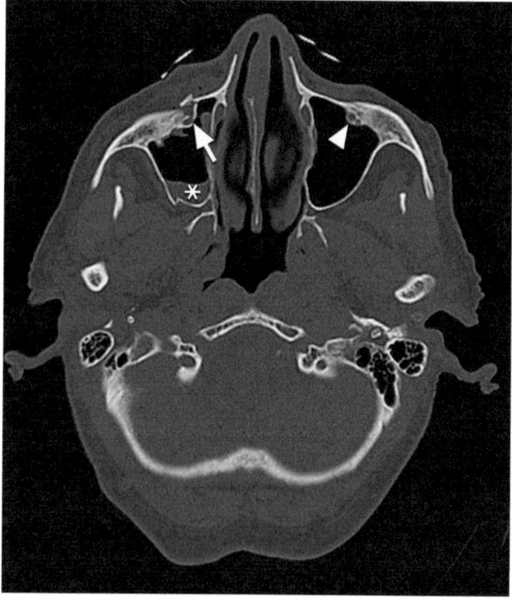

Fig. 2.7 Maxillary fracture. Axial CT. Fracture of the maxilla on the right side with air-fluid level in the right maxillary sinus (white asterisk). The infraorbital canal is also affected (arrow), while the canal is intact on the left side (arrowhead)

From the foramen rotundum to the infraorbital canal, CT depicts the bony walls of the pathway and MRI of the soft tissue. Leaving the infraorbital canal, the branches of the infraorbital nerve course into the soft tissue of the face, where the nerve branches can be assessed directly with high-resolution ultrasound.

3. The mandibular branch (V3) does not enter the cavernous sinus. Instead, the nerve passes through the foramen ovale into the masticatory space, where it supplies the motor branches for the pterygoid muscles and the muscle of the soft palate. For the passage through the skull base, CT is the best modality. Below the base of the skull direct visualization of the mandibular nerve branches is not possible. However, the anatomical surroundings of the known nerve branch pathways can be assessed with MRI. Peripheral branches, which may be directly visualized, are branches on the surface of the head, such as the auriculotemporal masseteric nerve. The bony canal and the inferior alveolar nerve itself can be visualized by CT and MRI, respectively. The superficial segment of the auriculotemporal nerve and of the masseteric nerve can be examined with high-resolution ultrasound [8].

Trigeminal neuralgia: Blood vessels with contact to the trigeminal nerve are visualized best with high-resolution MRI [9].

Inflammation: Local infections can be visualized with MRI and contrast enhancement.

Cranial Nerve VI: Abducens Nerve

Originating from the abducens nuclei in the pons, the nerve leaves the brain stem in a groove between the pons and the medulla oblongata. For assessing the pons, MRI is the imaging modality of choice.

In the prepontine cistern and cavernous sinus, the nerve lies in the center, lateral to the internal carotid artery. Here, the nerve is visualized best by MRI, where in most cases due to the anatomical course of the nerve, 3D reconstructions might be necessary (Fig. 2.8). Passing through the superior orbital fissure and orbit, the nerve may be depicted directly by MRI and CT, with the latter for the bony walls adjacent to the nerve.

Petrous apicitis/Gradenigo syndrome: The inflammatory changes, which extend from the middle ear into the pneumatized petrous apex, might also affect the trochlear nerve. CT depicts the bony destruction, whereas MRI proves the meningeal thickening [10] (Fig. 2.9).

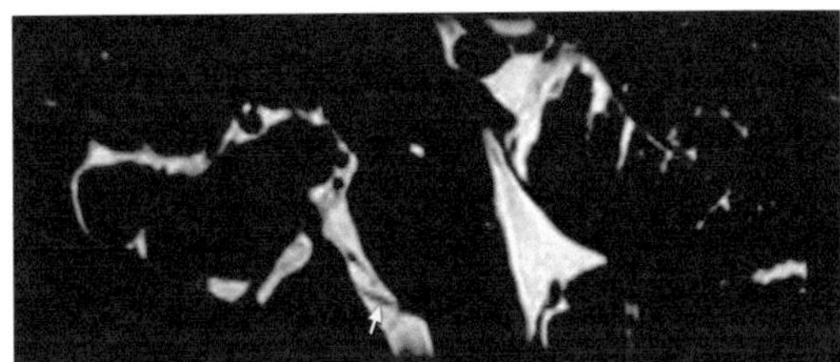

Fig. 2.8 Regular abducens nerve. Sagittal space MRI reconstruction. As the course of the nerve (arrow) is not aligned to the typical axial, sagittal, or coronal scanning plane, 3D reconstructions are often necessary to visualize the nerve longitudinally

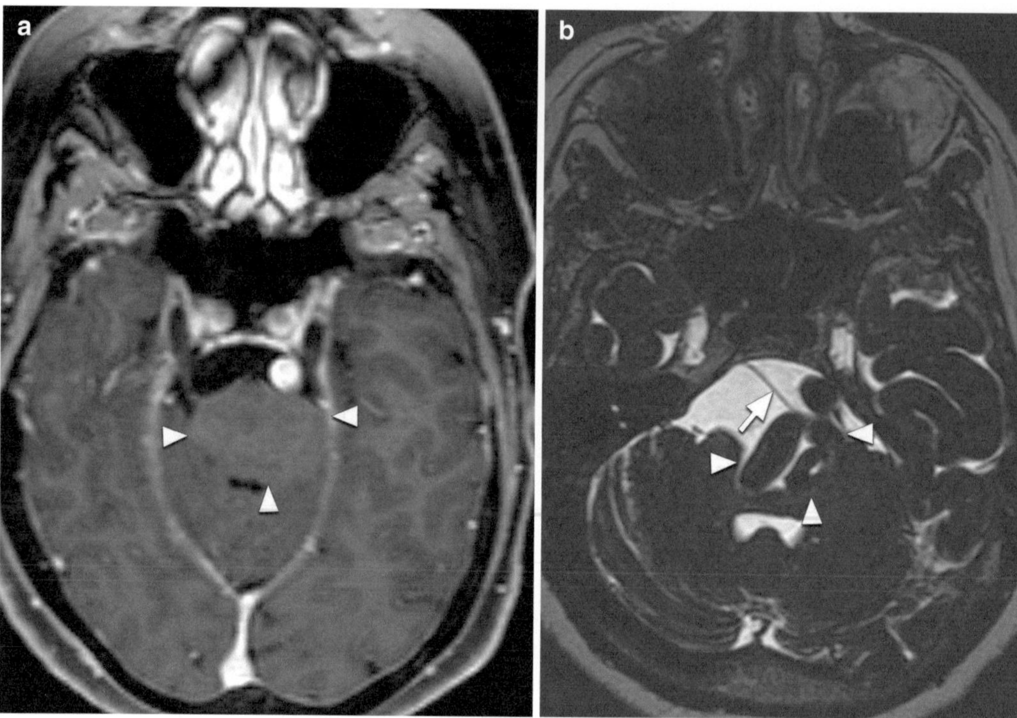

Fig. 2.9 Bulging of the abducens nerve by a vascular malformation. (**a**) Axial T1w MRI with contrast. (**b**) Axial space MRI. A voluminous vascular malformation (arrowheads) leads to a bulging of the right abducens nerve (arrow) to the left side

Cranial Nerve VII: Facial Nerve

The intra-axial origins of the facial nerve lie in the pons and medulla oblongata. The facial nerve leaves the brain stem at the cerebellopontine angle. In the cisternal segment, the larger motor root lies anterior and the smaller sensory posterior. Together with the vestibulocochlear nerve, the facial nerve enters the internal auditory canal. MRI is the best imaging modality for the segments from the brain stem to the internal auditory canal. In the latter, CT may be used to depict the bony boundaries. In the temporal bone, the course of the facial nerve can be divided into internal auditory canal, labyrinthine, tympanic, and mastoid segment. After application of contrast agent, the nerve may be depicted directly by MRI. Leaving the skull base at the stylomastoid foramen, the facial nerve gives off its motor branches in the parotid gland. The chorda tympani joins the lingual nerve.

Starting at about 1 cm below the opening of the stylomastoid foramen, the motor branches of the facial nerve in the parotid gland can be directly visualized with high-frequency ultrasound and high-resolution MRI. Depicting the tiny branches into the periphery of the nerve well outside the parotid gland is feasible with high-resolution ultrasound (Fig. 2.10) [11].

Bell's Palsy: MRI may depict contrast enhancement of the facial nerve on the symptomatic side. Ultrasound may depict thickening of the facial nerve in the parotid gland (Fig. 2.11).

Schwannoma: Both MRI and ultrasound depict the well-circumscribed tumor. To assess the tumor extent at the stylomastoid foramen, MRI is the best imaging modality (Fig. 2.12).

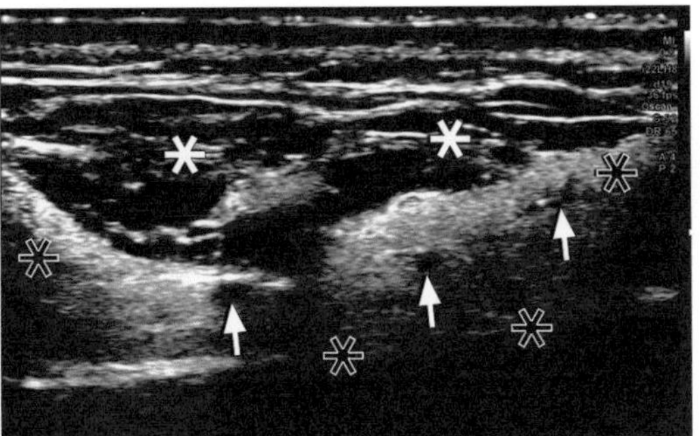

Fig. 2.10 Hyaluronic acid depositions in the parotid gland. Coronal ultrasound of the parotid gland. The patient originally underwent hyaluronic acid filler injections for cosmetic reasons. The original target region was the dermis. Inside the parotid gland (black asterisks), hypoechoic hyaluronic acid depositions (white asterisks) can be seen. Close to these depositions are the peripheral branches of the facial nerve (arrows)

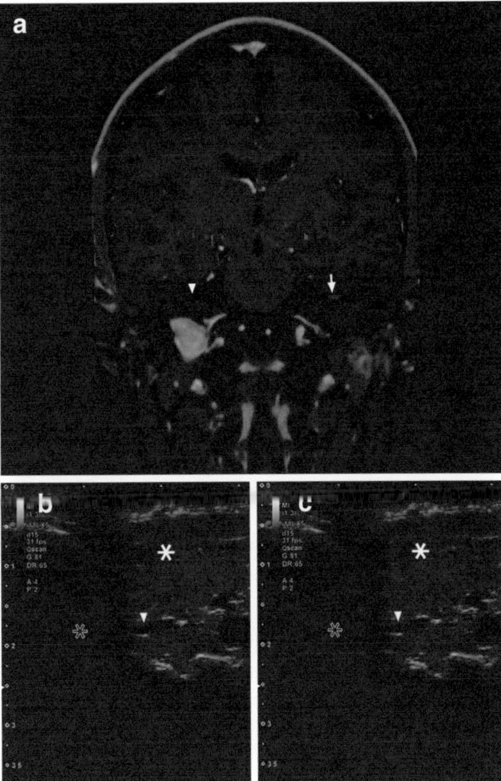

Fig. 2.11 Bell's palsy. (**a**) Coronal T1w MRI with contrast. On the symptomatic left side, contrast enhancement of the facial nerve (arrow) in the temporal bone is markedly stronger compared to the asymptomatic right side (arrowhead). (**b**) Para-axial ultrasound of the parotid gland. The facial nerve on the symptomatic side is swollen (arrow) compared to the asymptomatic side (arrowhead). (**c**) Mastoid process (Back asterix), parotid gland (white asterisk)

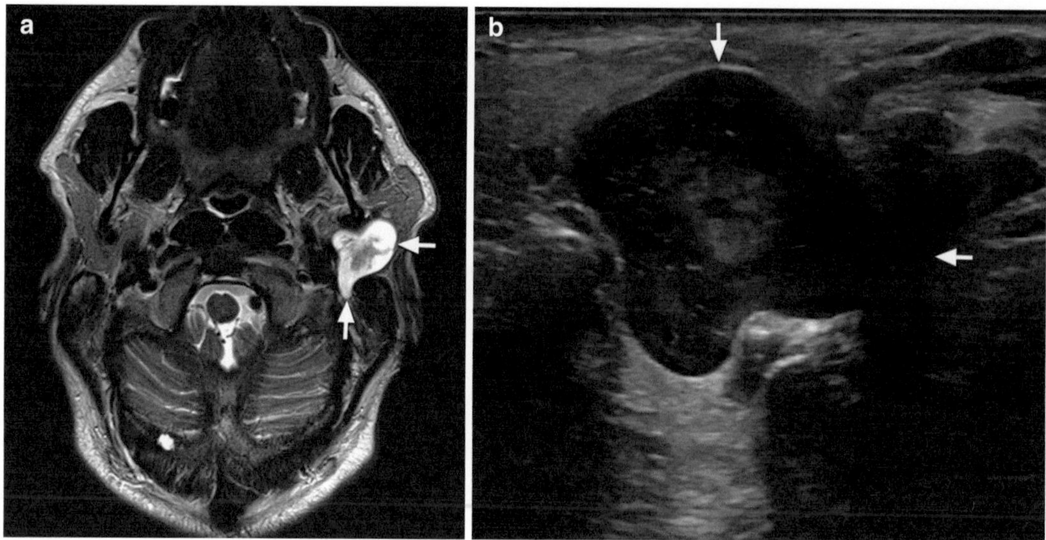

Fig. 2.12 Facial nerve schwannoma. (**a**) Axial T2w MRI, (**b**) para-axial ultrasound of the parotid gland. Large schwannoma (arrows) in the parotid gland of the left side

Cranial Nerve VIII: Vestibulocochlear Nerve

The first cochlear nuclei lie in the inferior cerebellar peduncle. The cochlear part of the vestibulocochlear nerve enters the brain stem at the cerebellopontine angle. In the cerebellopontine angle, the cochlear nerve forms the vestibulocochlear nerve with the vestibular nerve. In the temporal bone, the cochlear part lies in the anterior inferior quadrant of the internal auditory canal, which the nerve enters from the cochlea, where it is situated in the central axis of the spiral.

The vestibular fibers enter the brain stem at the cerebellopontine angle. In the cerebellopontine cistern, the vestibular part of the vestibulocochlear nerve lies posterior to the cochlear nerve.

The brain stem and the cisternal section of the nerve are visualized with MRI. The entire temporal section of the nerve can be examined with CT and MRI, depending on the suspected pathology. Contrast agent application is recommended.

Schwannoma: High-resolution MRI depicts the nerve in the entire segment form the cerebellopontine angle into the internal auditory canal (Fig. 2.13) [12].

Ramsay Hunt syndrome: With MRI the contrast enhancement of the vestibulocochlear nerve can be detected.

Metastases: Local metastases may also be visualized best with MRI with contrast. Alternatively, CT with contrast may be used.

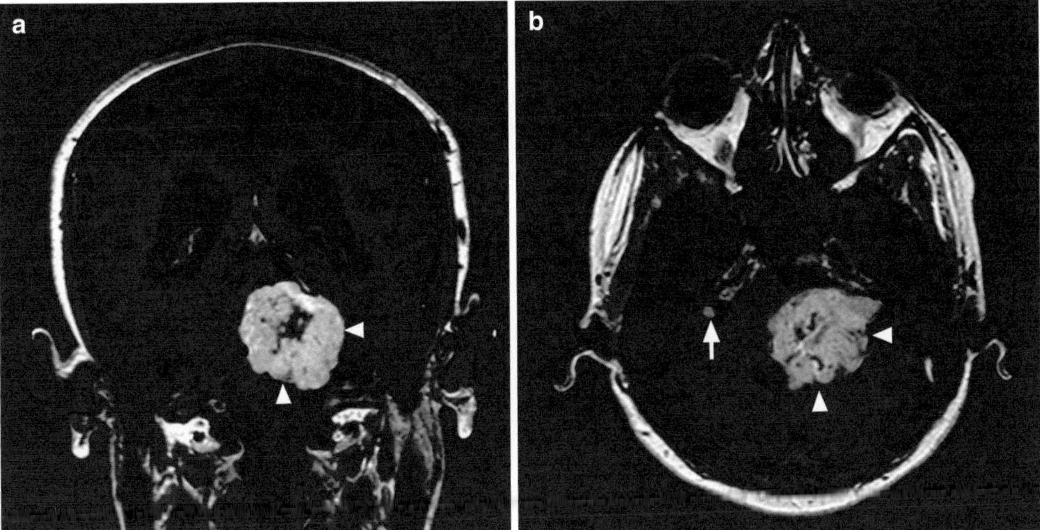

Fig. 2.13 Schwannoma and meningioma. (**a**) Coronal T1w MRI with contrast, (**b**) Axial T1w MRI with contrast. Large meningioma on the left side (arrowheads). Schwannoma of the vestibulocochlear nerve on the right side (arrow)

Cranial Nerve IX: Glossopharyngeal Nerve

The nuclei of the glossopharyngeal nerve lie in the medulla oblongata. In the retroolivary sulcus, the nerve leaves the brain stem and enters the basal cistern with the vagus nerve and the bulbar part of the accessory nerve (Fig. 2.14) In the anterior part of the jugular foramen, the nerve has its superior and inferior sensory ganglia. In the anterior part of the carotid space, the nerve passes lateral to the internal carotid artery to the neck and gives off branches to the lingual nerve, to the tympanic branch, to the stylopharyngeus branch, to the carotid sinus, and to the pharynx.

For visualization of the intracranial part, MRI and CT are necessary. The extracranial part of the glossopharyngeal nerve cannot be depicted directly. Unfortunately, the examination is limited to the visualization of the assumed regular course of the nerve [13] (Fig. 2.15).

Glossopharyngeal compression: Vascular compression by the posterior inferior cerebellar artery and anterior inferior cerebellar artery are examined best by high-resolution MRI.

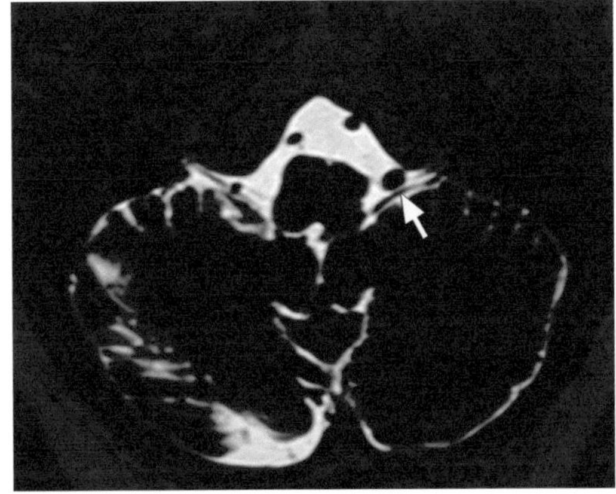

Fig. 2.14 Regular glossopharyngeal nerve. Axial space MRI. Regular course of the glossopharyngeal nerve on the left side (arrow)

Eagle syndrome: For this rare syndrome with compression of the glossopharyngeal nerve by an elongated styloid process, CT depicts the osseous situation (Fig. 2.16).

Schwannoma jugular foramen: For delineation of the soft tissue, MRI is the best imaging modality, and for the osseous borders, CT is the best imaging modality.

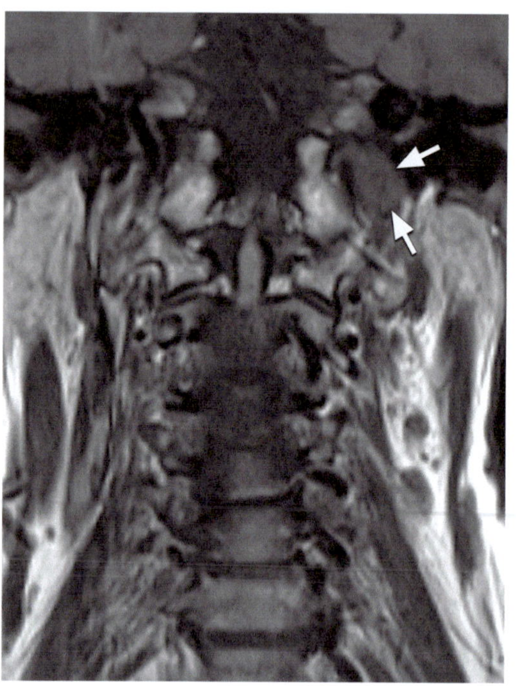

Fig. 2.15 Glomus tumor. Coronal T1w MRI. Ovoid-shaped, glomus jugulare tumor (arrows) right below the jugular foramen on the left side

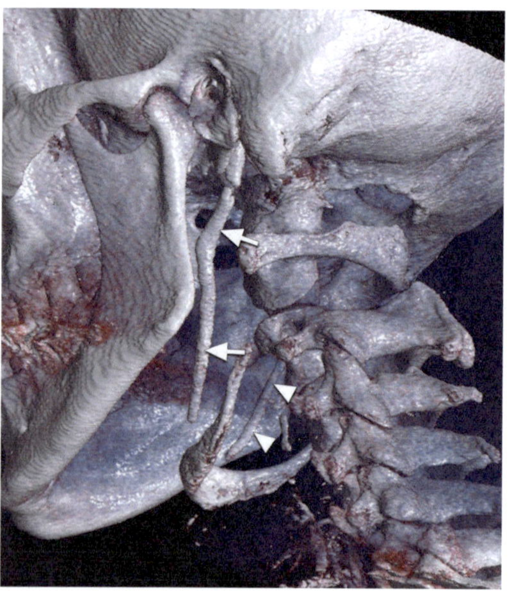

Fig. 2.16 Eagle syndrome. 3D reconstruction of a CT scan. The excessively long styloid processes on both sides (arrows) almost come in contact with the hyoid bone

Cranial Nerve X: Vagus Nerve

The nuclei of the vagus nerve lie in the medulla oblongata. Along with the glossopharyngeal nerve, the vagus nerve exits the brain stem at the retroolivary sulcus. Via the jugular foramen, the vagus nerve passes through the skull base. Below the skull base, the nerve lies in the carotid space. Along the posterior side of the carotid artery, the nerve enters the thorax, where the right nerve is located anterior to the right subclavian artery and the left nerve anterior to the aortic arch. Via a plexus around the bronchi, the nerve fibers enter the lungs, and around blood vessels, the nerve innervates the heart. The nerve also forms a plexus around the esophagus. Via this plexus, the nerve also reaches the abdomen and provides innervation for the intestines, from the stomach to the left colon flexure.

For the nerve segments in the brain, the subrachnoidal space, and skull base, MRI is the best imaging modality. In the neck, the main trunk of the vagus nerve can be partially visualized with ultrasound. The segments in the thorax and abdomen cannot be directly depicted. CT or MRI may visualize the regular pathway and surrounding of the nerve [14].

Glomus vagal paraganglioma: In the region 1–2 cm below the jugular foramen equally contrast-enhanced CT and MRI are recommended.

Schwannoma: If the location of the tumor is accessible, ultrasound is the best imaging modality. If the location is 1–2 cm below the jugular foramen MRI with contrast is recommended. With CT the scalloping of the jugular foramen may be detected (Fig. 2.17).

Neurofibroma: MRI with contrast is the best imaging modality. If accessible ultrasound can be used to directly visualized the neurogenic origin of the tumor. Sequences with strong T2-weighted signal and low signal from fat tissue may be used to search for neurofibromas.

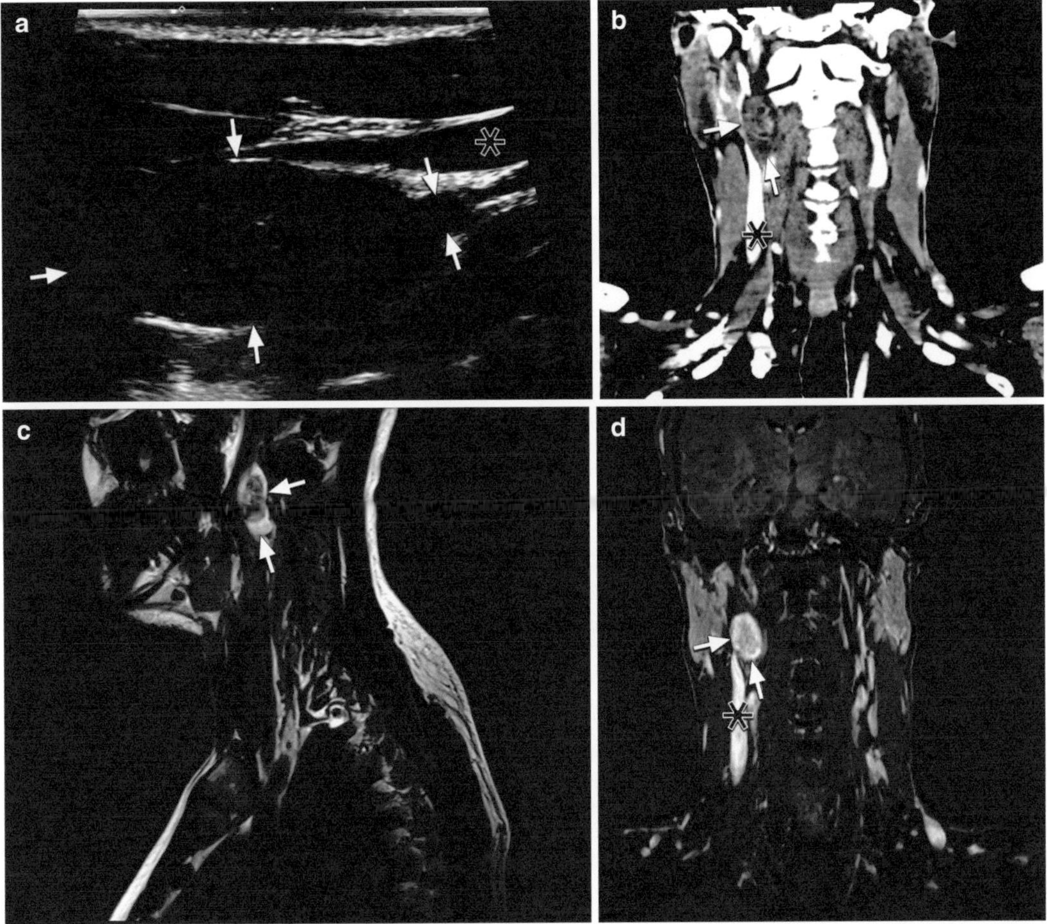

Fig. 2.17 Vagus nerve schwannoma. (**a**) Coronal ultrasound of the schwannoma at the neck, (**b**) coronal CT with contrast of the neck, (**c**) sagittal T2w MR, (**d**) coronal T1w with fat saturation MRI with contrast. Schwannoma (arrows) of the vagus nerve in the cranial part of the neck. Partially compressed internal jugular vein (black asterisks)

Cranial Nerve XI: Accessory Nerve

For the intra-axial and subarachnoidal segments, MRI is the best imaging modality. The accessory nerve originates from the medulla oblongata and from the cervical spinal cord. The fibers from the medulla oblongata exit the brain stem at the retroolivary sulcus. The fibers from the cervical spine exit the cervical cord between the ventral and dorsal roots and course cranially in the spinal canal.

CT provides depiction of the skull base. In the foramen magnum, the fibers unite and merge with the fibers from the medulla oblongata. Via the basal cistern and the jugular foramen, the accessory nerve leaves the skull. The fibers originating from the medulla oblongata merge with the vagus nerve, and the branches from the cervical spinal cord go to the sternocleidomastoid and trapezius muscle.

Extracranial segments of the nerve may be examined indirectly with MRI and directly with high-resolution ultrasound. With MRI, the supposed, regular nerve pathway and the specific target muscles of the nerve may be assessed, whereas high-resolution ultrasound visualizes the nerve directly from 1–2 cm below the inferior surface of the skull base to branches of the nerve within the muscles [15].

Injury: Ultrasound is the best imaging modality to visualize the nerve in the neck region. From 1–2 cm below the jugular foramen to the trapezius muscle, the nerve and its surround can be assessed with superior spatial resolution. High-resolution MRI may also be used to examine the course of the nerve (Figs. 2.18 and 2.19).

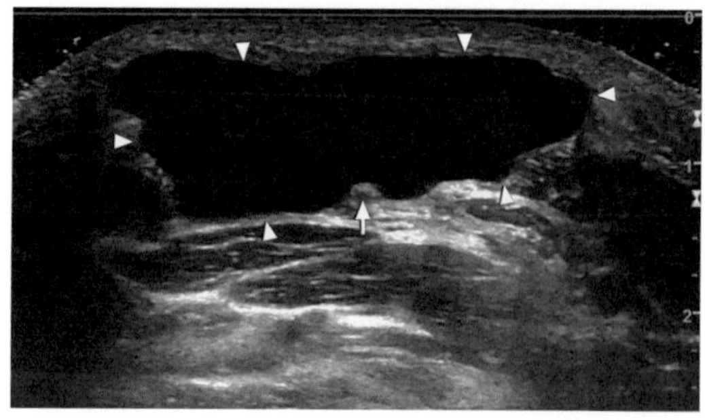

Fig. 2.18 Nerve compression by a seroma. Axial ultrasound of the accessory nerve at the lateral side of the neck. Compression of the accessory nerve (arrow) by a postoperative seroma (arrowheads) following a diagnostic excision of a lymph node

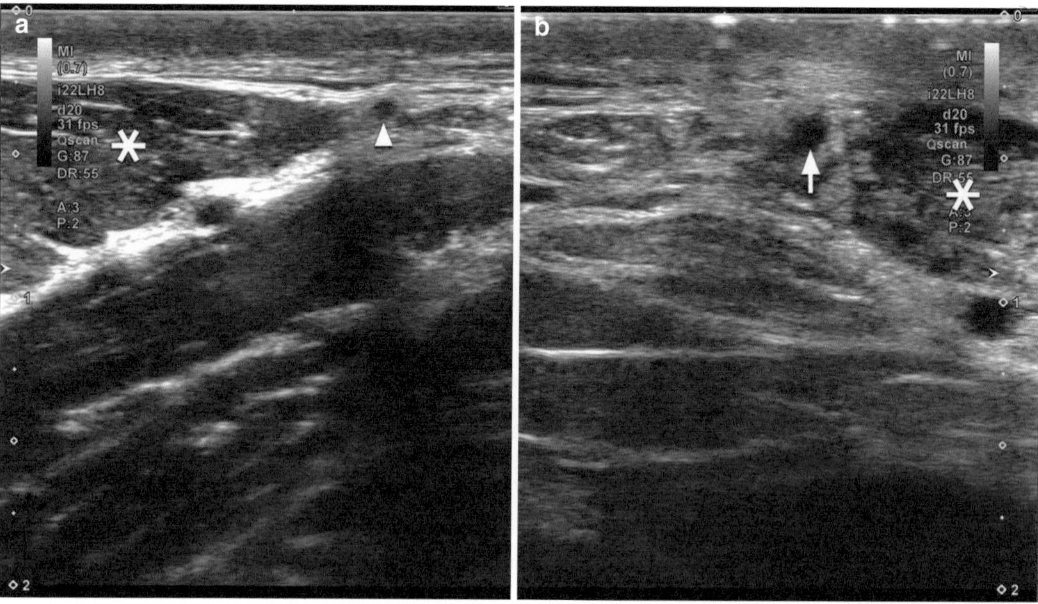

Fig. 2.19 Postoperative neuroma. Axial ultrasound of the accessory nerve (**a**) at the asymptomatic lateral side of the neck and (**b**) at the symptomatic lateral side of the neck. After surgical removal of a lipoma, the accessory nerve is swollen over a segment of several centimeters resulting in a severe shoulder lift weakness

Cranial Nerve XII: Hypoglossal Nerve

For the medullary origin, MRI is the modality of choice. The hypoglossal nuclei lie in the medulla oblongata in a posterior, paramedian position.

In the subarachnoid segment, MRI is also standard. Leaving the brain stem anterolaterally, multiple rootlets of the hypoglossal nerve converge to one nerve in the subarachnoid space. Close to the hypoglossal canal, the hypoglossal nerve is adjacent to the course of the vertebral artery, which is located medial to the nerve.

The hypoglossal canals are directed laterally. The canals may have osseous spurs or may be divided unilaterally. For the assessment of the bony structure of the skull base, the use of CT is advised. MRI might pick up pathologic contrast enhancement of the nerve (Fig. 2.20).

Outside the skull, MRI provides visualization of the supposed pathway of the nerve. High-resolution ultrasound picks up the nerve directly, although ultrasound cannot routinely reach the nerve close to the inferior side of skull base. In the submental and oral region, visualization of the hypoglossal nerve is excellent with high-resolution ultrasound. Beginning at the carotid sheath, the course of the nerve can be picked up by ultrasound and tracked into the body of the tongue. Inside the tongue, branching of the hypoglossal nerve can be partly visualized (Figs. 2.21 and 2.22).

Visualization of the tongue muscles facilitates adapting the diagnostic algorithm. Denervation edema and atrophy may direct the clinical focus to the hypoglossal nerve [16].

Malignant tumor progression: Entrapment or Infiltration by neoplastic processes in the neck can be examined best by MRI for the cervical region below the skull base. Especially in the lower region at the jaw and tongue, ultrasound has superior spatial resolution.

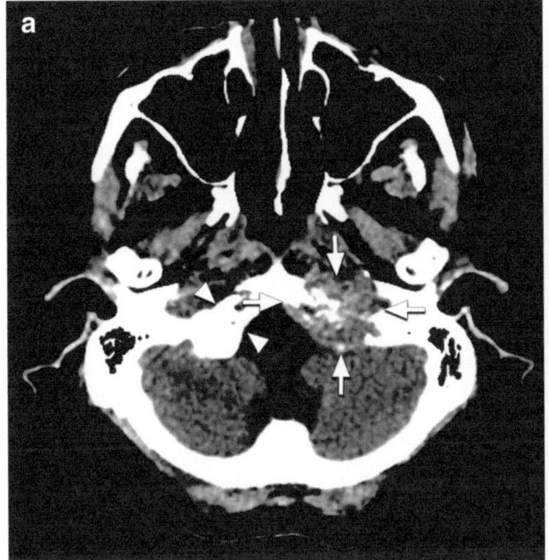
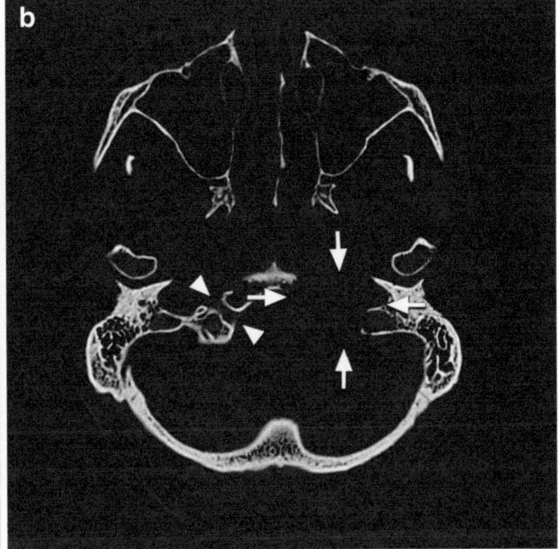

Fig. 2.20 Skull base destruction. Axial CT with (**a**) soft tissue window setting and (**b**) bone window setting. In a patient with known bronchial carcinoma, the skull base on the left side is infiltrated by a lytic bone metastasis (arrows). On the contralateral side, the intact hypoglossal canal (arrowheads) can be seen

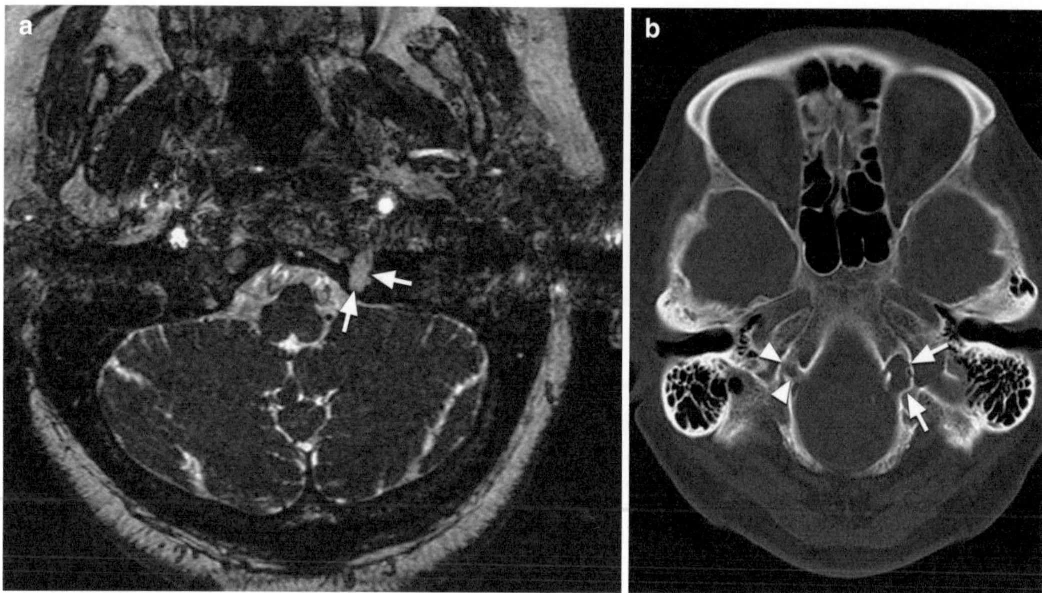

Fig. 2.21 Schwannoma. (**a**) Axial T2w MRI, (**b**) axial CT. Schwannoma of the hypoglossal nerve with scalloping of the hypoglossal canal (arrows). Regular hypoglossal canal on the asymptomatic side (arrowheads)

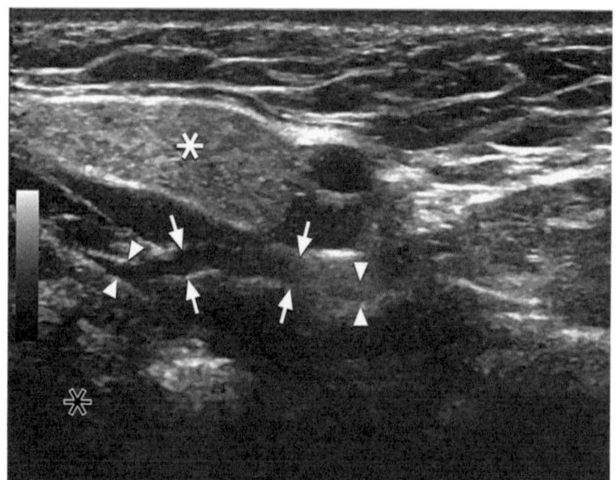

Fig. 2.22 Neurofibroma of the hypoglossal nerve. Longitudinal scan of the hypoglossal nerve at the mandibula. Marked thickening of the hypoglossal nerve due to a neurofibroma (arrows) in a patient with neurofibromatosis. Note the regular nerve caliber (arrowheads). Submandibular gland (white asterisk) and body of the tongue (black asterisk)

Cavernous Sinus/Cavernous Sinus Region/Parasellar Region

The region around the sella, and the parasellar region, contains a plethora of structures that are profoundly covered in the anatomy section of this book: the plexus of cavernous sinus veins; cranial nerves III, IV, V, and VI; sympathetic fibers; and the internal carotid artery.

As mapped out for each cranial nerve, selecting the best imaging modality depends on the clinical problem and the selected anatomical target.

In general, MRI with contrast—ideally in a high resolution—ensures a good overview.

For osseous, destructive processes, high-resolution CT with multiplanar reconstructions is recommended.

Regarding pathologies of the internal carotid artery, CT angiograms and MRI angiograms are the best modalities. In cases of suspected internal carotid artery fistulas, conventional angiography provides the insight of the vascular situation necessary for percutaneous interventional treatment.

Gasserian Ganglion/Semilunar Ganglion/Trigeminal Ganglion/ Meckel's Cave

The trigeminal ganglion is located in the lateral wall of the above mentioned parasellar region. From here, the three branches of the trigeminal nerve leave in different directions. MRI with contrast is the best imaging modality to assess this region, granting a good overview.

MRI also plays a decisive role in detecting perineural spread of tumors from the masticatory space. CT may provide additional information on the aggressiveness of the tumor spread by assessment of potential bone destruction.

In the diagnostic workup of trigeminal neuralgia, MRI may confirm clinical suspicions, such as by depicting contrast enhancement in viral etiologies or deformation of the cisternal root by vascular loops [17] (Fig. 2.23).

Orbit

The orbit contains a multitude of different structures. By imaging of the orbit, a pathology should

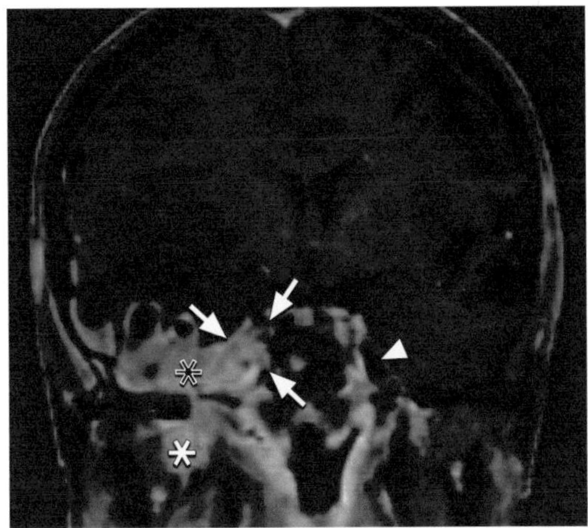

Fig. 2.23 Perineural tumor spread with infiltration of the trigeminal ganglion. Coronal T1w MRI with contrast. Squamous cell carcinoma tumor progression from below the skull base (white asterisk) into the neurocranium (black asterisk) infiltrating Meckel's cave (arrows). Here, the trigeminal ganglion is infiltrated and entirely contrast enhanced, while the ganglion can be seen as a hypointense structure (arrowhead)

first be assigned to a region, such as regarding the globe, the optic nerve, the myofascial cone, and the lacrimal gland.

MRI provides the best soft tissue contrast and allows a suppression of the fat tissue signal intensity (Fig. 2.24).

With ultrasound, it is easy to visualize the entire orbit, while CT depicts the osseous structures of the orbit, especially the bony orbital openings.

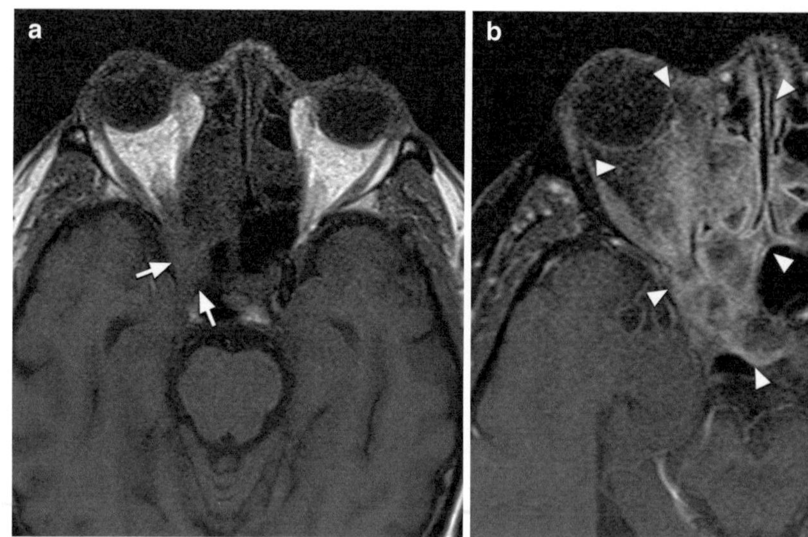

Fig. 2.24 Aspergilloma infiltration. (**a**) Axial T1w precontrast enhancement MRI, (**b**) Axial T1w MRI with contrast. Note the true extent of the aspergilloma infiltration (arrowheads) after application of a contrast agent and the smaller visual impression before contrast (arrows)

References

1. Meng S, Platzgummer H, Loizides A, Chang KV, Gruber H. Ultrasound of small nerves. Ultraschall Med. 2022;43(1):12–33.
2. Abolmaali N, Gudziol V, Hummel T. Pathology of the olfactory nerve. Neuroimaging Clin N Am. 2008;18(2):233–42. preceding x
3. Duprez TP, Rombaux P. Imaging the olfactory tract (cranial nerve #1). Eur J Radiol. 2010;74(2):288–98.
4. Kendall CJ, Prager TC, Cheng H, Gombos D, Tang RA, Schiffman JS. Diagnostic ophthalmic ultrasound for radiologists. Neuroimaging Clin N Am. 2015;25(3):327–65.
5. Becker M, Masterson K, Delavelle J, Viallon M, Vargas MI, Becker CD. Imaging of the optic nerve. Eur J Radiol. 2010;74(2):299–313.
6. Liang C, Du Y, Lin X, Wu L, Wu D, Wang X. Anatomical features of the cisternal segment of the oculomotor nerve: neurovascular relationships and abnormal compression on magnetic resonance imaging. J Neurosurg. 2009;111(6):1193–200.
7. Agarwal N, Ahmed AK, Wiggins RH 3rd, McCulley TJ, Kontzialis M, Macedo LL, et al. Segmental imaging of the trochlear nerve: anatomic and pathologic considerations. J Neuroophthalmol. 2021;41(1):e7–e15.
8. Seeburg DP, Northcutt B, Aygun N, Blitz AM. The role of imaging for trigeminal neuralgia: a segmental approach to high-resolution MRI. Neurosurg Clin N Am. 2016;27(3):315–26.
9. Haller S, Etienne L, Kovari E, Varoquaux AD, Urbach H, Becker M. Imaging of neurovascular compression syndromes: trigeminal neuralgia, hemifacial spasm, vestibular paroxysmia, and glossopharyngeal neuralgia. AJNR Am J Neuroradiol. 2016;37(8):1384–92.
10. Price T, Fayad G. Abducens nerve palsy as the sole presenting symptom of petrous apicitis. J Laryngol Otol. 2002;116(9):726–9.
11. Singh AK, Bathla G, Altmeyer W, Tiwari R, Valencia MP, Bazan C 3rd, et al. Imaging spectrum of facial nerve lesions. Curr Probl Diagn Radiol. 2015;44(1):60–75.
12. Skolnik AD, Loevner LA, Sampathu DM, Newman JG, Lee JY, Bagley LJ, et al. Cranial nerve Schwannomas: diagnostic imaging approach. Radiographics. 2016;36(5):1463–77.
13. Garcia Santos JM, Sanchez Jimenez S, Tovar Perez M, Moreno Cascales M, Lailhacar Marty J, Fernandez-Villacanas Marin MA. Tracking the glossopharyngeal nerve pathway through anatomical references in cross-sectional imaging techniques: a pictorial review. Insights Imaging. 2018;9(4):559–69.
14. Sniezek JC, Netterville JL, Sabri AN. Vagal paragangliomas. Otolaryngol Clin North Am. 2001;34(5):925–39. vi
15. Ong CK, Chong VF. The glossopharyngeal, vagus and spinal accessory nerves. Eur J Radiol. 2010;74(2):359–67.
16. Meng S, Reissig LF, Tzou CH, Meng K, Grisold W, Weninger W. Ultrasound of the hypoglossal nerve in the neck: visualization and initial clinical experience with patients. AJNR Am J Neuroradiol. 2016;37(2):354–9.
17. Malhotra A, Tu L, Kalra VB, Wu X, Mian A, Mangla R, et al. Neuroimaging of Meckel's cave in normal and disease conditions. Insights Imaging. 2018;9(4):499–510.

Bullet Points

- Electrodiagnosis in certain cranial nerve lesions may be of useful diagnostic and prognostic value.
- Knowledge about clinical implications is an important feature in managing patients with cranial neuropathies.

Introduction

Medical history and clinical examination are the most important diagnostic steps in diagnosing cranial nerve lesions and localizing the site of lesion in most cases. Depending on the affected nerve and the medical history, additional laboratory tests and neuroradiological images, particularly magnetic resonance tomography (MRT) of the brain stem, CT of the base of the skull, and ultrasound for soft tissue regions, will detect the cause of the nerve lesion.

What is the role of electrophysiology in testing cranial nerves? First, electrophysiology is a valuable, reliable, and easily obtainable method for providing prognosis of cranial nerve lesions within the first 3 weeks after onset of paresis, such as for facial nerve palsy or accessory nerve lesions (Table 3.1). Second, tests of cranial nerves

may be of essential value in the diagnosis of neuromuscular diseases, such as bulbar types of myasthenia gravis and motor neuron disease (Table 3.2). Follow-up studies in chronic diseases, such as multiple sclerosis-related optic neuritis with visual evoked potentials (VEPs), and various central nervous system disorders are also part of electrodiagnosis (Table 3.3). Finally, the below-described techniques may confirm clinically suspected nerve lesions and may provide further information on the location of lesion.

However, a number of cranial nerves, such as the olfactory nerve; the oculomotor nerve; cranial nerves III, IV, VI; and the glossopharyngeal nerve, cannot be examined electrophysiologically in routine laboratories.

Electrodiagnosis cannot replace the clinical examination. Informative interpretation of electrodiagnostic findings require knowledge of the history and clinical findings.

Written assignment to a neurophysiological lab is recommended. Before starting the electrodiagnostic test, the patient has to be informed precisely of the planned examination, possible unpleasant sensations during the test, and possible side effects, particularly if performing needle EMG, as an assessment of possible anticoagulant therapies is needed.

Subsequently, the most important and regularly performed techniques are described in this chapter. Neurophysiological techniques not routinely used in examining cranial nerves are only mentioned.

Author of this chapter: Udo A Zifko.

Table 3.1 Cranial nerve lesions and valuable electrodiagnostic methods

Nerve	NCV	EMG	EP	TMS	Reflex tests	Other
I			++			
II			++		+	
III, IV, VI						
V		+	+	+	+	
VII	++	++		+	+	
VIII			+			
IX						
X						RR interval
XI	++	++				
XII	+	++				

+ technically sophisticated, not used routinely, ++ routinely performed examination with high diagnostic and/or prognostic value

Table 3.2 Generalized neuromuscular diseases and electrodiagnosis of cranial nerves

Disease	NCV	EMG	Repetitive nerve stimulation	Blink reflex
AIDP, CIDP				+
MND		++		
MG, LEMS			++	+?

+ technically sophisticated, not used routinely, ++ routinely performed examination with high diagnostic and/or prognostic value

AIDP acute inflammatory demyelinating polyneuropathy, *CIDP* chronic inflammatory demyelinating polyneuropathy, *EMG* electromyography, *LEMS* Lambert Eaton myasthenic syndrome, *NCV* nerve conduction velocity, *MG* myasthenia gravis, *MND* motor neuron disease

Table 3.3 Central nervous system disorders and electrodiagnosis of cranial nerves

Disease	VEP	TMS	Reflex tests	EP
Brain stem disorders			+	+
Hemispheric lesions		+	+	+
Multiple sclerosis	++			+
Movement disorders			+	

+ technically sophisticated, not used routinely, ++ routinely performed examination with high diagnostic and/or prognostic value

Optic Nerve

Visual Evoked Potentials

VEPs provide a qualitative and quantitative measure of the whole optical pathway from retinal cells to the visual cortex.

Technique:
- Patient in sitting position.
- Pattern reversal studies with standardized checkerboard pattern.
- Recording with EEG electrodes according to the EEG 10–20 system from O1 and O2.
- Referred to Fz and ground electrode at Cz.
- Each eye is tested separately.
- Stimulation rate: 2 Hz.
- In VEP, pattern reversal stimuli are more routinely used rather than flash stimuli, as results are more variable with the latter [1].

Normal values: The waveform has three separate phases, including an initial negative deflection (N1 or N75), a prominent positive deflection (P1 or P100), and a later negative deflection (N2 or N145). The values depend on the size of the checkerboard pattern used [2].

Clinical applications: VEPs are used to detect an optic nerve lesion, such as optic neuritis, ischemic optic neuropathy, and others. VEPs are also a reliable neurophysiological method for follow-up studies in patients suffering from optic neuritis.

Pitfalls: Absent or severely reduced visual optic function may result in a wrong interpretation of an absent VEP signal.

Trigeminal Nerve

Electrical Blink Reflex

Technique:
- Patient lying with eyes open.
- Electrical stimulation of supraorbital nerve with the cathode placed over the supraorbital notch. To minimize habituation, shocks should be delivered at intervals of 7 s or more [3].
- Blink reflex may also be performed by triggered visual and/or acoustic stimulation.
- Recording with surface electrodes from both orbicularis oculi muscles simultaneously, with the active electrode on the mid third of the infraorbital rim and the reference electrode on the lateral surface of the nose.

Normal Values:
- Ipsilateral R1 latency: R1: 10 ms; delay >13 ms or difference more than 1.5 ms between the two sides.
- Ipsilateral R2 latency: R2: 30 ms; delay >41 ms or difference more than 8 ms between the two sides.
- Difference between ipsilateral and contralateral R2 should not exceed 8 ms [4, 5].
- Amplitudes vary considerably and should be documented in the report; diagnostic information due to "abnormal amplitude" alone should be done with high precaution.
- In lesions of the trigeminal nerve, ipsilateral R1 and bilateral R2 responses can be delayed or absent, depending on the severity of the lesion, but both R1 and bilateral R2 responses will be normal with stimulation of the unaffected side [1].

Clinical Applications:
- Trigeminal nerve lesion, of either the ophthalmic division of the trigeminal nerve or the supraorbital nerve branch, results in ipsilateral delayed or absent R1.
- The early ipsilateral response (R1) is mediated by the main sensory nucleus of the fifth nerve in the pons, and the bilateral R2 responses by the spinal nucleus and tract of the fifth nerve through polysynaptic pathways in the pons and medulla.
- Blink reflex may also provide information in facial nerve palsy [4]; see below.
- Lesions affecting the lower pons and /or the dorsolateral medulla oblongata cause electrical blink reflex abnormalities; lesions affecting the mesencephalon are detected by visual evoked blink reflex.

Motor function: The masseteric muscle is well accessible to needle examination and less uncomfortable to examine for patients than the temporalis or medial and lateral pterygoid muscle. The masseteric muscle is examined with the needle electrode between the anterior edge of the muscle and the lower edge of mandible when the patient clenches their teeth.

Transcranial Magnetic Stimulation

Technique:
- The coil is positioned flat over the parietooccipital surface, behind and just superior and anterior to the ear.
- Recording with surface electrodes from the masseter muscle.

Normal values: Mean latency – 6.9 ms (±0.3 ms) [5].

Clinical applications: Detection of abnormalities in the central pathway toward the masseteric muscle may be of particular interest in critically ill patients, where both the central and peripheral lesions may impair the patient's neuromuscular function.

Other Methods

Corneal reflex, jaw-jerk reflex, masseter-inhibitory reflex, and trigeminal somatosensory evoked potentials are technically more sophisticated and usually not used in routine electrophysiological departments.

Facial Nerve

Nerve Conduction Study (NCV)

Technique (Fig. 3.1):
- Patient lying or sitting.
- Electrical stimulation with bipolar surface stimulating electrode at the stylomastoid foramen.
- Recordings from the following muscles are possible: frontal, nasalis, mentalis, and orbicularis oculi.

Normal Values:
- -Latency: 1.5–4.0 ms (distance 8–14 cm); side-to side latency difference < 0.6 ms.
- Amplitude: 1.8–4 mV [1].
- Amplitude reduction to more than 50% of the response on the unaffected side suggests distal degeneration [5]; amplitude reduction less than 30% within the first 3 weeks after onset of palsy argues for a good prognosis; amplitude reduction more than 70–80% gives evidence for poor prognosis.

Clinical applications: To confirm clinical diagnosis of peripheral facial nerve palsy and inform prognosis.

Pitfalls:
- Volume conduction from nearby muscles, mainly the masseteric, alters the waveform of compound muscle action potentials and may result in wrong interpretation in case of absent facial nerve amplitude.
- Normal compound muscle action potentials are typical within the first 4–7 days. Hence, the first facial NCV study should be performed after the first week of onset of nerve palsy, except for forensic reasons.

Repetitive Facial Nerve Stimulation

With the same stimulation and recording technique as described above, a stimulation frequency of <5 Hz allows for the detection of myasthenia gravis, and a stimulation frequency of 20 or

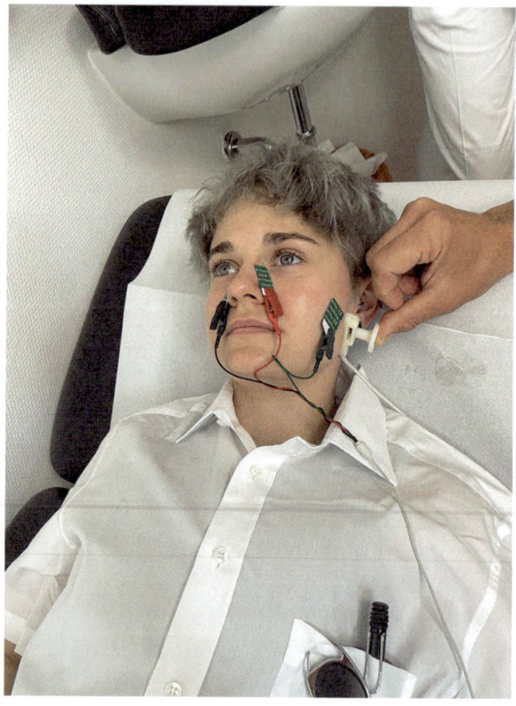

Fig. 3.1 Electrical facial nerve stimulation with bipolar surface stimulating electrode at the stylomastoid foramen. Recording with surface electrodes from the ipsilateral nasalis muscle with the active (red) and from the contralateral nasalis muscle with the reference electrode (black). Ground electrode (green) positioned between stimulation and recording site

30 Hz allows for the detection of Lambert Eaton syndrome (see Chap. 11, section "Cranial Nerve VII: Facial Nerve").

Recordings can be made from the nasalis (most common), frontalis, orbicularis oculus, orbicularis oris, and mentalis muscles.

For identifying a neuromuscular junction defect, a decrement of at least 10%, usually from potential 1–5, is expected [6].

Needle Electromyography (EMG)

Needle EMG may be useful for estimating prognosis in affected muscles showing abnormal spontaneous activity after 3 weeks of symptom onset. In the course analysis of motor units, needle EMG may give further evidence regarding neurogenic lesions or ongoing regeneration.

Facial muscles are characterized by more numerous, short-duration, smaller amplitude motor unit potentials than is the case for limb muscles. The motor unit action potentials are more difficult to analyze, because their higher firing rates make it difficult to distinguish from myopathic potentials or from the fibrillation potentials and positive sharp waves seen in axonal degeneration [7].

Single fiber electromyography (SFEMG) is a sensitive technique for detecting a neuromuscular transmission defect and is used for comparison with the edrophonium chloride (Tensilon) test, conventional repetitive stimulation, and acetylcholine receptor antibody testing [8].

SFEMG is not specific and may also be abnormal in other myopathic and neuropathic disorders. Increased jitter values are also seen during the early stage of reinnervation, motor neuron disease, polyneuropathies, polymyositis, facioscapulohumeral dystrophy, and others. However, if SFEMG is normal in a weak muscle, it almost excludes the diagnosis of myasthenia. The technique of SFEMG needs considerable experience and technical expertise and demands patient cooperation [7].

Transcranial Magnetic Stimulation

Technique:
- The coil is positioned flat over the parietooccipital surface, behind and above the ear.
- Recording similar to electrical stimulation.

Normal Values:
- Latency: 6.5 ms (±0.5 ms).
- Central conduction time: Transosseous conduction time (latency difference between transcranial and electrical stimulation) – 1.25 ± 0.2 ms [5, 7].

Clinical Applications:
- In the acute stage (first 4–7 days) of Bell's palsy, transcranial magnetic stimulation shows an absent response due to conduction block, whereas the M-wave is normal.
- After day 7 of Bell's palsy, the side-to-side comparison of the compound muscle action potential gives evidence of the severity of the facial nerve lesion.
- At the chronic stage of facial nerve palsy, the side-to-side latency comparison and the needle EMG of the facial nerve branches innervating the frontalis, orbicularis oculi, and orbicularis oris muscles may detect axonal degeneration of the facial nerve [8].

Other Methods

Blink reflex: See technique details noted above under the trigeminal nerve. Blink reflex gives valuable information from the early onset of the palsy, with absent R1 and R2 ipsilaterally or delayed response in patients without distal degeneration.

Vestibulocochlear Nerve

Brain Stem Auditory Evoked Potentials (BAEPs)

BAEPs represent the successive components of the auditory pathway. In general, they are performed by otolaryngologists and are not described in detail in this chapter. Further tests, such as the acoustically evoked blink reflex and others, are not performed routinely in neurophysiological laboratories and are usually part of an otolaryngological diagnosis.

Vagus Nerve

The various techniques for examining the autonomic nerve fibers mediated by the vagus nerve are described in Chap. 15, section "Cranial Nerve X: Vagus Nerve".

Accessory Nerve

Nerve Conduction Study (NCV)

Technique:
- Patient lying or sitting.
- Electrical stimulation with bipolar surface stimulating electrode 1–2 cm posteriorly to the border of the sternocleidomastoid muscle at the level of the upper margin of the thyroid cartilage.
- Recording from the motor end plate of the trapezius muscle [9].

Normal Values:
- Latency: 1.8–3.0 ms.
- Amplitude: Compared to the unaffected side, a difference of more than 50% is abnormal.

Clinical applications: To confirm clinical diagnosis of accessory nerve lesion and also inform prognosis.

Needle Electromyography (EMG)

Needle EMG of all three parts of the trapezius muscle and the sternocleidomastoid muscle is a reliable technique to confirm the clinical diagnosis of an accessory nerve lesion.

Hypoglossal Nerve

Nerve Conduction Study (NCV)

The electrical stimulation is performed at the base of the mandible, but recording is only possible with a specially designed orthoplast bite. Hence, this technique is not used in routine neurophysiological labs [10].

Needle EMG

Analysis of needle EMG is mainly limited to the analysis of pathological spontaneous activity. Analysis of motor units with moderate and forced stimulation is difficult and quite inconvenient for the patient.

The tongue may be examined with an opened mouth at the lateral part of the genioglossus muscle, or with a closed mouth by inserting the needle just medial to the mandible. In our experience, the closed-mouth technique seems to be less painful. Observation of abnormal spontaneous activity and firing pattern are valuable parameters; analysis of motor units of the tongue muscle is not reliable.

References

1. Kenelly KD. Electrophysiological evaluation of cranial neuropathies. Neurologist. 2006;12:188–203.
2. Lee HJ, Delisa JA. Manual of nerve conduction velocity and surface anatomy for needle electromyography. Baltimore: Lippincott Williams and Wilkins; 2004.
3. Jaaskelainen SK. Blink reflex with stimulation of the mental nerve: methodology, reference values, and some clinical vignettes. Acta Neurol Scand. 1995;91:477–82.
4. Kimura J. Conduction abnormalities of the facial and trigeminal nerves in polyneuropathy. Muscle Nerve. 1982;5:139–44.
5. Muzyka IM, Estephan B. Electrophysiology of cranial nerve testing: trigeminal and facial nerves. J Clin Neurophysiol. 2018;35:16–24.
6. Mansukhani KA, Khadilkar SV. EMG simplified, repetitive nerve stimulation (RNS) study; 2020. p. 202–16. ISBN: 978-93-83989
7. Sarrigiannis PG, Kennet RP, Read S, Farrugia ME. Single fiber EMG with a concentric needle evaluation in myasthenia gravis. Muscle Nerve. 2006;33:61–5.
8. Brown WF, Bolton CF. Clinical electromyography. 2nd ed. Boston: Butterworth-Heinemann; 1993.
9. Daube JR. Compound muscle action potentials. In: Daube JR, editor. Clinical neurophysiology. Oxford: Oxford University Press; 1996. p. 199–234.
10. Redmond MD, DiBenedetto M. Hypoglossal nerve conduction in normal subjects. Muscle Nerve. 1988;11:447–52.

Cranial Nerve Examinations

See Table 4.1.

Table 4.1 Cranial nerve examinations

Cranial nerve	Standard assessment	Extended testing
CN I Olfactory nerve	Patient is asked to identify odors at each nostril with eyes closed When malingering is suspected, use ammonia (testing nociceptive receptors of trigeminal nerve)	"Sniffin' sticks"/Screening 12 Test [1] Olfactory evoked potentials [2] Odor detection threshold test [3]
CN II Optic nerve	Testing visual acuity using a pocket chart for near vision [4], or counting fingers or hand movements Visual fields are tested by direct confrontation in all four quadrants for each eye (specificity 97%) Using two moving red points (i.e., pen) (sensitivity 77%), both monocular and binocular In comatose patients: blink to threat reflex [5] Color perception is tested by using Ishihara charts Pupil: observe size, shape, and symmetry Pupillary light response (afferent limb), consensual reflex, accommodation reflex Swinging flashlight test (afferent)	Direct ophthalmoscopy [6], pocket ophthalmoscope Testing visual acuity using Snellen chart (distance vision) [4] Visual evoked potentials [2] Slit lamp examination [6] Perimetry using tangent screen, Goldmann perimeter, or computerized automated perimeters [6] Optical coherence tomography (OCT) [6, 7] Scanning laser polarimetry and scanning laser tomography [6] Optic nerve sheath diameter ultrasound (ONSD) [8]
CN III Oculomotor nerve	Inspect for ptosis and miosis (Horner syndrome), mydriasis (parasympathetic) Pupillary light response (efferent limb) Swinging flashlight test (efferent limb) Pupil: observe size, shape, and symmetry Convergence reaction Usually CN III, CN IV, and CN VI are tested together: move fingers or tip of pen in H shape; observe eye movements and possible nystagmus Check if gaze to each side, gaze upwards, and gaze downwards is possible (medial rectus, inferior rectus, and inferior oblique muscle)	Pupillometry Pharmacological pupil testing Pupillography (automated swinging flashlight test) EMG of eye muscles Electrooculography (EOG) Video oculography [9] Binocular infrared oculography [9] Hess charts [9]

(continued)

Authors of this chapter: Naela Alhani and Walter Struhal.

Table 4.1 (continued)

Cranial nerve	Standard assessment	Extended testing
CN IV Trochlear nerve	Check intorsion and depression in adducted position (superior oblique muscle) ("look down and in") Head tilt test (Bielschowsky test) [6]	Refer to CN III Maddox rod for testing manifest deviation [6]
CN V Trigeminal nerve	Test sensation in ophthalmic (V1), maxillary (V2), and mandibular (V3) sensory branches in the face using cotton wool Check corneal reflex Inspect masseter and temporal muscle while clenching teeth Jaw jerk	Trigeminal somatosensory-evoked potentials [2] Blink reflex Masseter reflex Masseter inhibitory reflex [2] EMG of the masseter, temporalis, and pterygoid muscle Motor evoked potentials from masseter muscle
CN VI Abducens nerve	Check abduction on both sides for function of lateral rectus muscle	Refer to CN III
CN VII Facial nerve	Evaluation of asymmetry of facial movements (raise eyebrows, close eyes, puff out cheek, reveal teeth) Corneal reflex Schirmer test of lacrimation [10] Taste in the anterior two thirds of the tongue Stethoscope test [11]	Facial motor nerve conduction studies Motor evoked potential EMG of innervated muscles Repetitive nerve stimulation Nerve excitability test (NET) [12] Maximal stimulation test (MST) [12] Blink reflex Acoustic (stapedius) reflex test [13] Impedance audiometry Electrogustometry [14]
CN VIII Vestibulocochlear nerve	Rubbing fingers by each ear Weber test, Rinne's test Check for nystagmus, also using Frenzel lenses (for fixation) Rhomberg's test, Unterberger's test Pointing test of Bàrany [11] Repositioning maneuvers: Dix-Hallpike, Epley canalith repositioning maneuver, Semont Head-thrust-test	Pure tone audiometry Brainstem evoked auditory potential Electronystagmography Vestibular evoked myogenic potentials (VEMP) testing
CN IX Glossopharyngeal nerve	Taste in the posterior third of the tongue Inspect for palatal asymmetry and uvular deviation Check for abnormal palatal sensation Test gag reflex separately on each side Valsalva maneuver Carotid sinus pressure test	Electrogustometry [14] EMG of soft palate
CN X Vagus nerve	Inspect for palatal asymmetry and uvular deviation Check for abnormal palatal sensation Check speech for hoarseness Valsalva maneuver	Laryngoscopy [15] Stroboscopy [15] Tilt table test, heart rate variability Laryngeal electromyography Barium swallow
CN XI Accessory nerve	Patient should shrug shoulders (testing for trapezius muscle) and turn head against resistance (test for sternocleidomastoid muscle)	EMG trapezius muscle Repetitive nerve stimulation Motor evoked potential Accessory motor nerve conduction studies
CN XII Hypoglossal nerve	Inspect tongue at rest in mouth and while sticking it out (check for atrophy and fasciculation) Test strength by pushing the patient's tongue against a tongue blade	EMG of the tongue Corticobulbar motor evoked potentials from tongue muscles [16] Sonography of the tongue

CN cranial nerve, *EMG* electromyography, *EOG* electrooculography, *MST* maximal stimulation test, *NET* nerve excitability test, *OCT* optical coherence tomography, *ONSD* optic nerve sheath diameter ultrasound, *VEMP* vestibular evoked myogenic potentials

References

1. Hummel T, Sekinger B, Wolf SR, Pauli E, Kobal G. 'Sniffin' sticks': olfactory performance assessed by the combined testing of odor identification, odor discrimination and olfactory threshold. Chem Senses. 1997;22(1):39–52. https://doi.org/10.1093/chemse/22.1.39.

2. Urban P. Neurophysiologische Diagnostik bei Hirnnervenerkrankungen. J Neurol Neurochir Psychiatr. 2009;10(1):60–73.

3. Xian LLS, Nallaluthan V, De Jun Y, Lin-Wei O, Halim SA, Chuan CY, Idris Z, Ghani ARI, Abdullah JM. Examination techniques of the first cranial nerve: what neurosurgical residents should know. Malays J Med Sci. 2020;27(5):124–9. https://doi.org/10.21315/mjms2020.27.5.12.

4. Hufschmidt A, Rauer S, Glocker F, Hrsg. Neurologie compact. 9. vollständig überarbeitete Auflage. Stuttgart: Thieme; 2022.

5. Zakaria Z, Abdullah MM, Abdul Halim S, Ghani ARI, Idris Z, Abdullah JM. The neurological exam of a comatose patient: an essential practical guide. Malays J Med Sci. 2020;27(5):108–23. https://doi.org/10.21315/mjms2020.27.5.11.

6. Riordan-Eva P, Augsburger JJ. Vaughan & Asbury's general ophthalmology. McGraw Hill; 2017. 19e

7. Kroll P, Küchle HJ, Küchle M, Hrsg. Augenärztliche Untersuchungsmethoden, 3., vollständig überarbeitete und erweiterte Auflage. Stuttgart: Thieme; 2008.

8. Chen L, Wang L, Hu Y, et al. Br J Ophthalmol. 2019;103:437–41.

9. Kanski J reiterate, Bowling B, Klinische Ophthalmoskopie, 7. Auflage. München: Urban & Fischer; 2021.

10. Hanson J, Fikertscher R, Roseburg B. Schirmer test of lacrimation. Its clinical importance. Arch Otolaryngol. 1975;101(5):293–5. https://doi.org/10.1001/archotol.1975.00780340025005.

11. Berlit P. (Hrsg.) Klinische Neurologie. 4 Auflage. Berlin: Springer; 2020.

12. Guntinas-Lichius O, Volk GF, Olsen KD, Mäkitie AA, Silver CE, Zafereo ME, Rinaldo A, Randolph GW, Simo R, Shaha AR, Vander Poorten V, Ferlito A. Facial nerve electrodiagnostics for patients with facial palsy: a clinical practice guideline. Eur Arch Otorhinolaryngol. 2020;277(7):1855–74. https://doi.org/10.1007/s00405-020-05949-1.

13. Kopala W, Kukwa A. Evaluation of the acoustic (stapedius) reflex test in children and adolescents with peripheral facial nerve palsy. Int J Pediatr Otorhinolaryngol. 2016;89:102–6. https://doi.org/10.1016/j.ijporl.2016.08.001.

14. Tomita H, Ikeda M. Clinical use of electro-gustometry: strengths and limitations. Acta Otolaryngol Suppl. 2002;546:27–38. https://doi.org/10.1080/00016480260046391.

15. Strutz J, Mann W, Hrsg. Praxis der HNO-Heilkunde, Kopf- und Halschirurgie. 3., unveränderte Auflage. Stuttgart: Thieme; 2017.

16. Urban P, Hrsg. Klinisch-neurologische Untersuchungstechniken. 2., überarbeitete Auflage. Stuttgart: Thieme; 2016.

Part II of this book is intended to serve as a practical summary for CN examination. The chapters are structured in a similar fashion, with sections including symptoms, signs, and specific qualities. Lesions are considered topographically during the course of the individual CNs.

This comprises the intraparenchymal and intracranial course, the point of exit of the skull, and the course outside of the skull to reach the final destinations (end organs). If appropriate, the importance of anastomoses is also mentioned.

Detailed anatomical considerations, as well as neuroimaging and electrophysiology, and a list of the most useful and available investigations are discussed in Part I.

Each CN is discussed in regard to possible lesions and causes.

The main investigations and possible therapies are mentioned, which of course cannot cover all causes.

Chapter 18 summarizes functions that cannot be attributed to an individual CN but are always executed in synergy of several CNs. Examples are the pupil, the eyelid function, and others.

We hope this structured approach to CN examination and diagnosis is useful, and practical as intended. The complexity of CN functions often requires searches for additional references. Although not peer reviewed, video presentations, such as those on YouTube, are often a useful source of practical information.

All chapters in Part II are authored by Wolfgang Grisold, MD, Prof., FAAN (Ludwig Boltzmann Institute for Experimental und Clinical Traumatology, Donaueschingenstraße 13, A-1200 Vienna, Austria). 18 is also co-authored by Stacey A. Sakowski, PhD (Department of Neurology, University of Michigan, Ann Arbor, MI 48109, USA).

One sentence: The olfactory nerve is the afferent nerve for the sense of smell (it is the only CN where the afferents into the brain do not reach the brain via the thalamus) (Fig. 5.1).

Genetic testing	NCV/ EMG	Laboratory	Imaging	Clinical testing
		+	+	+, smell charts

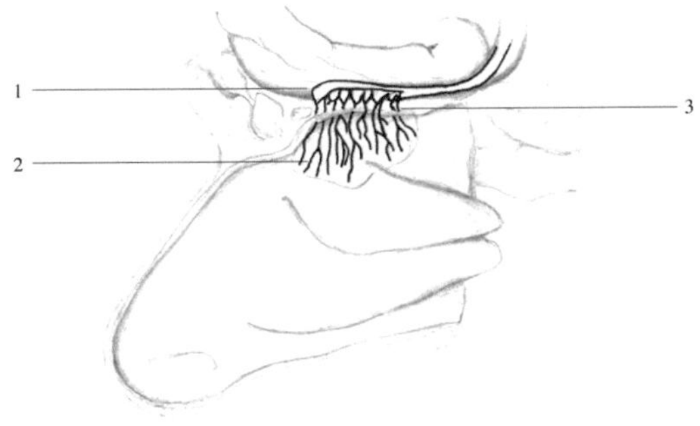

Fig. 5.1 Olfactory nerve. (1) Olfactory bulb, (2) fila olfactoria, (3) lamina cribrosa

Symptoms

The ability to smell varies individually (hypoosmic to normo-osmic).

Disorders of smell can develop rapidly (*e.g.*, trauma) or insidiously. Often taste is also impaired.

The term parosmia describes a qualitative change in smell, while anosmia is the total loss of smell. Other phenomena can be dysosmia, phantosmia [1], cacosmia, and olfactory illusions, among others.

"Nose blindness" describes the inability to detect one's own smell and also that of one's own surroundings.

(Also see "Hallucinations," Chap. 35).

Signs

Altered smell is difficult to quantify by a clinical examination (see "Main Investigations" below).

Age reduces the ability to smell.

Anatomists also discuss a CN "zero", or terminal nerve, receiving inputs from the vomeronasal organ [2].

Specific Qualities

Motor:
Sensory:
Autonomic:
Special senses: +.
Other:

Location of Lesions

Central: Neurodegenerative disorders, Alzheimer's and Parkinson's disease.

Intracranial within the skull: Olfactory tumors, neuroblastoma, meningioma.

Exit of the skull: Via the cribriform plate; trauma, tumors [3].

Outside of the skull: Nasal polyps, local cancer; other factors: colds, infections, medications and recreational drugs, airborne toxins [4], zinc.

Combination with Other CN

Frontobasal tumors.

Causes and Frequency

Causes for loss of smell.

Aging: Aging is a predominant cause of olfactory decline [5, 6]. The etiology of age-related olfactory loss is unclear.

Congenital anosmia: Isolated congenital anosmia is a rare condition; *e.g.*, Kallman syndrome (a form of hypogonadotropic hypogonadism that is distinguished from other forms by the unique symptom of anosmia).

Creutzfeldt-Jakob disease (CJD): [7].
Neurodegenerative diseases:

Alzheimer disease.
Down syndrome.

Huntington disease.
Parkinson disease.

Depression: [8].
Drugs: Allopurinol, analgesics, antibiotics (amphotericin B, ampicillin, ethambutol, lincomycin, tetracycline) [9], anthelmintics, local anesthetics, chemotherapy (carmustine, doxorubicin, methotrexate, vincristine), colchicine, diuretics, immunosuppressants (azathioprine), muscle relaxants, opiates, and statins [10].
Iatrogenic: Anterior base of the skull surgery.
Infections:

Common cold.
Covid-19 [11–14].
Meningitis, herpes, tuberculosis, syphilis.
Rhinitis.
Sinonasal disease, sinusitis.
Viral infections.

Inflammatory: Granulomatosis, Wegener, Sjögren.
Metabolic: Diabetes, renal insufficiency, Korsakoff syndrome.
Neoplastic:
Extracranial: Carcinoma, esthesioneuroblastoma, lymphoma, meningioma.
Salivary gland tumor (meningioma: Foster Kennedy).
Radiation therapy.
Smoking: Chronic.
Stroke: Chronic [15].
Toxic: Chemicals—benzene, carbon disulfide, heavy metals, menthol, sulfur dioxide, solvents, zinc, and occupational exposures [16].
Trauma: [17].

Closed head injury, anteroposterior skull fracture, post-concussion.
Fiber damage at cribriform palate.
Hemorrhages bulb and olfactory cortex.
Missile injuries.
Subarachnoidal hemorrhage.

Vaccination: [1].
Vitamin A deficiency.

Main Investigations

Diagnosis is based on history, signs upon clinical testing, and rarely olfactory on evoked potentials. If loss of taste accompanies loss of smell, electro-gustometry is rarely used.

Unilateral or bilateral testing.

Olfactory testing, *e.g.*, "smell identification test." Each nostril is tested separately for the patient's ability to smell coffee, peppermint oil, oil of cloves, and/or camphorated oil. Ammonia provokes a painful sensation and can be used to diagnose fictitious anosmia. Smell charts can be used.

Smell charts can also be used for the assessment of neurodegenerative disorders; *e.g.*, testing in persons with suspected dementia [18].

MRI can demonstrate the olfactory bulb and tract, demonstrating inflammation or atrophy [19, 20].

In acute trauma, nasal bleeding and swelling may hamper examination (see Chap. 32).

Differential diagnosis: The perception of lost or altered smell may also be due to altered taste secondary to dysfunction of CN IX.

Therapy

No specific therapies.

Therapy depends upon etiology and in cases of trauma is usually supportive.

When the loss of smell is due to trauma, more than 1/3 of individuals have full recovery within 3 months.

References

1. Keir G, Maria NI, Kirsch CFE. Unique imaging findings of neurologic phantosmia following Pfizer-BioNtech COVID-19 vaccination: a case report. Top Magn Reson Imaging. 2021;30(3):133–7.
2. Sonne J, Reddy V, Lopez-Ojeda W. Neuroanatomy, cranial nerve 0 (terminal nerve). Treasure Island, FL: StatPearls; 2022.
3. Thompson LD. Olfactory neuroblastoma. Head Neck Pathol. 2009;3(3):252–9.
4. Doty RL. Neurotoxic exposure and impairment of the chemical senses of taste and smell. Handb Clin Neurol. 2015;131:299–324.
5. Attems J, Walker L, Jellinger KA. Olfaction and aging: a mini-review. Gerontology. 2015;61(6):485–90.
6. Olofsson JK, Ekstrom I, Larsson M, Nordin S. Olfaction and aging: a review of the current state of research and future directions. Iperception. 2021;12(3):20416695211020331.
7. Reuber M, Al-Din AS, Baborie A, Chakrabarty A. New variant Creutzfeldt-Jakob disease presenting with loss of taste and smell. J Neurol Neurosurg Psychiatry. 2001;71(3):412–3.
8. Kohli P, Soler ZM, Nguyen SA, Muus JS, Schlosser RJ. The Association between olfaction and depression: a systematic review. Chem Senses. 2016;41(6):479–86.
9. Ferraro S, Convertino I, Leonardi L, Blandizzi C, Tuccori M. Unresolved gustatory, olfactory and auditory adverse drug reactions to antibiotic drugs: a survey of spontaneous reporting to Eudravigilance. Expert Opin Drug Saf. 2019;18(12):1245–53.
10. Ackerman BH, Kasbekar N. Disturbances of taste and smell induced by drugs. Pharmacotherapy. 1997;17(3):482–96.
11. Xydakis MS, Albers MW, Holbrook EH, Lyon DM, Shih RY, Frasnelli JA, et al. Post-viral effects of COVID-19 in the olfactory system and their implications. Lancet Neurol. 2021;20(9):753–61.
12. Konstantinidis I, Tsakiropoulou E, Hahner A, de With K, Poulas K, Hummel T. Olfactory dysfunction after coronavirus disease 2019 (COVID-19) vaccination. Int Forum Allergy Rhinol. 2021;11(9):1399–401.
13. Hiraga A, Muto M, Kuwabara S. Loss of taste as an initial symptom of a "Facial Diplegia and Paresthesia" Variant of Guillain-Barre Syndrome. Intern Med. 2022;61(19):2957–9.
14. Han AY, Mukdad L, Long JL, Lopez IA. Anosmia in COVID-19: mechanisms and significance. Chem Senses. 2020;45(6):423–8.
15. Wehling E, Naess H, Wollschlaeger D, Hofstad H, Bramerson A, Bende M, et al. Olfactory dysfunction in chronic stroke patients. BMC Neurol. 2015;15:199.
16. Genter MB, Doty RL. Toxic exposures and the senses of taste and smell. Handb Clin Neurol. 2019;164:389–408.
17. Peter W, Schofield RLD. Smell and taste. In: Doty RL, editor. Handbook of clinical neurology, vol. 164; 2019. p. 2–490.
18. Christensen IT, Larsson EM, Holm IE, Nielsen OBF, Andersen S. Olfactory testing in consecutive patients referred with suspected dementia. BMC Geriatr. 2017;17(1):129.
19. Keshavarz P, Haseli S, Yazdanpanah F, Bagheri F, Raygani N, Karimi-Galougahi M. A systematic review of imaging studies in olfactory dysfunction secondary to COVID-19. Acad Radiol. 2021;28(11):1530–40.
20. Kandemirli SG, Altundag A, Yildirim D, Tekcan Sanli DE, Saatci O. Olfactory bulb MRI and paranasal sinus CT findings in persistent COVID-19 anosmia. Acad Radiol. 2021;28(1):28–35.

One sentence: The optic nerve is considered a part of the brain and serves the special sense of vision and is essential for visual reflexes.

Genetic testing	NCV/ EMG	Laboratory	Imaging	Clinical testing
+	+ EP	+	+ MR, US (partly)_	+

Symptoms

Variable loss of vision, ranging to blindness.

Signs

The major function is the reflex reaction of the pupil, directly and indirectly.

Specific Qualities

Motor:
   Sensory:
   Autonomic:
   Special senses: Information, such as brightness and color perception and contrast (visual acuity). Reflex pathways for lightning and accommodation. Visual field defects.
   Other:

Location of Lesions: (Fig. 6.1)

Lesions of the optic nerve can be divided into three categories:

- Anterior to the chiasm (monocular field defect or blindness).
- Medial and temporal compression of the chiasm (hemianopia).
- Posterior to the chiasm.

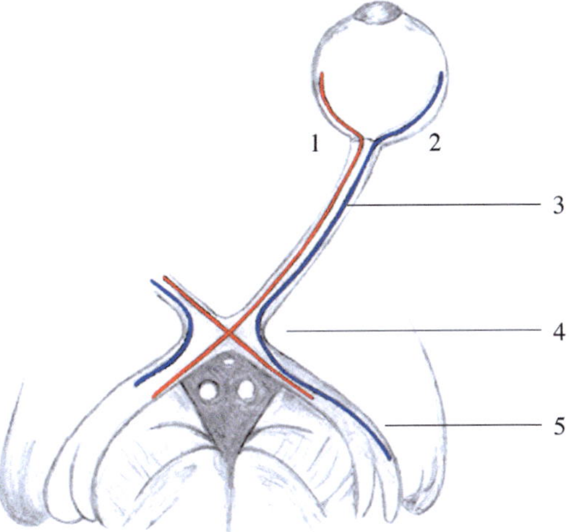

Fig. 6.1 Optic nerve. (*1*) medial fibers, (*2*) lateral fibers, (*3*) optic nerve, (*4*) optic chiasm, (*5*) optic tract

Central:
Tumors: glioma, infarction; multiple sclerosis and others.

Most axons of the optic nerve terminate at the lateral geniculate body.

From there, they relay to the visual cortex in the occipital lobe. Other fibers relate to the pretectal area (for reflexes) and the suprachiasmatic nucleus.

Intracranial within the skull:
Prechiasmatic lesions.

Chiasmatic lesions [1]: Aneurysm, craniopharyngioma, meningioma, optic glioma, pituitary adenoma, Rathke cleft cyst.

Retrochiasmatic pathways: [2].

Type of lesion: Compression, infiltration, arachnoid thickening (e.g., tabes dorsalis) [3].

Exit of the skull:
Optic canal.

Cavernous hemangioma [4], cysticercosis [5], meningioma [6], mucocele, orbital fasciitis resulting in visual loss, proptosis, and visual defects.

Neoplasm: Optic glioma, cancer [7].

Pressure: *e.g.,* acute in trauma [8].

Outside of the skull: Within the orbit, e.g., neoplasm or other space-occupying lesion.

For practical purposes, the length of the parts of the optic nerve can be assumed as noted in Table 6.1, and the vascular supply of the optic nerve is as noted in Table 6.2.

Table 6.1 Length of optic nerve parts in adults

	Length (mm)	Location
Intracranial	14–16	From the chiasm to the optic nerve canal
Intracanalicular	9	Optic nerve channel
Intraorbital	25	Intraorbital
Intraocular	1	Optic head

Table 6.2 Vascular supply of the optic nerve

Optic nerve	Proximal part: ophthalmic artery Distal part: small branches from internal carotid artery (ICA) and anterior carotid artery (ACA)
Optic chiasm	Superior: perforators from ACA Interior part: ICA, posterior communicating cerebral artery (PCommA), posterior cerebral artery (PCA)
Optic tract	PCommA, PCA, anterior choroidal artery

Combination with Other CN

Frontal tumors, trauma.

Causes and Frequency

Compression: Apoplexy of the pituitary (associated with headache), carotid aneurysm, endocrine orbitopathy. *Tumors in the sella result in visual field defects and a swollen optic disc.* Compression occurs in 50% of pituitary adenomas. Other causes include craniopharyngioma (in childhood), meningioma of the tuberculum sellae, aneurysm, and tumors of the chiasm itself (e.g., meningioma, neurinoma, or retinoblastoma).

Hereditary: Friedreich's ataxia, Leber's hereditary optic neuropathy, lysosomal disease, mitochondrial myopathy, Kearns-Sayre syndrome, neuropathy, ataxia, retinitis pigmentosa (NARP), storage disease (Tay-Sachs disease), optic atrophy 1, spinocerebellar disease. The optic nerve can also be damaged in genetic neuropathies: Autosomal dominant optic atrophy with cataract (ADOAC), cerebral dysgenesis-neuropathy-ichthyosis-keratoderma syndrome (CEDNIK) [9], Charcot-Marie-Tooth disease type 4 (CMT4; HMSN VI), *OPA1* and *OPA3* mutations.

Iatrogenic: Pressure on the eye bulb caused by anesthesia (ischemic optic nerve neuropathy), blepharoplasty, fractures of the orbit, or surgery of the nasal sinus.

Infectious: Meningitis, sarcoid, syphilis, tuberculosis. *Focal*: Granulomatous disease, orbital tumors, sinusitis. Chronic sinusitis [10].

Inflammatory: Optochiasmatic arachnoiditis.

Immune mediated: Optic neuritis in Devic's syndrome and multiple sclerosis, aquaporin 4 [11].

Metabolic: Diabetes, thyrotoxicosis, uremia.

Nutritive: Alcohol ingestion, B1 deficiency, B12 anemia, Cuban neuropathy, folic acid, methylol toxicity, Strachan's syndrome.

Paraneoplastic: Rarely involved in paraneoplastic dysfunction – carcinomatous retinopathy (CRMP5 and CAR) antibodies [12].

Radiation: Radiation therapy of brain tumors, pituitary tumors, metastases, or ENT tumors can cause unilateral or bilateral loss of vision with long latencies. Progressive optic nerve atrophy is seen within 6 weeks of exposure to 70 Gy.

Toxic optic neuropathy:

Alcohol: Methyl alcohol [13].

Drugs: Table 6.3.

Other causes: Heavy metals (arsenic, lead, mercury, thallium), aniline dye, carbon monoxide, carbon tetrachloride, tobacco [14], nitrous oxide.

Ethambutol: Color perception [15].

Trauma: Several mechanisms have been implicated:

- "Blowout" fractures, gunshot wounds, penetrating trauma, trauma of the orbit, traumatic optic neuropathy. Directly by objects: Penetrating trauma, transaction, avulsion, bleeding, air and gases.
- Indirect trauma (blow combined with commotion or concussion).
- Lesion in the intracanalicular part: Contusion of nerve axons and edema.

Tumors: Metastasis, melanocytoma, meningeal carcinomatosis (Fig. 6.2), nasopharyngeal tumor compresses the nerve and chiasm, neurofibromatosis (NF1, NF2), orbital tumors, optic nerve glioma, retinal infiltration (leukemia).

*Vascular:*Vascular diseases of the optic nerve: [16].

Aneurysms, giant cell arteritis, herpes zoster, ischemic optic neuropathy retrobulbar optic neuropathy, systematic lupus, temporal arteritis.

Table 6.3 Drugs causing optic nerve toxicity (see also toxic)

Drug class	Drugs
Antibiotics	Chloramphenicol, ethambutol, isoniazid, linezolid, streptomycin sulfonamides
Anticancer drugs	Chlorambucil, methotrexate, tamoxifen vincristine
Antimalarial drugs	Chloroquine, hydroxychloroquine, quinine
Antiarrhythmics	Amiodarone, digitalis
Phosphodiesterase inhibitors	Sildenafil

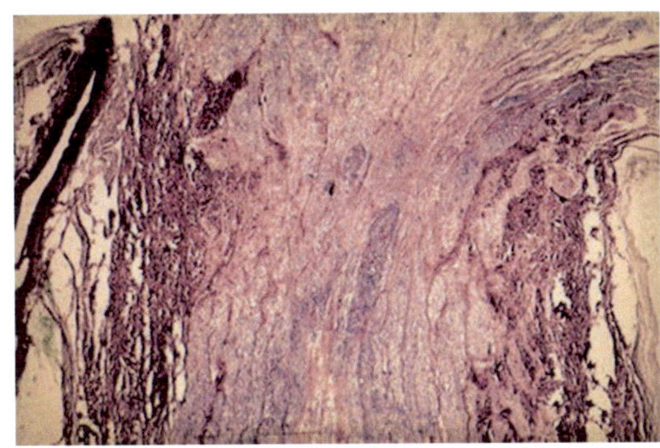

Fig. 6.2 Optic neuropathy. A photomicrograph of an optic nerve that is compressed by tumor cells ("cuffed") in meningeal carcinomatosis, resulting in blindness of the patient

Ischemia: Anterior ischemic optic neuropathy (AION), nonarteritic (NAION) and arteritic (AAION) forms.

Main Investigations

Diagnosis is based on clinical test, on X-ray, CT, or MR imaging, optical coherence tomography, visual function and color discrimination tests, ophthalmoscopic exam, visual evoked potentials, and electroretinogram.

Special ultrasound techniques also allow a partial identification of the infraorbital optic nerve.

Differential diagnosis: Other causes of papilledema need to be considered, including increased intracranial pressure and pseudotumor cerebri.

Therapy

Treatment depends upon the cause of the lesion.

Prognosis is presently subject to research [17].

References

1. Acheson J. Optic nerve and chiasmal disease. J Neurol. 2000;247(8):587–96.
2. Zhang X, Kedar S, Lynn MJ, Newman NJ, Biousse V. Homonymous hemianopia in stroke. J Neuroophthalmol. 2006;26(3):180–3.

3. Igersheimer J. Atrophy of the optic nerve in tabes and dementia paralytica. Arch Ophthalmol. 1949;42(2):170–7.

4. Chan AT, Micieli JA. Complete unilateral vision loss and optic nerve cupping from metastatic prostate cancer to the optic canal. BMJ Case Rep. 2021;14(1):e236685.

5. Gurha N, Sood A, Dhar J, Gupta S. Optic nerve cysticercosis in the optic canal. Acta Ophthalmol Scand. 1999;77(1):107–9.

6. Cristante L. Surgical treatment of meningiomas of the orbit and optic canal: a retrospective study with particular attention to the visual outcome. Acta Neurochir. 1994;126(1):27–32.

7. Christmas NJ, Mead MD, Richardson EP, Albert DM. Secondary optic nerve tumors. Surv Ophthalmol. 1991;36(3):196–206.

8. Tayal VS, Neulander M, Norton HJ, Foster T, Saunders T, Blaivas M. Emergency department sonographic measurement of optic nerve sheath diameter to detect findings of increased intracranial pressure in adult head injury patients. Ann Emerg Med. 2007;49(4):508–14.

9. Lenaers G, Neutzner A, Le Dantec Y, Juschke C, Xiao T, Decembrini S, et al. Dominant optic atrophy: culprit mitochondria in the optic nerve. Prog Retin Eye Res. 2021;83:100935.

10. Kim YH, Kim J, Kang MG, Lee DH, Chin HS, Jang TY, et al. Optic nerve changes in chronic sinusitis patients: correlation with disease severity and relevant sinus location. PLoS One. 2018;13(7):e0199875.

11. Kitley J, Leite MI, Nakashima I, Waters P, McNeillis B, Brown R, et al. Prognostic factors and disease course in aquaporin-4 antibody-positive patients with neuromyelitis optica spectrum disorder from the United Kingdom and Japan. Brain. 2012;135(Pt 6):1834–49.

12. Khan Y, Khan W, Thalambedu N, Ashfaq AA, Ullah W. Optic neuritis: a rare paraneoplastic phenomenon of Hodgkin's lymphoma. Cureus. 2019;11(7):e5181.

13. Bennett IL Jr, Cary FH, Mitchell GL Jr, Cooper MN. Acute methyl alcohol poisoning: a review based on experiences in an outbreak of 323 cases. Medicine (Baltimore). 1953;32(4):431–63.

14. Grzybowski A, Zulsdorff M, Wilhelm H, Tonagel F. Toxic optic neuropathies: an updated review. Acta Ophthalmol. 2015;93(5):402–10.

15. Nasemann J, Zrenner E, Riedel KG. Recovery after severe ethambutol intoxication—psychophysical and electrophysiological correlations. Doc Ophthalmol. 1989;71(3):279–92.

16. Patel HR, Margo CE. Pathology of ischemic optic neuropathy. Arch Pathol Lab Med. 2017;141(1):162–6.

17. Gokoffski KK, Lam P, Alas BF, Peng MG, Ansorge HRR. Optic nerve regeneration: how will we get there? J Neuroophthalmol. 2020;40(2):234–42.

Cranial Nerve III: Oculomotor Nerve

One sentence: The oculomotor nerve supports motor nerve innervation of most extraocular muscles and main lid elevator, while the autonomic part is responsible for the pupillary reflex and accommodation (Fig. 7.1).

Genetic testing	NCV/ EMG	Laboratory	Imaging	Clinical testing
		+	+	+

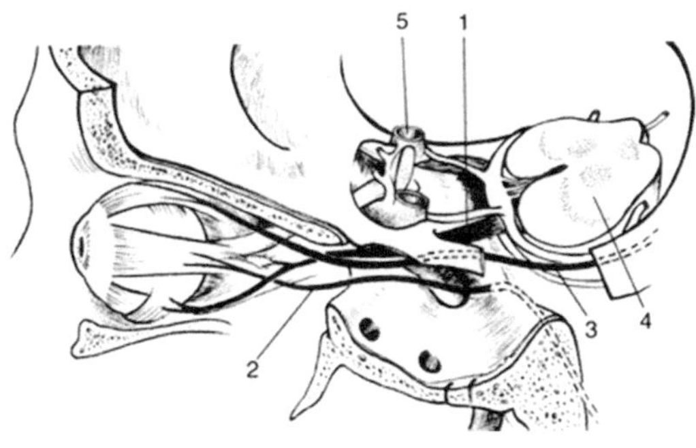

Fig. 7.1 Anatomy of oculomotor nerve: (*1*) oculomotor nerve, (*2*) abducens nerve, (*3*) trochlear nerve, (*4*) cross section through brain stem, (*5*) internal carotid artery

Symptoms

Patients with third nerve palsies have diplopia and unilateral ptosis. Complete ptosis may alleviate diplopia. Patients have difficulty viewing near objects because convergence is impaired.

Signs

Partial or complete ipsilateral ptosis. Examination of eye movements reveals ipsilateral adduction, elevation, and depression deficit of the eye. If the deficit of adduction is significant, there will be a primary position exotropia that is worse when the gaze is directed toward the paretic medial rectus muscle. If the levator muscles (e.g., superior rectus or inferior oblique muscles) are involved, ipsilateral hypotropia occurs. External ophthalmoplegia involves only the extraocular eye muscles while sparing the pupillary parasympathetic fibers.

© The Author(s), under exclusive license to Springer Nature Switzerland AG 2023
W. Grisold et al., *The Cranial Nerves in Neurology*, https://doi.org/10.1007/978-3-031-43081-7_7

The pupil can be dilated and poorly reactive or nonreactive to light and accommodation. Internal ophthalmoplegia involves the parasympathetic pupillary fibers exclusively. Pupil-sparing oculomotor lesions [1] exist.

In a complete oculomotor nerve palsy, the eye is fixed in a lateral and downward position, the pupil is dilated due to the unopposed action of dilator papillae, and the upper eyelid droops down (ptosis) due to paralysis of levator palpebrae superioris (Figs. 7.2 and 7.3).

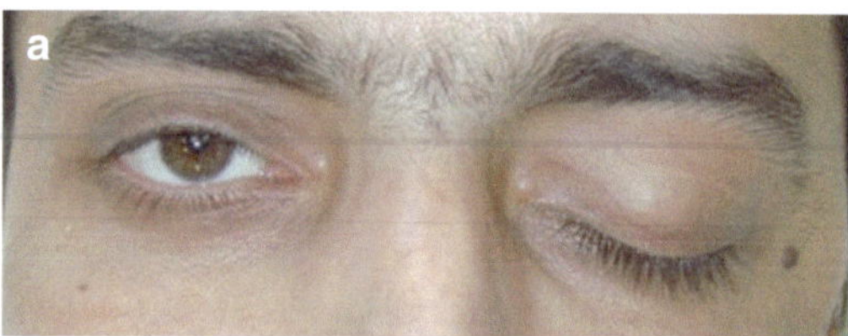
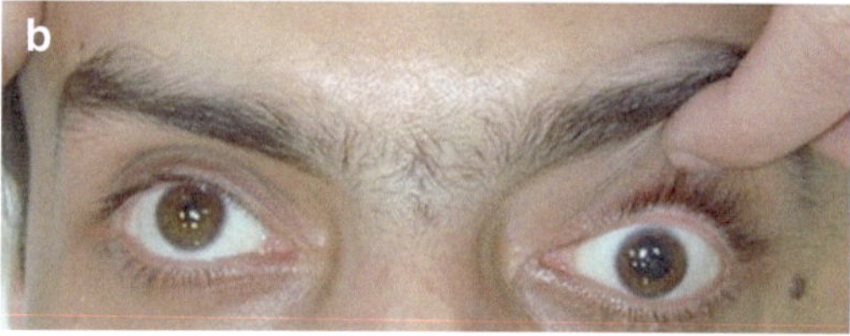

Fig. 7.2 Oculomotor nerve paresis. (**a**) Complete ptosis. (**b**) Upon lifting of the lid, lateral deviation of the left eye with an enlarged pupil (mydriasis) secondary to dysfunction of the parasympathetic fibers to the sphincter pupillae

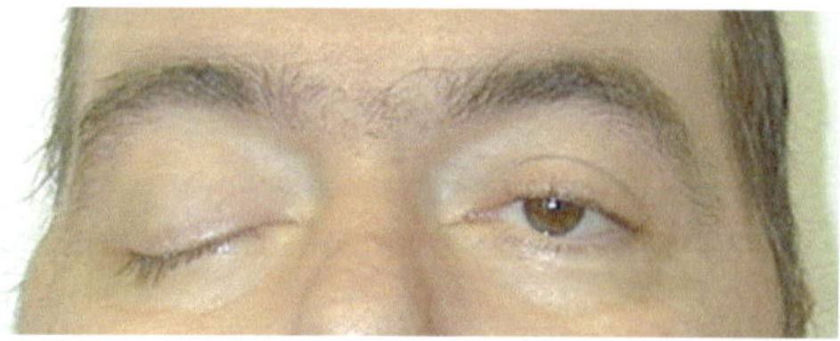

Fig. 7.3 Right-sided ptosis, caused by glioma infiltration of the cavernous sinus, in a patient with glioma. Neuralgic pain due to trigeminal nerve involvement was also associated

Specific Qualities

Motor: +.
 Sensory:
 Autonomic: +.
 Special senses:
 Other:

Location of Lesions

Oculomotor nerve structures from the nuclei to the orbit are outlined in Table 7.1.

Several types of lesions: [2].

Central: Central (brain stem: nuclear and fascicular) lesions are usually not isolated and include long tract or medial longitudinal fascicle (MLF) signs. In addition to the complex nuclear nerve lesions [3], there are also fascicular oculomotor brain stem lesions.

Vascular lesions: Vascular brain stem syndromes (e.g., Benedikt, Claude, Nothnagel, Weber syndrome).

Other intraparenchymal lesions can be caused by tumors, infections, and metabolic disease (e.g., Wernicke's encephalopathy).

Intracranial within the skull: Subarachnoidal space.

The nerve arises from medial aspect of cerebral peduncle and continues in the interpeduncular cistern between the posterior cerebral and superior cerebellar arteries. It enters the cavernous sinus. Positioned above the trochlear nerve in the lateral wall. It is divided into an upper and lower division in the ventral cavernous sinus (Fig. 7.4).

Lesions at the clivus and plica petroclinoidea: Occur in herniation or local tumors.

Compression (e.g., aneurysm), herniation, tumors (Schwannoma), meningeal carcinomatosis, infection, inflammation.

Table 7.1 Oculomotor nerve structures from the nuclei to the orbit

CN III	Brain parenchyma	Intracranial and subarachnoid	Cranial exit	Extracranial lesion
III	Anatomy of complex nuclear structure	Clivus (pressure)	Fissura orbitalis superior	Orbital
	Fascicular intraparenchymal lesion	Meningeal carcinomatosis, infections, granulomatous tissue, osteoporosis		Orbital neuroma
	Vascular brain stem syndromes	Cavernous sinus tumors, aneurysms		Ciliary ganglion lesion
Autonomic	Edinger-Westphal nucleus	Inferior portion of the nerve		

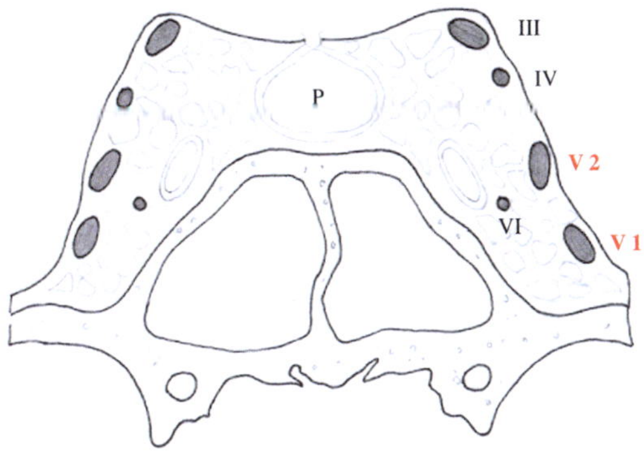

Fig. 7.4 Cavernous sinus. *III* oculomotor nerve, *IV* trochlear nerve, *VI* abducens nerve, *V 1* ophthalmic nerve, *V 2* maxillary nerve, *P* pituitary gland

Iatrogenic lesions caused by radiation therapy [4], base of the skull surgery.

Exit of the Skull: Both divisions of the oculomotor nerve enter the orbit through the middle part of the superior orbital fissure, within the tendinous ring of Zinn.

Lesions of the superior orbital fissure syndrome, bony lesions, and local tumors, e.g., metastasis.

Outside of the skull: Within the orbit:

Superior division: Superior rectus and levator palpebrae superioris.

Inferior division: Inferior rectus, inferior oblique, medial rectus, and presynaptic parasympathetic fibers.

The parasympathetic fibers terminate in the ciliary ganglion. Postganglionic fibers form the ciliary nerves, which join the nasociliary nerve (V 1) to reach the ciliary body and iris. They control the sphincter papillae and ciliary muscles.

The oculomotor nerve receives sympathetic fibers in the cavernous sinus from the sympathetic plexus around the internal carotid artery. The sympathetic fibers supply the muscle dilatator pupillae and smooth muscles, which are part of the levator palpebrae superioris (muscle of Mueller).

Lesions: Oculomotor nerve lesions in the orbit are rare, caused by infraorbital *metastasis and perineuronal spread, among other space-occupying lesions* [5].

Combination with Other CN

If the superior orbital fissure and cavernous sinus are affected [6].

Causes and Frequency

Congenital: Nucleus usually unilateral.

Compressive: Herniation of the temporal lobe, neurosurgical procedures, pathologic conditions in the cavernous sinus.

Idiopathic: In adults, 20–25% of cases; in pediatric cases, up to 40%.

Infections: Botulinum, herpes zoster, mumps, syphilis [7], tuberculosis, or tetanus. Case reports: varicella zoster encephalitis [8], herpes zoster [9].

Inflammation: Guillain-Barré syndrome (GBS; rare), meningitis – with other CN involvement. Chronic ataxic neuropathy ophthalmoplegia M-protein agglutination disialosyl antibodies syndrome (CANOMAD), Miller Fisher (MLF), Tolosa Hunt syndrome.

Metabolic causes: Diabetes – often painful with sparing of the pupil; usually self-limiting with recovery in 4 months.

Myotonia ocular: [10].

Myopathy ocular.

Myasthenia gravis.

Osteopetrosis: [11].

Toxic: Alcohol, arsenic, carbon monoxide, and lead; carbon disulfide or dinitrophenol poisoning.

Neoplastic: Leptomeningeal carcinomatosis, multiple myeloma, neurinoma. Muscle metastasis, perineurial spread [5].

Neuropathy: Nerve thickening [12].

Nuclear, fascicular: In combination with brain stem infarcts.

Synkinesis upon regeneration: [13].

Tumors of CN III: Neurinoma, schwannoma, and cancer-associated.

Trauma: Cranial trauma with or without fracture, blowout fractures, traumatic aneurysm, war and combat injury. Regeneration after trauma may be aberrant, and posttraumatic reinnervation can cause erroneous innervation of adjacent muscles, resulting in unusual movements; e.g., upper lid may retract on attempted downward gaze (pseudo-von Graefe sign), etc. The pupil can also restrict during adduction.

Vascular:

Aneurysm: Often painful and involves the pupil.

Pituitary apoplexy [14, 15].

Ischemic vascular, often painful [16].

Others:

Migraine: Ophthalmoplegic migraine [17].

Pediatric oculomotor lesions: Congenital, traumatic, and inflammatory causes are most common. Isolated third nerve palsy in adults may be due to aneurysm, vascular, or undetermined causes.

Main Investigations

Ophthalmology, Leigh screen.

Laboratory to exclude diabetes.

Imaging to exclude aneurysm, MR techniques identify nerve lesions.

Differential diagnosis: Botulism (additional involvement of pupil), brain stem disorders, CANOMAD syndrome, chronic progressive external ophthalmoplegia, congenital lesions, Miller Fisher syndrome, myasthenia gravis, and myopathy.

Therapy

Long duration of defects may require prism therapy or strabismus surgery.

Prognosis depends on the treatment of the underlying pathology. If the lesion is of vascular etiology, resolution occurs usually within 4–6 months.

References

1. Jacobson DM. Relative pupil-sparing third nerve palsy: etiology and clinical variables predictive of a mass. Neurology. 2001;56(6):797–8.
2. Condos A, Sullivan MA, Hawley D, Cho A, Cathey M. Not just down and out: oculomotor nerve pathologic spectrum. Curr Probl Diagn Radiol. 2022;51(2):217–24.
3. Zee DS. The organization of the brainstem ocular motor subnuclei. Ann Neurol. 1978;4(4):384–5.
4. Grassmeyer JJ, Fernandes JA, Helvey JT, Kedar S. Radiation-induced bilateral oculomotor nerve palsy 20 years after radiation treatment. Neurology. 2021;96(20):955–7.
5. McNab AA, Francis IC, Benger R, Crompton JL. Perineural spread of cutaneous squamous cell carcinoma via the orbit. Clinical features and outcome in 21 cases. Ophthalmology. 1997;104(9):1457–62.
6. Rush JA, Younge BR. Paralysis of cranial nerves III, IV, and VI. Cause and prognosis in 1000 cases. Arch Ophthalmol. 1981;99(1):76–9.
7. Corr P, Bhigjee A, Lockhat F. Oculomotor nerve root enhancement in meningovascular syphilis. Clin Radiol. 2004;59(3):294–6.
8. Quan SC, Skondra D. Case report: varicella-zoster encephalitis with acute retinal necrosis and oculomotor nerve palsy. Optom Vis Sci. 2019;96(5):367–71.
9. Marsh RJ, Dulley B, Kelly V. External ocular motor palsies in ophthalmic zoster: a review. Br J Ophthalmol. 1977;61(11):677–82.
10. Nahar VK, Wilkerson AH, Ghafari G, Martin B, Black WH, Boyas JF, et al. Skin cancer knowledge, attitudes, beliefs, and prevention practices among

medical students: a systematic search and literature review. Int J Womens Dermatol. 2018;4(3):139–49.

11. Vrabec F, Sedlackova J. Neuro-histological findings in osteopetrosis (Albers-Schoenberg disease). Br J Ophthalmol. 1964;48:218–22.

12. Alwan AA, Mejico LJ. Ophthalmoplegia, proptosis, and lid retraction caused by cranial nerve hypertrophy in chronic inflammatory demyelinating polyradiculo-neuropathy. J Neuroophthalmol. 2007;27(2):99–103.

13. Lepore FE, Glaser JS, Misdirection revisited. A critical appraisal of acquired oculomotor nerve synkinesis. Arch Ophthalmol. 1980;98(12):2206–9.

14. Rosso M, Ramaswamy S, Sucharew H, Vagal A, Anziska Y, Levine SR. Isolated third cranial nerve palsy in pituitary apoplexy: case report and systematic review. J Stroke Cerebrovasc Dis. 2021;30(9):105969.

15. Keane JR. Aneurysms and third nerve palsies. Ann Neurol. 1983;14(6):696–7.

16. Wilker SC, Rucker JC, Newman NJ, Biousse V, Tomsak RL. Pain in ischaemic ocular motor cranial nerve palsies. Br J Ophthalmol. 2009;93(12):1657–9.

17. Geraud G. Rare and atypical forms of migraine. Rev Neurol (Paris). 2000;156(Suppl. 4):4S42–6.

One sentence: The trochlear nerve (Fig. 8.1) is a pure motor nerve, and its lesions result in vertical diplopia, which increases when the gaze is directed downward and medially.

Genetic testing	NCV/ EMG	Laboratory	Imaging	Biopsy
			+	

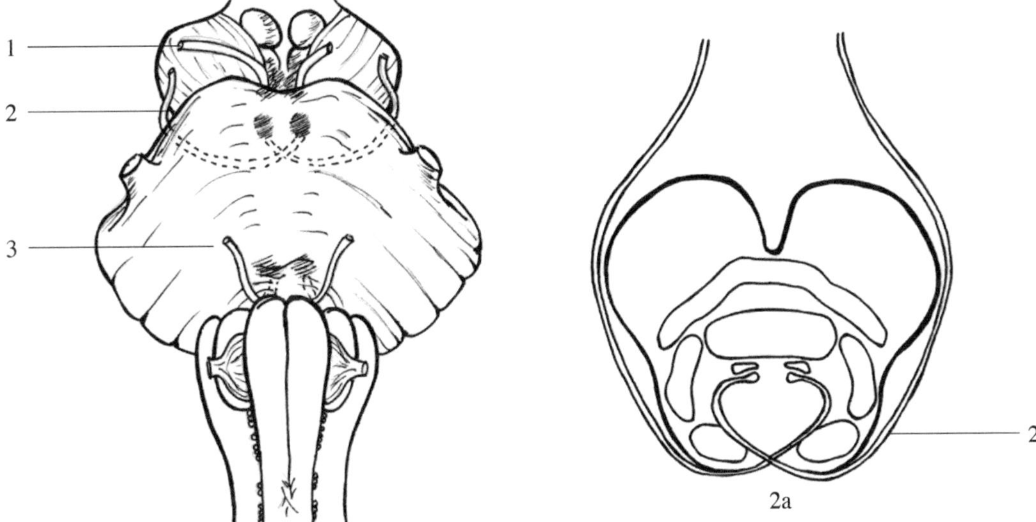

Fig. 8.1 Trochlear nerve. (*1*) Oculomotor nerve, (*2*) *a* fiber crossing, (*3*) abducens nerve

Symptoms

Diplopia: Patients experience vertical diplopia that increases when the gaze is directed downward and medially.

"Torsional diplopia": Trochlear nerve palsy affects the torsion of the eyeball in the plane of the face. Physiologically, the torsion of the eyeball is a normal response to tilting the head sideways.

Signs

The affected eye is sometimes deviated (although this may not be visible to the examiner) and displays less depression during adduction. Hypertropia occurs in severe weakness.

Patients adapt by tilting the head forward to bring the visual fields together. This posture of the head gives a "dejected" appearance ("pathetic nerve" palsies).

Specific Qualities

Motor: +.
Sensory:
Autonomic:
Special senses:
Other:

Location

Central:
Nuclear/fascicular lesion results in a contralateral superior oblique palsy. Lesions distal to the decussation cause an ipsilateral palsy.

Brain stem nuclear or fascicular lesions are not isolated and usually involve the medial longitudinal fascicle (MLF), the sympathetic pathway, or cause afferent pupillary defects (lesion of pretectal fibers).

Central causes include vascular, demyelinating disease, glioma, trauma, and infections.

Intracranial Within the Skull:

The trochlear nerve is the longest intracranial nerve with a length between 60–75 mm, and it decussates before emerging from the brain stem [1].

Lesions occur in the cisternal and subarachnoidal part and also in the cavernous sinus.

Lesions occur due to diabetes, iatrogenic, infection, inflammation, neoplastic, pituitary apoplexy, raised intracranial pressure, and trauma.

Exit of the skull: The nerve exits through the superior orbital fissure outside of the annulus of Zinn.

Outside of the Skull:
Orbital nerve lesions are rare. Signs and symptoms are associated with concomitant lesions of CN II, III, V, and VI. Mechanical restrictions by rheumatoid disease, tendons, trauma.

In orbital lesions proptosis, chemosis and orbital edema are often associated.

Bilateral trochlear nerve lesions present with alternating hypertropia on horizontal gaze or tilt and positive Bielschowsky head tilt test to either side. They are rare, usually observed in trauma [2].

Combination with Other CN

Lesion at the cavernous sinus and in the orbital apex.

Causes and Frequency

Trochlear nerve palsies are well described: [3–6].

Congenital: Rare [7].

Compression: Cavernous sinus, orbital fissure lesions, inflammatory aneurysms (posterior cerebral artery, anterior superior cerebellar artery), tentorial herniation.

Infection: Mastoiditis, meningitis. Herpes zoster [8].

Inflammatory: Ophthalmoplegia or diplopia associated with giant cell arteritis. Local anesthesia [9].

Metabolic: Diabetes.

Myokymia: Superior oblique myokymia.

Neoplastic: Carcinomatous meningitis, cerebellar hemangioblastoma, ependymoma, meningioma, metastasis, neurilemmoma, neurofibroma [2], pineal tumors, trochlear nerve sheath tumors, *e.g.,* schwannoma [10] and others. Orbital apex tumors, cancer metastasis [11].

Pediatric: Congenital, traumatic, and idiopathic.

Trauma: Head trauma causing compression at the tentorial edge, lumbar puncture or spinal anesthesia, subarachnoid hemorrhage, surgery. The trochlear nerve is the most commonly injured CN in head trauma.

Vascular: Arteriosclerosis, diabetes (painless diplopia), hypertension. Rarely in vascular brain stem lesion. Bilateral [12, 13].

Main Investigations

Diagnosis includes clinical optomotor examination and imaging. The diagnosis can be facilitated by the Bielschowsky test.

Suggestive of a trochlear nerve lesion:

Hypertropia of the affected eye.

Diplopia is exacerbated by gazing downward.

Diplopia can be improved by tilting the head away from the affected eye.

Imaging: [14].

Differential diagnosis: Skew deviation, a disparity in the vertical positioning of the eyes of supranuclear origin, can mimic trochlear palsy. Myasthenia gravis, disorders of the extraocular muscles, thyroid disease, and oculomotor palsy that affect the superior rectus can also cause similar signs.

Therapy

The vertical diplopia may be alleviated by the patching of one eye or the use of prisms or sight training. Surgery could be indicated to remove compression or repair trauma.

Prognosis: The recovery rate over a 6-month time period is higher in cases of diabetic etiology than in other nonselected cases.

References

1. Joo W, Rhoton AL Jr. Microsurgical anatomy of the trochlear nerve. Clin Anat. 2015;28(7):857–64.
2. Lekskul A, Wuthisiri W, Tangtammaruk P. The etiologies of isolated fourth cranial nerve palsy: a 10-year review of 158 cases. Int Ophthalmol. 2021;41(10):3437–42.
3. Morillon P, Bremner F. Trochlear nerve palsy. Br J Hosp Med (Lond). 2017;78(3):C38–40.
4. Abkur TM. Trochlear nerve palsy. Pract Neurol. 2017;17(6):474–5.
5. Brazis PW. Palsies of the trochlear nerve: diagnosis and localization—recent concepts. Mayo Clin Proc. 1993;68(5):501–9.
6. Keane JR. Fourth nerve palsy: historical review and study of 215 inpatients. Neurology. 1993;43(12):2439–43.
7. Orphanet. The portal for rare diseases and orphan drugs (Available from: https://www.orpha.net/consor/cgi-bin/OC_Exp.php?lng=EN&Expert=91498).
8. Grimson BS, Glaser JS. Isolated trochlear nerve palsies in herpes zoster ophthalmicus. Arch Ophthalmol. 1978;96(7):1233–5.
9. Chisci G, Chisci C, Chisci V, Chisci E. Ocular complications after posterior superior alveolar nerve block: a case of trochlear nerve palsy. Int J Oral Maxillofac Surg. 2013;42(12):1562–5.
10. Maurice-Williams RS. Isolated schwannoma of the fourth cranial nerve: case report. J Neurol Neurosurg Psychiatry. 1989;52(12):1442–3.
11. Kong E, Koh SA, Kim WJ. Rapid progression from trochlear nerve palsy to orbital apex syndrome as an initial presentation of advanced gastric cancer. Yeungnam Univ J Med. 2019;36(2):159–62.
12. Murray RS, Ajax ET. Bilateral trochlear nerve palsies. A clinicoanatomic correlate. J Clin Neuroophthalmol. 1985;5(1):57–8.
13. Simon S, Sandhu A, Selva D, Crompton JL. Bilateral trochlear nerve palsies following dorsal midbrain haemorrhage. N Z Med J. 2009;122(1300):72–5.
14. Agarwal N, Ahmed AK, Wiggins RH 3rd, McCulley TJ, Kontzialis M, Macedo LL, et al. Segmental imaging of the trochlear nerve: anatomic and pathologic considerations. J Neuroophthalmol. 2021;41(1):e7–e15.

One sentence: The trigeminal nerve is predominately sensory with a smaller motor portion and several autonomic fibers that travel via nerve anastomosis and blood vessels.

Genetic testing	NCV/ EMG	Laboratory	Imaging	Biopsy
	+		+	

Symptoms

The symptoms of trigeminal nerve lesions are predominately sensory and rarely motor. Pain in the distribution of the trigeminal nerve can vary widely from symptomatic pain to neuralgia. Motor lesions are rare and affect chewing and biting.

The distribution of sensory symptoms can be central (as in supranuclear and brain stem lesions) and then follow a hemi- or "onion skin" pattern, or peripheral, from the individual branches toward isolated peripheral nerve twigs.

Trigeminal neuralgia is a complex pain disorder, which can be symptomatic or idiopathic (see Chap. 33).

Signs

The corneal reflex may be absent. Complete sensory loss, or loss of pain and temperature, may cause ulcers on the skin, mucous membranes, and the cornea. Sensory lesions in the trigeminal nerve distribution may be also caused by central (brain stem) lesions and then follow an "onion skin" pattern in distribution.

Several neuralgic trigeminal pain syndromes may be associated with autonomic symptoms, such as redness of the eye or abnormal tearing during the attack.

Motor lesions are rarely symptomatic and could cause a mono- or diplegia with difficulty chewing. When the patient opens the mouth widely, the jaw will deviate to the affected side.

Specific Qualities

Motor: +.

  Sensory: ++.

  Autonomic: The trigeminal nerve is accompanied by both sympathetic and parasympathetic fibers. A trophic syndrome can appear [1–3].

  Special senses:

  Other:

Location of Lesions: [4]

Central: See **Table 9.1**.

  Hemispheric, in particular thalamic lesions.
  Lateral pons: Pain and temperature loss.
  Midpons: Motor and loss of pain sensation.

Medulla oblongata: Spinal tract and spinal tract nucleus ipsilaterally affected. Spinothalamic tract and occasionally ventral trigeminal tract contralaterally. Sometimes associated with pain [5].

Intracranial Within the Skull:

In the subarachnoid space, preganglionic lesions cause motor dysfunction and ipsilateral sensory loss in the face. Also, other CNs, such as VII and VIII, are likely to be involved. Causes include local tumors, tumor spread, infections, and trauma.

Lesions at the petrous apex and Meckel's cave: Lesions of the main trunk or ganglion lesions result in numbness or pain. Causes include infections, trauma, and tumors.

Specific syndromes:

Gradenigo syndrome: Inflammation of the petrosal apex and associated CN VI nerve lesion caused by *infections* e.g., otitis.

Raeder's paratrigeminal syndrome.

Herpes zoster ophthalmicus.

Lesions at the cavernous sinus: Involve other CNs, such as III, IV, and VI; Horner syndrome. Often associated with pain and ophthalmoplegia.

Exit of the Skull: (Fig. 9.1)

V1, the ophthalmic nerve exits at the superior orbital fissure: "Superior orbital fissure syndrome." Although located distally from the cavernous sinus, it may have similar symptoms as the cavernous sinus syndrome, involving CN III, IV, and VI and causing oculosympathetic paresis, pain, and exophthalmos via venous blockage.

Table 9.1 Trigeminal lesions at various levels of the pons and medulla oblongata

Location	Affected structures	Functional loss
Lateral rostral pons and upward	Spinothalamic ventral trigeminal tracts	Pain, temperature, touch over entire body, including face ipsilaterally and body contra laterally
Midpons	Main sensory trigeminal nucleus, motor nucleus, and entering root fibers ipsilaterally	Pain, temperature, touch over face ipsilaterally. Motor trigeminal
Lateral inferior pons or lateral medulla oblongata	Spinal tract and spinal tract nucleus ipsilaterally; spinothalamic tract and occasionally ventral trigeminal tract contralaterally	Pain, temperature over face ipsilaterally; pain, temperature over body contralaterally

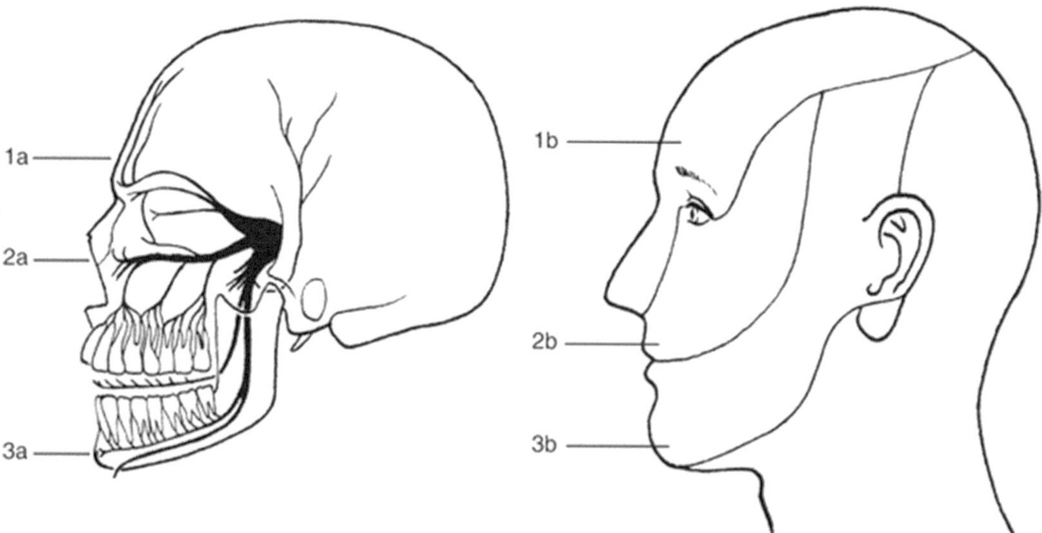

Fig. 9.1 Trigeminal nerve: 3 branches: *1a* Ophthalmic nerve, *2a* maxillary nerve, *3a* mandibular nerve, *1b–3b* sensory distribution

V2, the maxillary nerve, exits at the *foramen rotundum*. This foramen is also used for therapeutic approaches [6]. Also, retrograde perineurial spread via this foramen has been described [7].

V3, the mandibular nerve, exits at the *foramen ovale*. Interventions for trigeminal neuralgia are performed through this orifice. Nerve thickening can be inflammatory or neoplastic [8, 9].

Outside of the skull: For practical clinical purposes, the clinical syndromes are usually attributed to the three branches, which are to a large extent available for clinical investigation. Below is a list of further branching. This clinical practical view does not consider the numerous anastomoses.

- *V1, ophthalmic nerve* (Fig. 9.2): It has three major branches, the frontal, lacrimal, and nasociliary nerves. Intracranially, V1 sends a sensory branch to the tentorium cerebelli. The frontal nerve and its branches can be damaged during surgery and fractures. It provides sensory innervation to the face at a level above the orbits, the superior portion of the nasal cavity, the frontal sinus and inside the skull the dura mater, and portions of the anterior cranial fossa. The ophthalmic nerve also innervates the ciliary body, iris, lacrimal gland, conjunctiva, and cornea.

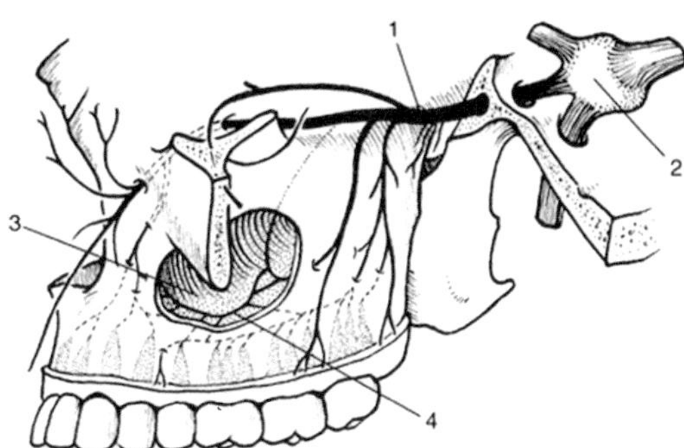

Fig. 9.3 Trigeminal nerve: sensory innervation of the maxilla. (*1*) Maxillary nerve, (*2*) trigeminal ganglion, (*3*) the maxilla (bone removed), (*4*) branch of superior alveolar nerve

- Branches:
  - Frontal: Within the orbit, the frontal nerve branches into the supraorbital and supratrochlear nerve.
  - Lacrimal: The lacrimal nerve supplies the lacrimal gland and part of the upper eyelid (anastomoses with CN VII).
  - Nasociliary nerve: The nasociliary nerve enters the orbit via the annulus of Zinn and supplies sensory innervation for the skin of the forehead and scalp through the supraorbital nerve and the supratrochlear nerve.
- *V2, maxillary nerve* (Fig. 9.3): The maxillary nerve has three branches: the infraorbital, zygomatic, and pterygopalatine nerves. V2 is most frequently affected in trauma. Sensory loss of the cheek and lip appear. V2 can also be injured in facial surgery and dental surgery.
- The maxillary nerve supplies the region between the orbit and the mouth, including the inferior portion of the nasal cavity and the maxillary teeth.
- The middle meningeal nerve arises from the trigeminal ganglion at the inferior wall of the cavernous sinus and exits at the foramen ovale.
- *V3, mandibular nerve* (Fig. 9.4): The mandibular nerve's major branches are the auriculotemporal, inferior alveolar, and lingual nerves. A separate motor division innervates the temporal and masseteric muscles and the tensor tympani, pterygoid, mylohyoid, and

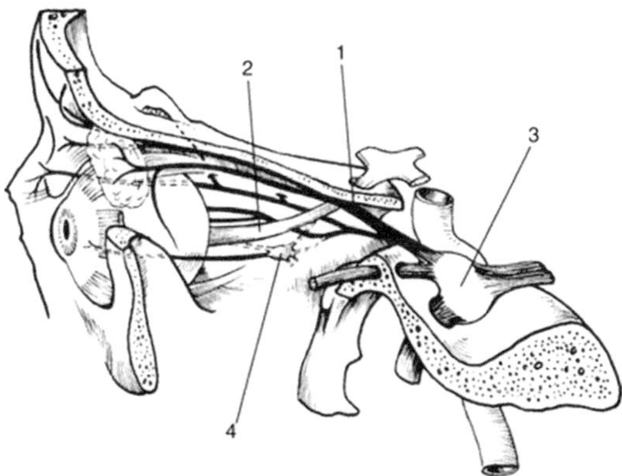

Fig. 9.2 Trigeminal nerve: sensory innervation of the eye and orbit (*1*). Ophthalmic nerve, (*2*) optic nerve, (*3*) trigeminal ganglion, (*4*) ciliary ganglion

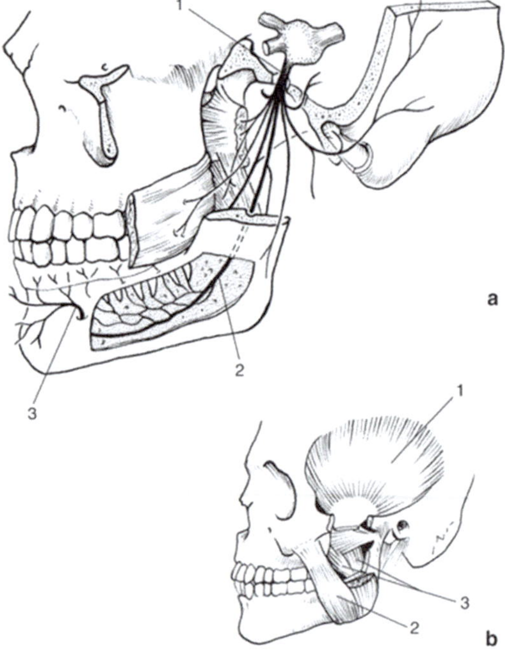

Fig. 9.4 Trigeminal nerve: motor and sensory innervation. (**a**) *1* mandibular nerve, *2* inferior alveolar nerve, *3* mental nerve. (**b**) *1* temporal muscle, *2* masseteric muscle, *3* pterygoid muscles

tensor veli palatini muscles. Lesions of V3 result from dentistry, implantation [11], infection, mandible resection, hematoma of the lower lip, or bites. The lingual nerve is most frequently damaged at the site of the third molar [12] nerve in dentistry. Pure motor lesions (usually unilateral) are rarely described [13] (see Fig. 9.7).

Examples of anastomosis of the trigeminal nerve:

- Anastomosis of the greater superficial petrosal nerve (GSPN) via the pterygoid canal, linking to the geniculate ganglion (cranial nerve VII) and the pterygopalatine ganglion (V2). This can explain the symptom complex of loss of taste sensation, hyperacusis, loss of sensation of ear structures, and absence of tearing (Fig. 9.5).
- Anastomosis between the auriculotemporal nerve (V3) and the lesser superficial petrosal nerve (VII) near the stylomastoid foramen. These anastomotic connections are also

Fig. 9.5 Anastomosis between the trigeminal and facial nerve. *SOF* superior orbital fissure, *PG* ganglion pterygopalatinum, *PPF* pterygopalatine fossa, *FO* foramen ovale, *FR* foramen rotundum, *GSPN* greater sphenopalatine nerve. V1, V2 trigeminal nerves. Vidian nerve, greater palatine nerve, lesser palatine nerve

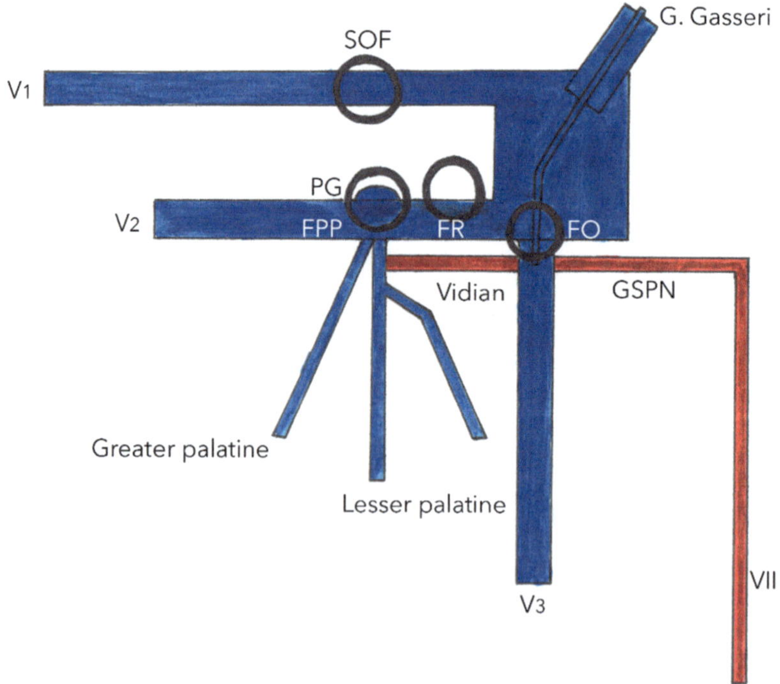

thought to provide a conduit for perineural spread in tumors.

- The chorda tympani innervates the anterior 2/3 of the tongue for taste sensations. The *nerve* arises from the facial nerve. It runs in the superior and anterior direction and perforates the *tympanic cavity*. It exits the skull through the petrotympanic fissure and descends into the *infratemporal fossa*, and medial to the *lateral pterygoid muscle* joins the lingual nerve.
- The chorda tympani contains two types of fibers:
  - For taste from the anterior 2/3 of the tongue and from the soft palate.
  - Preganglionic secretory and vasodilatory fibers, synapsing in the submandibular ganglion and supplying the submandibular, sublingual, and lingual glands.
  - The chorda tympani also communicates with the *otic ganglion.*
- Otic ganglion: Anastomosis with glossopharyngeal, facial, and auriculotemporal nerve. Frey syndrome appears with gustatory sweating [10] as a sign of misregeneration after surgical intervention (e.g., Parotid surgery).
- Artificial anastomosis for face reanimation: Hypoglossal-trigeminal-facial anastomoses [11]. Used in surgery to enable facial reanimation.

Combination with Other CN

Disorders of the base of skull and cavernous sinus.

Causes and Frequency

Compressive: Compressive lesions of the trigeminal nerve in the intracranial portion can be caused by vascular loops (posterior inferior cerebellar artery, superior cerebellar artery, arteriovenous malformation) and are considered to be a major cause of trigeminal neuralgia. Compressive lesions can occur in bone disease (Paget), local destruction base of the skull, and osteopetrosis.

Dental procedures: See iatrogenic.

Facial onset sensory and motor neuropathy (FOSMN): [12].

Genetic: [13].

Hypertrophic neuropathy: [14].

Iatrogenic: Pressure and compression of infra- and supraorbital nerves by oxygen masks during operations. Excessive pressure during operating procedures on the mandibular joint may affect the lingual nerve. The infraorbital nerve can also be damaged by maxillary surgery.

The lingual nerve can be affected by dental surgery (extraction of the second or third molars from the medial side or wisdom teeth).

Abscesses and osteosynthetic procedures of the mandibula can also damage the lingual nerve. Clinically, patients suffer from hypesthesia and hypalgesia of the tongue, floor of the mouth, and lingual gingiva. Patients have difficulties with eating, drinking, and taste perception.

Infections: Herpes zoster ophthalmicus may rarely be associated with corneal ulcer, iridocyclitis, retinal and arterial occlusions, optic nerve lesions, and oculomotor nerve lesions. Herpes zoster is usually located in V1 (Fig. 9.6); it is rarely in V3 [15] and even more rarely in V2 [16,

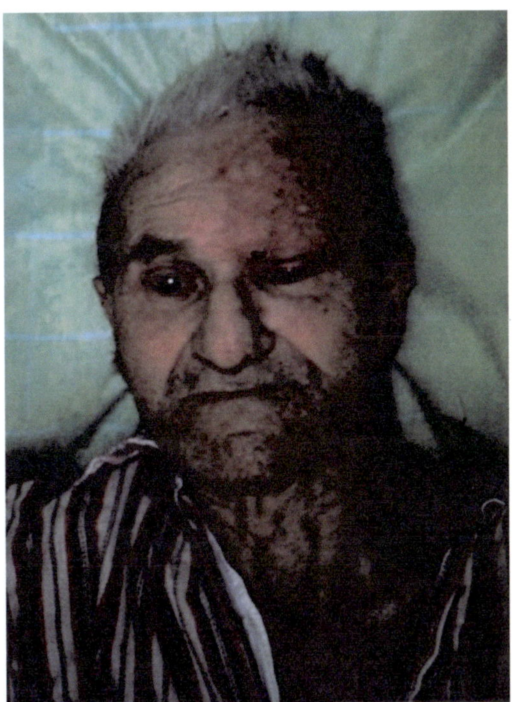

Fig. 9.6 Some features of trigeminal neuropathy. Left ophthalmic zoster

17]. The skin manifestations of *herpes zoster ophthalmicus* with involvement of one or more branches of the ophthalmic division of the trigeminal nerves, such as the supraorbital, lacrimal, and nasociliary branches, are characteristic. Involvement of the tip of the nose (Hutchinson's sign) indicates a lesion of the nasociliary branch and is a sign of ocular involvement [18, 19].

Trigeminal nerve enhancement in MR in listeriosis [20] and leprosy [21].

Adjacent infections of the sinus [22].

Inflammatory/immune mediated: Often abrupt onset, usually affecting one or two trigeminal branches unilaterally and frequently associated with pain. Etiologies: sensory trigeminal neuropathy, subacute sensory neuronopathy, sensory trigeminal neuropathy (connective tissue disease), Sjögren's syndrome [23, 24], scleroderma, systemic lupus erythematosus (SLE), and progressive sclerosis.

Masticatory muscles: Familial hypertrophy of masticatory muscles [25]. Hemifacial myohyperplasia [26]. Masseteric muscle calcification in ultrasound.

Motor trigeminal neuropathy: Pure motor trigeminal neuropathy [27, 28] (Fig. 9.7). Muscle

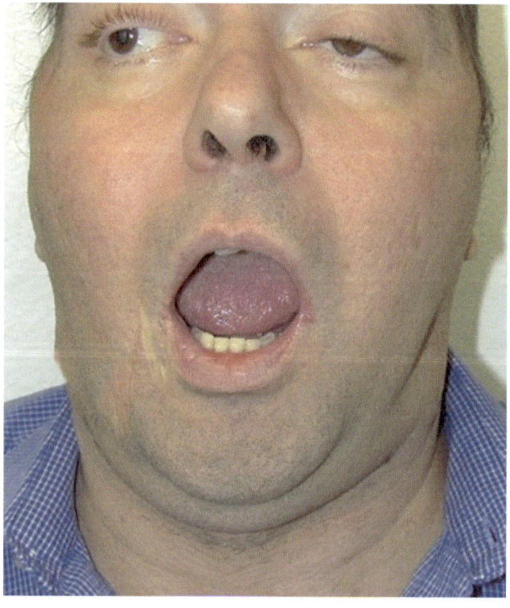

Fig. 9.7 Features of trigeminal neuropathy. Motor lesion of the right trigeminal nerve. The jaw deviates to the ipsilateral side upon opening the mouth

infiltration by chloroma [29]. Trismus following RT [30].

Neurofibromatosis: Bilateral involvement in NF [31, 32].

Neoplastic: Amyloidoma; Gasserian ganglion syndrome; cholesteatoma; chordoma; leptomeningeal carcinomatosis that may compress or invade the nerve or trigeminal ganglion, either intracranially or extracranially; metastasis to the base of the skull. Neurolymphomatosis and other tumors of the Gasserian ganglion. Infiltration of individual branches by tumors (Fig. 9.8).

Numb chin and cheek: "Numb chin syndrome" or mental neuropathy has been described as an idiopathic neuropathy or resulting from mandibular metastasis or focal nerve lesions. Numb chin syndrome can also occur due to metastasis, perineurial spread, mental nerve, odontogenic dental abscess, or amyloidosis [33].

"Numb cheek syndrome" involves a lesion of the infraorbital nerve.

Trauma: Lacerations, facial wounds and base of the skull fractures can damage the trigeminal nerve. Extensive sensory loss can interfere with communication and eating. Nerve branch lesions can result in neuralgia and hypersensitivity.

Tumors: Cerebellopontine angle tumors, chordoma, chondrosarcoma ependymoma, internal carotid artery aneurysm, perineural spread of metastasis, pituitary macroadenoma, skull base lesions such as vestibular schwannoma. Base of skull tumors [34] (Fig. 9.9). Amyloidoma [35].

Toxic: Trichloroethylene (trilene), solvents, pyridoxine toxicity, local injections: [36].

Radiation therapy: local RT, radiosurgery [37], thermal injury, post-RT trismus.

Trauma: Cranial fractures can cause local lesions of the supratrochlear, supraorbital, and infraorbital nerves (e.g., facial lacerations and orbital fractures). Trigeminal injury caused by fractures of the base of the skull is usually combined with injury of the abducens and facial nerves. Injury to the maxillary and ophthalmic divisions results in facial numbness, and involvement of the mandibular branch causes weakness of the mastication muscles.

Vascular: Medullary (brain stem) infarction may cause trigeminal sensory deficits in a char-

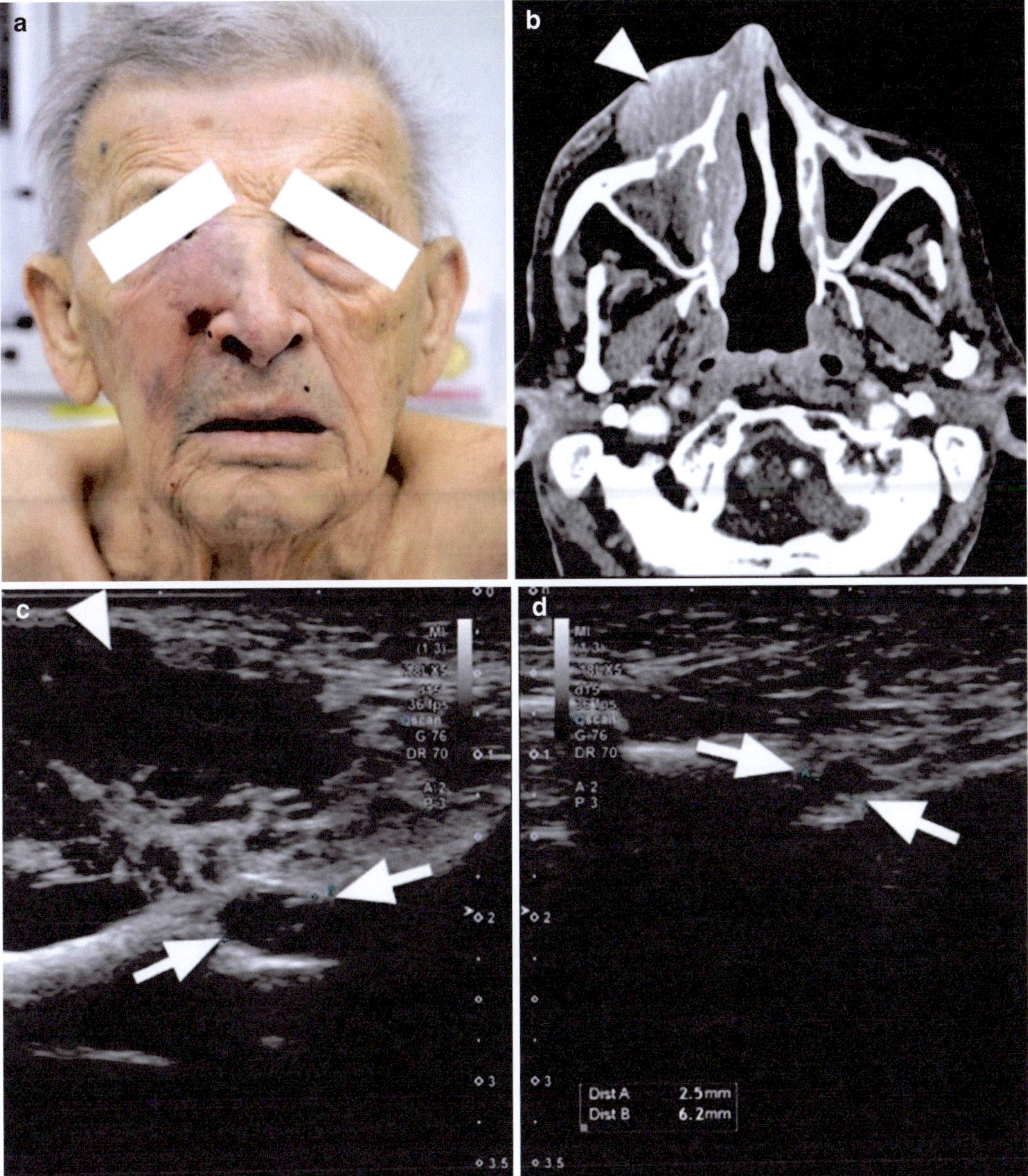

Fig. 9.8 Lymphoma infiltration in the infraorbital region affecting the infraorbital nerve. A 70-year-old patient with mantle cell lymphoma and chronic lymphocytic lymphoma: (**a**) pretherapeutic finding, (**b**) axial CT scan at the infraorbital level, (**c**) axial ultrasound scan at the infraor-bital level on the right side, and (**d**) axial ultrasound scan at the infraorbital level on the left side. *Arrowheads* = tumor mass (**b**, **c**), *arrows* = infraorbital nerve (**c**, **d**). Note the enlargement of the infraorbital foramen and increased size of the infraorbital nerve due to lymphoma infiltration

acteristic (e.g., "onion skin" pattern) and often involves pain usually not isolated but associated with long tract signs.

Aneurysm of the internal carotid artery can damage the cavernous sinus accompanied by concomitant headache, diplopia, and ptosis.

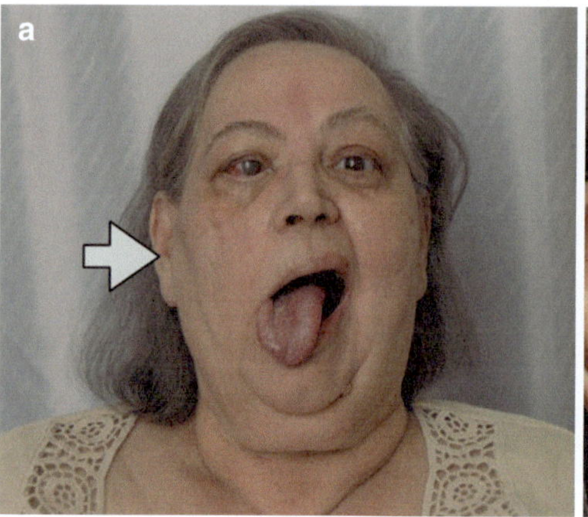
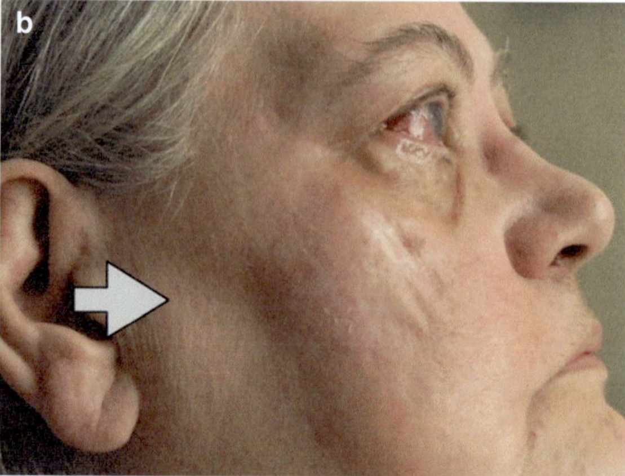

Fig. 9.9 Base of the skull metastasis with CN lesions and lesion of the trigeminal nerve. (**a**) Opening the mouth produces an ipsilateral deviation of the jaw. (**a, b**) *Arrows* points to atrophied masseteric muscle. In addition, CN VI, VII, and XII paresis also occurred due to the base of the skull metastasis

Pituitary apoplexy [38] is a rare occurrence.

Other Conditions:

Association of the trigeminal nerve with polyneuropathy, amyloidosis, diphtheria, leprosy, rheumatoid disease, syphilis, thallium neuropathies, and Waldenström's macroglobulinemia.

Sensory trigeminal neuropathy: Can occur idiopathically, in Sjögren's syndrome, and as part of paraneoplastic sensory neuronopathy [39, 40].

Cavernous sinus lesions: The ophthalmic nerve can be injured by all diseases of the cavernous sinus, such as local tumors, infections, and thrombosis. Neoplastic lesions can be caused by primary brain tumors, lymphoma, metastases, myeloma, sphenoid, and tumors of the nasopharynx. Typically, other CNs, particularly the oculomotor nerve, are also involved.

Gradenigo syndrome: Lesion of the apex of the pyramid (from middle ear infection) causes a combination of injury to CN V and VI and potentially VII.

Other conditions include Raeder's paratrigeminal syndrome, characterized by unilateral facial pain and sensory loss; Horner's syndrome; and oculomotor motility disturbances.

Trigeminal neuralgia (See also Chap. 33): Idiopathic trigeminal neuralgia has an incidence of 4 per 100,000. The average age of onset is 52–58 years. The neuralgia affects mostly the second and third divisions. Clinically, patients suffer from the typical "tic douloureux." Trigger mechanisms can vary but are often caused by specific movements, such as chewing, biting, or speaking. The neurologic examination is normal, and ancillary investigations show no specific changes. Vascular causes, like arterial loops in direct contact with the intracranial nerve roots, have been implicated as causal factors. Therapies include medication (anticonvulsants), decompression or lesion of the ganglion, vascular surgery in the posterior fossa, and medullary trigeminal tractotomy. Symptomatic trigeminal neuralgia may be caused by a structural lesion of the trigeminal nerve (Fig. 9.10) or ganglion and by surgical procedures, tumors of the cerebellopontine angle, meningitis, and MS. If the ophthalmic division is involved, causing neuroparalytic keratitis, hyperemia, ulcers, and perforation of the cornea occur.

Neuralgia: [41].

Facial pain syndromes: [42].

Neoplastic neuralgia: [43, 44].

Pain syndromes: see the trigeminocervical complex (TCC) [45].

Main Investigations

Imaging, MR, electrophysiology: blink reflex, EMG of motor portion, somatosensory evoked potential (SEP).

Neuroimaging is guided by the clinical symptoms and may include CT to detect bony changes

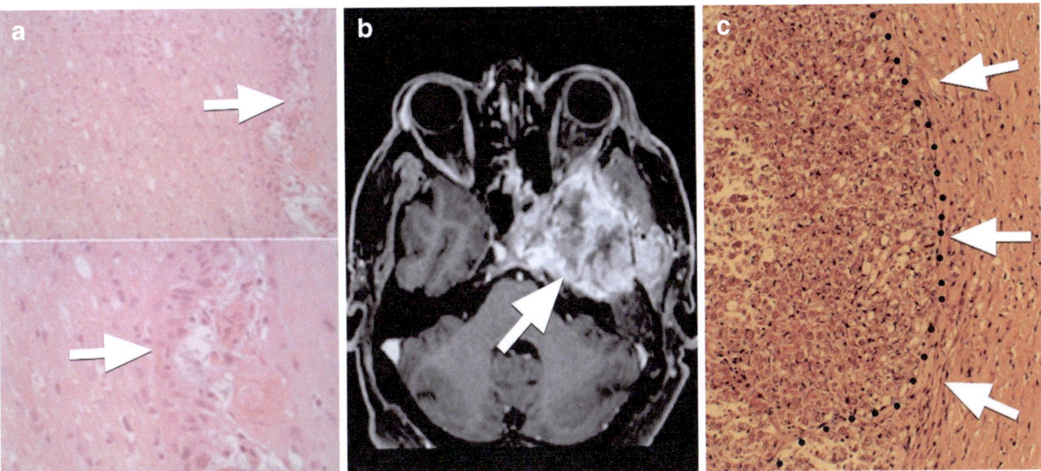

Fig. 9.10 (**a**) Invasion of the facial nerve via the skin and retrograde spread of the tumor (*arrows*). (**b**) Malignant glioma (arrow), with infiltration of the cavernous sinus. The patient experienced neuropathic trigeminal pain and ophthalmoplegia due to intrasinusoidal nerve infiltration. (**c**) Nerve infiltration of a CN by a glioma in the cavernous sinus: *dotted line,* circumference of the nerve; *arrows,* invasion

and MRI to investigate intracranial and extracranial tissue spaces [46].

Base of the skull: Imaging of denervated atrophic muscles is a useful indicator of motor trigeminal nerve lesions.

Neurophysiologic techniques rely on sensory conduction velocities and reflex studies (masseteric, blink reflex). Trigeminal SEP techniques can also be used. Motor impairment of the temporal and masseteric muscles can be confirmed by EMG.

Ultrasound of nerve and muscle can be used for the imaging of extracranial distribution and can also assess nerve continuity and thickening, muscle signs of denervation and atrophy, and distribution of muscle lesions.

Therapy

Treatment is dependent upon the underlying cause and symptoms. Neuralgias are usually treated with drugs and sometimes surgery or other interventions. Symptomatic care is required when protective reflexes, like the corneal reflex, are impaired and may lead to ulceration.

First-line treatment drugs are carbamazepine and oxcarbazepine. Other drugs, including gabapentin, pregabalin, lamotrigine and phenytoin, baclofen, and botulinum toxin type A, can be coadministered with carbamazepine or oxcarbazepine.

References

1. Curtis AR, Oaklander AL, Johnson A, Yosipovitch G. Trigeminal trophic syndrome from stroke: an under-recognized central neuropathic itch syndrome. Am J Clin Dermatol. 2012;13(2):125–8.
2. Margheim A, Spaulding R, Schadt CR. Trigeminal trophic syndrome: a cause of dysesthesia and persistent facial ulceration. Am J Med. 2020;133(6):685–6.
3. Nagel MA, Gilden D. The trigeminal trophic syndrome. Neurology. 2011;77(15):1499.
4. Walker HK, Dallas HW, Hurst JW, editors. Clinical methods: the history, physical, and laboratory examinations. 3rd ed; 1990. (https://www.ncbi.nlm.nih.gov/books/NBK384/)
5. Fitzek S, Baumgartner U, Fitzek C, Magerl W, Urban P, Thomke F, et al. Mechanisms and predictors of chronic facial pain in lateral medullary infarction. Ann Neurol. 2001;49(4):493–500.
6. Zeng F, Zhu M, Wan Q, Yan Y, Li C, Zhang Y. The treatment of V2+V3 idiopathic trigeminal neuralgia using peripheral nerve radiofrequency thermocoagulation via the foramen rotundum and foramen ovale compared with semilunar ganglion radiofrequency thermocoagulation. Clin Neurol Neurosurg. 2020;196:106025.

7. Martin-Duverneuil N, Sarrazin JL, Gayet-Delacroix M, Marsot-Dupuch K, Plantet MM. The foramen rotundum. Anatomy and radiological explorations. Pathology. J Neuroradiol. 2000;27(1):2–14.

8. Farran MZ, Kesserwani H. A case of Sjogren's syndrome associated with trigeminal neuropathy and enhancement of the mandibular nerve at the foramen Ovale: a case report and a review of the differential diagnosis and mechanisms of the disease. Cureus. 2021;13(11):e19463.

9. Hirota N, Fujimoto T, Takahashi M, Fukushima Y. Isolated trigeminal nerve metastases from breast cancer: an unusual cause of trigeminal mononeuropathy. Surg Neurol. 1998;49(5):558–61.

10. Drummond PD. Mechanism of gustatory flushing in Frey's syndrome. Clin Auton Res. 2002;12(3):144–6.

11. Jackler RK, Gralapp C. Hypoglossal-trigeminal-facial anastomoses 2019 [Available from: https://otosurgery-atlas.stanford.edu/otologic-surgery-atlas/facial-nerve/hypoglossal-trigeminal-facial-anastomoses/].

12. de Boer EMJ, Barritt AW, Elamin M, Anderson SJ, Broad R, Nisbet A, et al. Facial onset sensory and motor neuronopathy: new cases, cognitive changes, and pathophysiology. Neurol Clin Pract. 2021;11(2):147–57.

13. Butinar D, Zidar J, Leonardis L, Popovic M, Kalaydjieva L, Angelicheva D, et al. Hereditary auditory, vestibular, motor, and sensory neuropathy in a Slovenian Roma (gypsy) kindred. Ann Neurol. 1999;46(1):36–44.

14. Duvall ER, Pan J, Dinh KTT, Al Shaarani M, Pan G, Langford MP, et al. Trigeminal hypertrophic interstitial neuropathy presenting as unilateral proptosis, ptosis, tearing, and facial neuralgia. Am J Ophthalmol Case Rep. 2018;12:83–6.

15. Keskinruzgar A, Demirkol M, Ege B, Aras MH, Ay S. Rare involvement of herpes zoster in the mandibular branch of the trigeminal nerve: a case report and review of the literature. Quintessence Int. 2015;46(2):163–70.

16. Paquin R, Susin LF, Welch G, Barnes JB, Stevens MR, Tay FR. Herpes zoster involving the second division of the trigeminal nerve: case report and literature review. J Endod. 2017;43(9):1569–73.

17. Thada SR, Gadda R, Pai K. Nerve afflictions of maxillofacial region: a report of two cases. BMJ Case Rep. 2013;2013:bcr2013201002.

18. Zaal MJ, Volker-Dieben HJ, D'Amaro J. Prognostic value of Hutchinson's sign in acute herpes zoster ophthalmicus. Graefes Arch Clin Exp Ophthalmol. 2003;241(3):187–91.

19. Amano E, Machida A. Teaching NeuroImages: Hutchinson sign in herpes zoster Ophthalmicus. Neurology. 2021;96(15):e2033–4.

20. Karlsson WK, Harboe ZB, Roed C, Monrad JB, Lindelof M, Larsen VA, et al. Early trigeminal nerve involvement in listeria monocytogenes rhombencephalitis: case series and systematic review. J Neurol. 2017;264(9):1875–84.

21. Reichart PA, Srisuwan S, Metah D. Lesions of the facial and trigeminal nerve in leprosy. An evaluation of 43 cases. Int J Oral Surg. 1982;11(1):14–20.

22. Tewari S, Vashishth A. Painful trigeminal neuropathy in patients with invasive fungal sinusitis post COVID-19 infection. Pain Pract. 2022;22(2):295.

23. Kaltreider HB, Talal N. The neuropathy of Sjogren's syndrome. Trigeminal nerve involvement. Ann Intern Med. 1969;70(4):751–62.

24. Ozasa K, Noma N, Nakata J, Imamura Y. Unilateral trigeminal sensory neuropathy with Sjogren's syndrome with liver and renal impairment. Neurol Int. 2021;13(3):464–8.

25. Martinelli P, Fabbri R, Gabellini AS, Mazzini G, Rasi F. Familial hypertrophy of masticatory muscles. J Neurol. 1987;234(4):251–3.

26. Urban PP, Bruening R. Congenital isolated hemifacial hyperplasia. J Neurol. 2009;256(9):1566–9.

27. Kang YK, Lee EH, Hwang M. Pure trigeminal motor neuropathy: a case report. Arch Phys Med Rehabil. 2000;81(7):995–8.

28. Park KS, Chung JM, Jeon BS, Park SH, Lee KW. Unilateral trigeminal mandibular motor neuropathy caused by tumor in the foramen ovale. J Clin Neurol. 2006;2(3):194–7.

29. Bassichis B, McClay J, Wiatrak B. Chloroma of the masseteric muscle. Int J Pediatr Otorhinolaryngol. 2000;53(1):57–61.

30. Strojan P, Hutcheson KA, Eisbruch A, Beitler JJ, Langendijk JA, Lee AWM, et al. Treatment of late sequelae after radiotherapy for head and neck cancer. Cancer Treat Rev. 2017;59:79–92.

31. Nager GT. Neurinomas of the trigeminal nerve. Am J Otolaryngol. 1984;5(5):301–33.

32. Kchouk M, Aouidj L, Gouider R, Oueslati S, Touibi S, Khaldi M. Neurinomas of the trigeminal nerve in neurofibromatosis. Apropos of two cases and review of the literature. Ann Radiol (Paris). 1992;35(7–8):533–7.

33. Rabadi MH. Progressive lip numbness due to numb chin and cheek syndrome in a patient with prostate cancer. Radiol Case Rep. 2020;15(10):1996–8.

34. Greenberg HSDM, Vikram B. Metastasis to the base of the skull: clinical findings in 43 patients. Neurology. 1981;31(5):530–7.

35. Love S, Bateman DE, Hirschowitz L. Bilateral lambda light chain amyloidomas of the trigeminal ganglia, nerves and roots. Neuropathol Appl Neurobiol. 1997;23(6):512–5.

36. Hillerup S, Jensen RH, Ersboll BK. Trigeminal nerve injury associated with injection of local anesthetics: needle lesion or neurotoxicity? J Am Dent Assoc. 2011;142(5):531–9.

37. Al-Otaibi F, Alhindi H, Alhebshi A, Albloushi M, Baeesa S, Hodaie M. Histopathological effects of radiosurgery on a human trigeminal nerve. Surg Neurol Int. 2013;4(Suppl. 6):S462–7.

38. Salehi N, Firek A, Munir I. Pituitary apoplexy presenting as ophthalmoplegia and altered level of consciousness without headache. Case Rep Endocrinol. 2018;2018:7124364.

39. Misko AL, Batra A, Faquin WC, Cohen AB. An isolated trigeminal sensory neuropathy. Neurohospitalist. 2018;8(3):152–5.

40. Hagen NA, Stevens JC, Michet CJ Jr. Trigeminal sensory neuropathy associated with connective tissue diseases. Neurology. 1990;40(6):891–6.

41. Jones MR, Urits I, Ehrhardt KP, Cefalu JN, Kendrick JB, Park DJ, et al. A comprehensive review of trigeminal neuralgia. Curr Pain Headache Rep. 2019;23(10):74.

42. Aguggia M. Typical facial neuralgias. Neurol Sci. 2005;26(Suppl. 2):s68–70.

43. Berra LV, Armocida D, Mastino L, Rita AD, Norcia VD, Santoro A, et al. Trigeminal neuralgia secondary to intracranial neoplastic lesions: a case series and comprehensive review. J Neurol Surg A Cent Eur Neurosurg. 2021;82(2):118–24.

44. Chong VF. Trigeminal neuralgia in nasopharyngeal carcinoma. J Laryngol Otol. 1996;110(4):394–6.

45. Edvinsson JCA, Vigano A, Alekseeva A, Alieva E, Arruda R, De Luca C, et al. The fifth cranial nerve in headaches. J Headache Pain. 2020;21(1):65.

46. Gunes A, Bulut E, Akgoz A, Mocan B, Gocmen R, Oguz KK. Trigeminal nerve and pathologies in magnetic resonance imaging - a pictorial review. Pol J Radiol. 2018;83:e289–e96.

One sentence: The abducens or abducent nerve is CN VI and provides the motor innervation of the lateral rectus muscle.

Genetic testing	NCV/ EMG	Laboratory	Imaging	Biopsy	CSF
	0	+	+		+

Symptoms

A lesion results in diplopia in the horizontal gaze, looking in the direction of the paretic muscle, which is worse with distant objects. Rotation of the head toward the side of the unaffected muscle relieves the diplopia.

Signs

An isolated paralysis of the lateral rectus muscle causes the affected eye to be adducted at rest and results in a failure of eye abduction in the horizontal plane. Esotropia of the affected eye occurs due to unopposed action of the medial rectus muscle.

Specific Qualities

Motor: +.

Part of coordination of eye movements – abduction of the eye. In animals: includes "bulbus retractor "and" nictitating response"; rarely in humans [1].
Sensory:
Autonomic:
Special senses:
Other:

Location of Lesions

General summary: [2] (Fig. 10.1 and Table 10.1).

Central: Nuclear lesions: Can be caused by vascular events and appear rarely in isolation (associated with long tract signs or concomitant CN VII lesions).

Vascular brain stem lesions: Foville, Millard Gubler, Raymond syndromes [3], and "one and a half" syndrome as a mimic.

Internuclear ophthalmoplegia (INO) may be mistaken for abducens nerve weakness.

Genetic causes are rare and appear as Moebius and Duane's syndrome.

Intracranial Within the Skull: The long intracavitary pathway includes fixations and angulations. Knowledge of the relations of the nerve and the surrounding structures is important [4].

Lesions at the petrous apex and Dorello's canal [5]: Caused by mastoid infection, raised intracranial pressure (ICP), skull fracture, and local tumors, *e.g.*, trigeminal schwannoma.

Subarachnoid space lesions: Basilar aneurysm, cavernous sinus disorders, clivus tumor

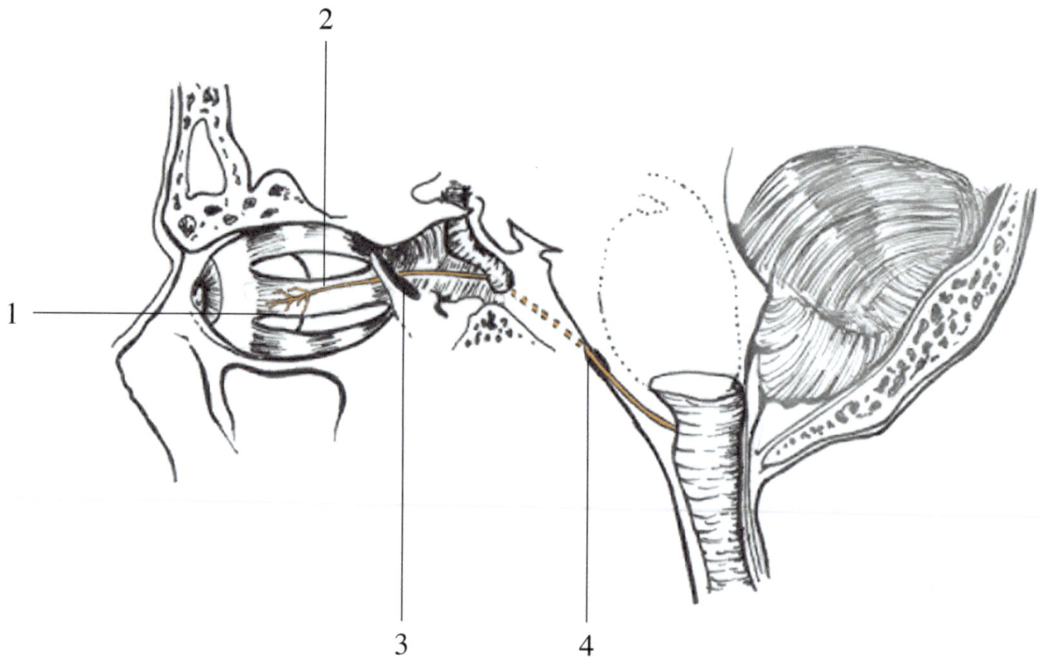

Fig. 10.1 Abducens nerve. (*1*) lateral rectus muscle, (*2*) abducens nerve, (*3*) superior orbital fissure, (*4*) Dorello's canal

Table 10.1 The site of CN VI lesions

Brain parenchyma	Intracranial and arachnoid space	Cranial vault exit	Extracranial lesion
Nucleus: pons, vicinity to VII fibers	Dorello's canal Clivus pressure Petrous apex	Superior orbital fissure	Orbit
Brain stem syndromes	Cavernous sinus Meningeal Carcinomatosis Aneurysms Rare: nerve tumors		

(chordoma, meningioma, metastasis), hemorrhage, leptomeningeal carcinomatosis, meningitis, trauma.

Uncertain location: Microvascular infarction, migraine.

In the cavernous sinus, the position of the nerve is between CN IV and V1 [6], which is important for surgical interventions. An isolated abducens nerve palsy at this site is unlikely.

Rare event as a cause: Cavernous sinus apoplexy [6–8].

Exit of the Skull: CN III, IV, and VI pass through the fissura orbitalis superior (superior orbital fissure). Local neoplastic lesions, aneu-rysms, or thrombosis of the carotid artery and trauma are causes, as well as inflammation and granulomatous inflammatory processes. Example: Tolosa Hunt syndrome [9].

Within the orbit: See anatomy of the orbit: [10]. The nerve travels through the annulus of Zinn to reach the lateral rectus muscle. An isolated CN VI paresis/palsy in the orbit is unlikely. Other local conditions that can cause an abduction paralysis are thyroid orbitopathy, local tumors, and rarely metastasis and orbital myositis [11].

Trauma: An abduction deficit can be produced by orbital disease, such as a blowout fracture.

Neuromuscular transmission disorders, such as MG, can cause lateral rectus paresis but are often combined with other cranial nerve dysfunctions, such as ptosis. The fluctuations are characteristic.

Combination with Other CN

Lateral rectus paralysis is the most frequently encountered paralysis of an extraocular muscle. Eighty percent of cases exhibit isolated paralysis of the lateral rectus, while 20% of cases are in association with lesions of other nerves serving the extraocular muscles (CN III or IV).

Causes and Frequency: (Table 10.2)

The most frequent causes are trauma, vascular causes, and diabetes. In pediatric cases, the most frequent causes are neoplasm (39%), trauma (20%), and inflammation (18%). Bilateral VI palsy causes include GBS, meningitis, pontine glioma, trauma, and Wernicke's encephalopathy. See table and series: [3].

Compressive: CN VI palsy is a common sign of increased cranial pressure caused by granuloma [12], hydrocephalus, pseudotumor cerebri, tumors, and lesions of the cavernous sinus (*e.g.*, thrombosis).

Congenital: Duane's syndrome.

IdiopathicInfections: Cytomegalovirus encephalitis, cryptococcal and other meningitis, cysticercosis, HIV, Lyme disease, syphilis, tuberculosis, ventriculitis of the IV ventricle [13], Covid-19 [14], Gradenigo's syndrome, herpes zoster [15].

Inflammatory/immune-mediated: Giant cell arteritis, sarcoidosis, systemic lupus erythematosus, vasculitis, Tolosa Hunt syndrome.

Table 10.2 Neurological conditions associated with CN VI

Associated condition	Comments
The brain stem syndrome	Does not occur isolated; other brain stem and long tract signs are associated
Elevated intracranial pressure syndrome	Brain edema and in pseudotumor cerebri
Petrous apex syndrome	Ipsilateral decreased hearing Ipsilateral facial pain in distribution of CN V and ipsilateral facial paralysis
Cavernous sinus syndrome	Distinct association with other CN lesions (III, IV, V). Often pain and additional signs
Orbital syndrome	Orbital swelling, chemosis, proptosis

Intracranial pressure: Either elevated or reduced.

Metabolic diseases: Rarely diabetes, endocrine (thyroid).

Microvascular/ischemic: [16, 17].

Migraine: Transient [18].

Myopathy: [19].

Neoplastic: Primary nerve tumor (*e.g.*, schwannoma), cerebellopontine angle tumor, clivus tumor, pontine glioma, leukemia, meningioma (Fig. 10.2), metastatic tumors, leptomeningeal carcinomatosis, myeloma [20].

Toxic: Vincristine therapy [21], pembrolizumab [22], immune checkpoint inhibitors, glufosinate herbicide [23].

Trauma: Fractures of the base of the skull [5, 24]. Bilateral lesions also occur (Fig. 10.3).

Vaccination: Recurrent sixth nerve palsy following measles mumps rubella vaccination [25–27].

Vascular: Aneurysms of the posterior inferior cerebelli or basilar or internal carotid arteries.

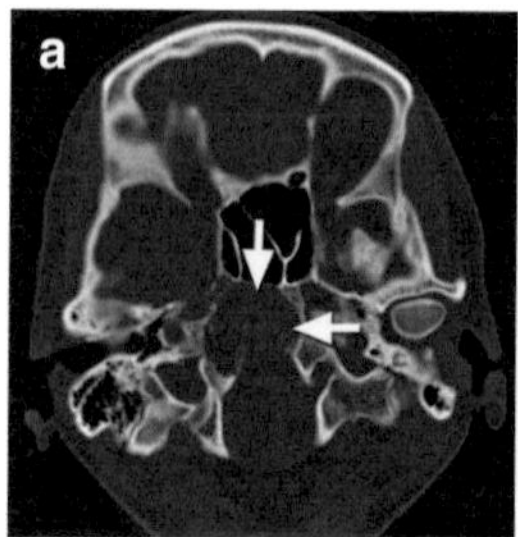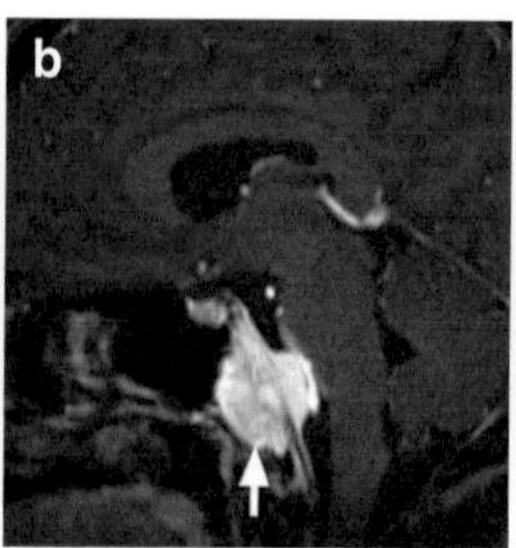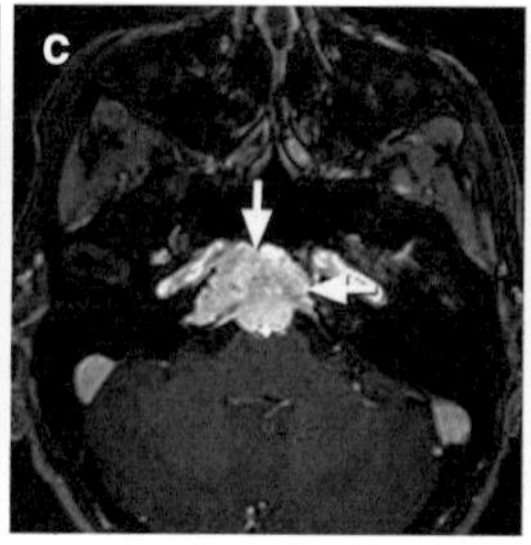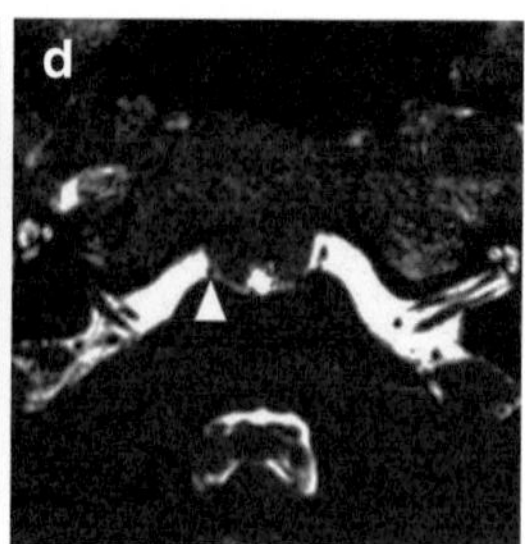

Fig. 10.2 (**a**) Axial CT, (**b**) sagittal, and (**c**) axial T1-weighted sequences after contrast agent injection, and (**d**) axial gradient echo sequence. Contrast-enhancing mass (arrow, **b** and **c**) of the clivus with intraosseous destruction and contacting the right abducens nerve (arrowhead, **d**). Histology revealed a meningioma

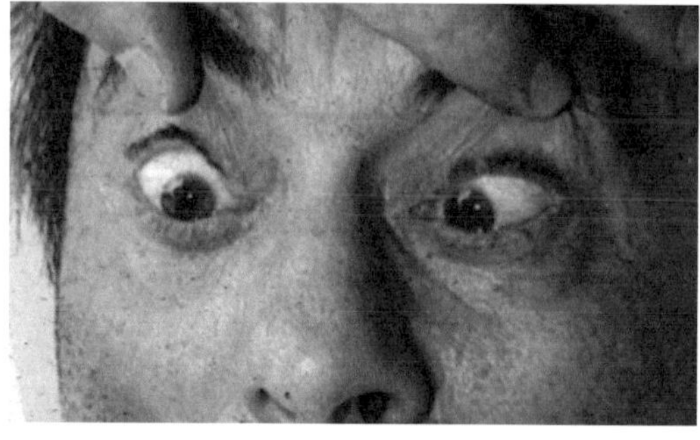

Fig. 10.3 Bilateral abducens nerve paresis. Inward gaze of both bulbi. This patient suffered a fall from a bicycle with a subsequent head trauma

Combination with Other CN

Meningitis, neoplastic meningitis, cavernous sinus lesions, orbital tumors.

Main Investigations [16]

Brain and orbital MRI.

Lee screen.

Assessing the patient's metabolic situation, imaging for tumors or vascular conditions, CSF for signs of infection.

Differential diagnosis: Convergence spasm, Duane's retraction syndrome, internuclear ophthalmoplegia, myasthenia gravis, pseudo-CN VI nerve palsy (lesion in the thalamic and subthalamic region) [28], thyroid disease.

Therapy

Treatment is dependent upon the underlying cause.

Prognosis: The most frequent "idiopathic" type in adults usually remits within 4–12 weeks.

References

1. Heralgi M, Thallangady A, Venkatachalam K, Vokuda H. Persistent unilateral nictitating membrane in a 9-year-old girl: a rare case report. Indian J Ophthalmol. 2017;65(3):253–5.
2. Rucker CW. The causes of paralysis of the third, fourth and sixth cranial nerves. Am J Ophthalmol. 1966;61(5 Pt 2):1293–8.
3. Azarmina M, Azarmina H. The six syndromes of the sixth cranial nerve. J Ophthalmic Vis Res. 2013;8(2):160–71.
4. Joo W, Yoshioka F, Funaki T, Rhoton AL Jr. Microsurgical anatomy of the abducens nerve. Clin Anat. 2012;25(8):1030–42.
5. Tubbs RS, Radcliff V, Shoja MM, Naftel RP, Mortazavi MM, Zurada A, et al. Dorello canal revisited: an observation that potentially explains the frequency of abducens nerve injury after head injury. World Neurosurg. 2012;77(1):119–21.
6. Kirici Y, Kilic C, Kocaoglu M. Location of the abducent nerve within the cavernous sinus. Turk Neurosurg. 2011;21(4):545–8.
7. Zoli M, Mazzatenta D, Pasquini E, Ambrosetto P, Frank G. Cavernous sinus apoplexy presenting isolated sixth cranial nerve palsy: case report. Pituitary. 2012;15(Suppl. 1):S37–40.
8. Kayayurt K, Gundogdu OL, Yavasi O, Metin Y, Ugras E. Isolated abducens nerve palsy due to pituitary apoplexy after mild head trauma. Am J Emerg Med. 2015;33(10):1539-e3.

9. Siddhanta KC, Shreeyanta KC, Kunwar P, Dhungana K. Tolosa-hunt syndrome: a case report. JNMA J Nepal Med Assoc. 2021;59(238):604–7.

10. Lieber S, Fernandez-Miranda JC. Anatomy of the orbit. J Neurol Surg B Skull Base. 2020;81(4):319–32.

11. Wazir M, FaisalUddin M, Tambunan D, Jain AG. Idiopathic lateral rectus myositis without signs of orbital inflammation VI. Cureus. 2019;11(6):e4859.

12. Roemer S, Maeder P, Daniel RT, Kawasaki A. Sixth nerve palsy from cholesterol granuloma of the petrous apex. Front Neurol. 2017;8:48.

13. Knoflach K, Holzapfel E, Roser T, Rudolph L, Paolini M, Muenchhoff M, et al. Case report: unilateral sixth cranial nerve palsy associated with COVID-19 in a 2-year-old child. Front Pediatr. 2021;9:756014.

14. Pereira A, Haslett RS. Acute abducens nerve palsy following the second dose of the AstraZeneca COVID-19 vaccine. J Pediatr Ophthalmol Strabismus. 2021;58(6):e49–50.

15. Hermann JS. Isolated abducens paresis complicating herpes zoster ophthalmicus. Am J Ophthalmol. 1962;54:298–301.

16. Elder C, Hainline C, Galetta SL, Balcer LJ, Rucker JC. Isolated abducens nerve palsy: update on evaluation and diagnosis. Curr Neurol Neurosci Rep. 2016;16(8):69.

17. Wilker SC, Rucker JC, Newman NJ, Biousse V, Tomsak RL. Pain in ischaemic ocular motor cranial nerve palsies. Br J Ophthalmol. 2009;93(12):1657–9.

18. Vasconcelos LP, Stancioli FG, Leal JC, da Silva A, Gomez RS, Teixeira AL. Ophthalmoplegic migraine: a case with recurrent palsy of the abducens nerve. Headache. 2008;48(6):961–4.

19. Wazir M, FaisalUddin M, Tambunan D, Jain AG. Idiopathic lateral rectus myositis without signs of orbital inflammation. Cureus. 2019;11(6):e4859.

20. Ibekwe E, Horsley NB, Jiang L, Achenjang NS, Anudu A, Akhtar Z, et al. Abducens nerve palsy as initial presentation of multiple myeloma and intracranial plasmacytoma. J Clin Med. 2018;7(9):253. https://doi.org/10.3390/jcm7090253.

21. Dixit G, Dhingra A, Kaushal D. Vincristine induced cranial neuropathy. J Assoc Phys India. 2012;60:56–8.

22. Jaben KA, Francis JH, Shoushtari AN, Abramson DH. Isolated abducens nerve palsy following pembrolizumab. Neuroophthalmology. 2020;44(3):182–5.

23. Park JS, Kwak SJ, Gil HW, Kim SY, Hong SY. Glufosinate herbicide intoxication causing unconsciousness, convulsion, and 6th cranial nerve palsy. J Korean Med Sci. 2013;28(11):1687–9.

24. Sam B, Ozveren MF, Akdemir I, Topsakal C, Cobanoglu B, Baydar CL, et al. The mechanism of injury of the abducens nerve in severe head trauma: a postmortem study. Forensic Sci Int. 2004;140(1):25–32.

25. Ng XL, Betzler BK, Testi I, Ho SL, Tien M, Ngo WK, et al. Ocular adverse events after COVID-19 vaccination. Ocul Immunol Inflamm. 2021;29(6):1216–24.

26. McCormick A, Dinakaran S, Bhola R, Rennie IG. Recurrent sixth nerve palsy following measles mumps rubella vaccination. Eye (Lond). 2001;15(Pt 3):356–7.

27. Bourtoulamaiou A, Yadav S, Nayak H. Benign recurrent sixth (abducens) nerve palsy following measles-mumps-rubella vaccination. Case Rep Pediatr. 2015;2015:734516.

28. Reid MS, DePoe SA, Darner RL, Reid JP, Slagle WS. Clinical presentation of pseudo-abducens palsy. Optom Vis Sci. 2015;92(4 Suppl. 1):S76–80.

One sentence: Predominate motor nerve for facial innervation with autonomic, sensory, and special senses functions.

Genetic testing	NCV/ EMG	Laboratory	Imaging	Clinical exam
	+	+	+	+

Major branches from the facial nerve (Fig. 11.1) include the chorda tympani for taste, the greater petrosal nerve for salivation and lacrimation, motor branches, and the nerve to the stapedius muscle. There is also sensory innervation of the pinna of the ear and external acoustic meatus by the auricular nerve, which occurs jointly with the vagus nerve.

The chorda tympani nerve exits the skull through the petrotympanic fissure, merges with the lingual nerve, and then synapses with neurons in the submandibular ganglion. These postganglionic neurons provide parasympathetic innervation to the submandibular and sublingual glands.

The nervus intermedius (or nerve of Wrisberg or glossopalatine nerve) is part of the facial nerve (CN VII) and is located between the motor component of the facial nerve and the vestibulocochlear nerve (CN VIII). The nerve contains sensory and parasympathetic fibers of the facial nerve [1].

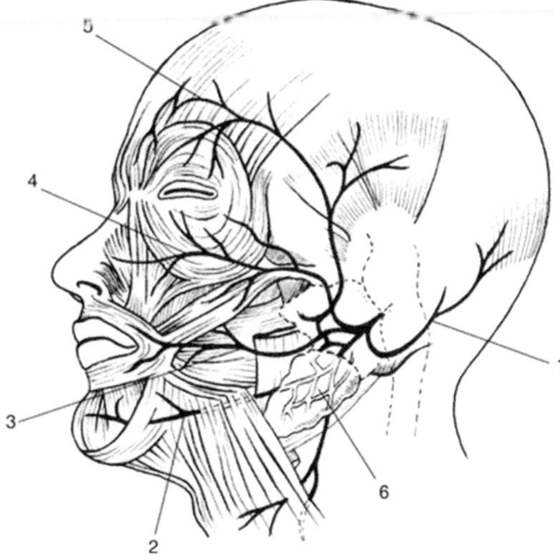

Fig. 11.1 Facial nerve: (*1*) posterior auricular nerve, (*2*) mandibular branch, (*3*) buccal branch, (*4*) zygomatic branch, (*5*) temporal branch, (*6*) parotid gland

Symptoms

Lesion of the facial nerve result predominantly in loss of motor function often characterized by acute onset of facial paresis, sometimes associated with pain and/or numbness around the ear. Loss of visceral functions results in

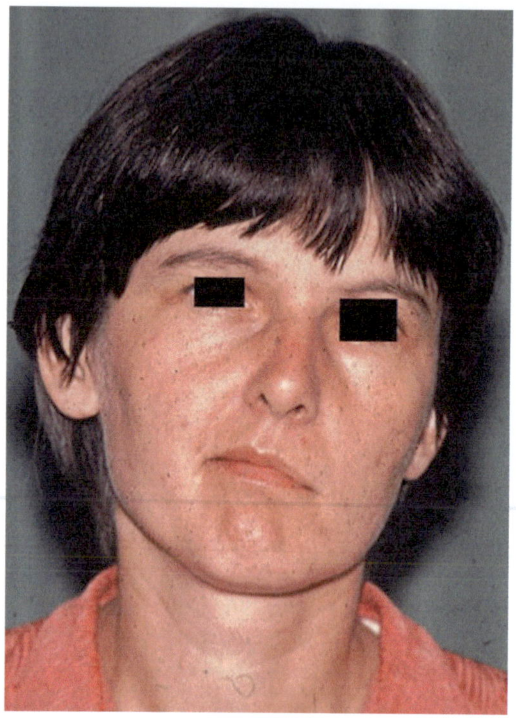

Fig. 11.2 Facial nerve palsy. This patient suffered from a left-sided Bell's palsy; note the deviation of facial muscles

loss of tearing or submandibular salivary flow (10% of cases), loss of taste (25%), and hyperacusis (although patients rarely complain of this).

Lesions of CN VII are significant for the individual in regard to eye protection, eating, drinking, and communication, speech, and emotional displays (Fig. 11.2).

Facial weakness occurs in muscle disease: Myopathic face (facies myopathica) occurs in several conditions (see Chap. 24).

Geniculate neuralgia is rare [2] (see Chap. 34).

Signs

Central Lesions

Supranuclear: As the facial motor nuclei receive cortical input concerning the upper facial muscles bilaterally but the lower face muscles unilaterally, a supranuclear lesion often results in paresis of a single lower quadrant of the face (contralateral to the lesion) [3].

Pyramidal facial weakness: Lower face paresis with voluntary motion.

Emotional: Facial paralysis with emotion (dorsolateral pons – anterior cerebellar artery).

Peripheral lesions: Mimic and voluntary movements of the facial muscles are impaired or absent. Drooping of the corner of the mouth, lagophthalmos. Patients are unable to whistle, frown, or show their teeth. Motor function is assessed by the symmetry and degree of various facial movements.

Partial peripheral lesion: Symptoms and signs depend upon the site of the lesion. Perifacial nerve branches can be damaged with trauma and surgical or neurosurgical procedures. Parotid surgery may damage one or several branches, and a paresis of the caudal perioral muscle can be seen in carotid surgery. Retrograde tumor nerve infiltration in parotid and skin tumors of the face can occur.

Specific Qualities

Motor: +.

Branchial motor innervation of facial muscles, stapedius, stylohyoid, and posterior belly of digastric muscle and platysma (Fig. 11.3).

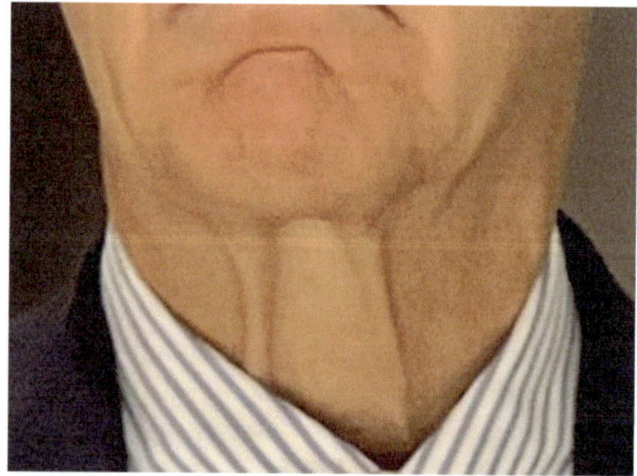

Fig. 11.3 Platysma. Innervation by the facial nerve and also the cervical plexus

Sensory: +.

External auditory meatus, auricle, and small retroauricular area.

Autonomic: +.

Visceral parasympathetic: Via greater superficial petrosal nerve (GSPN) – lacrimal gland, oral and nasal mucosa (GSPN), and submandibular and sublingual glands (via chorda tympani).

Special senses: +.

Anterior 2/3 of the tongue – taste, hard and soft palate (via chorda tympani).

Other:

Location of Lesions

See Table 11.1 for common sites of CN VII lesions.

Central Lesions:

Nuclear and brain stem: Pontine vascular lesions, e.g., Foville and Millard-Gubler syndrome.In vascular brain stem lesions, adjacent structures are affected causing additional lesion of CN as CN VI, impairment of conjugate ocular movements, hemiparesis, or long tract signs and Horner's syndrome.

Other causes include infection (*e.g.*, brain stem abscess), inflammatory disease (*e.g.*, multiple sclerosis), Moebius syndrome (congenital), and neoplastic causes (metastasis or brain stem glioma).

Intracranial lesions: Cerebellopontine angle tumors, infections, neoplastic lesions.

Peripheral Lesions:

Can be divided into complete or partial lesions:

Complete lesions:

Mimic and voluntary movements of the facial muscles are impaired or absent. Drooping of the corner of the mouth and lagophthalmos. Patients are unable to whistle, frown, or show their teeth. With paralysis of the posterior belly of the digastric muscle, the jaw is deviated to the healthy side. With pterygoid muscle paralysis, the opposite is true. The platysma sign appears in central hemiparesis and spinal lesions [4].

Partial lesions: Depending on the site of the lesions.

Numerous anastomoses exist with the cervical plexus/nerves [5].

Lesions Within the Temporal Bone:

Internal auditory meatus: Geniculate ganglion lesions cause reduced salivation and lacrimation. Loss of taste in the anterior 2/3 of tongue. Hyperacusis is rarely noted.

Between internal auditory meatus and stapedius nerve: Facial paralysis without impairment of lacrimation; however, loss of salivation, taste, and hyperacusis.

Between stapedius nerve and chorda tympani: Facial paralysis, intact lacrimation, reduced salivation, and taste. No hyperacusis.

Distal to the chorda tympani: Facial paralysis, no impairment of salivation, lacrimation, or hyperacusis.

Lesions After Exit From the Stylomastoid Foramen:

Facial nerve branches can be damaged with neurosurgical procedures. Parotid surgery may damage one or several branches, and paresis of the caudal perioral muscle can be seen in carotid surgery.

Table 11.1 Site of lesions

Brain parenchyma	Intracranial and CSF space	Exit of the cranial vault	Extracranial lesion	Multiple CN lesions
Central paresis: hemisphere Brain stem: pons (nuclear and fascicular)	Cerebellopontine angle, meninges Base of skull tumors	Facial canal Several possibilities	Parotid gland Each branch can be damaged by trauma or neoplastic process retrograde infiltration	Meningeal carcinomatosis Meningitis: granulomatous process and inflammation

Tumors: Retrograde nerve infiltration in parotid and skin tumors of the face occur rarely [6].

Muscle disease: Myopathic face (facies myopathica) occurs in several conditions (see Chap. 24).

Combination with Other CN

Cerebellopontine angle tumors (CPA) tumors, leptomeningeal carcinomatosis (LC), infections.

Causes and Frequency

Bell's palsy (idiopathic): Most frequent cause [7–10]. The prevalence is 6–7/100,000 to 23/100,000, increasing with age. Paralysis progresses within 3 h to 72 h. About half of patients have pain in the mastoid or ear, and some (30%) have excess tearing and dysgeusia. Facial weakness is complete in 70% of cases. Stapedius dysfunction occurs in 30% of cases, resulting in hyperacusis. Mild lacrimation and taste problems are rare. Some patients complain of ill-defined sensory symptoms in the trigeminal distribution. Improvement occurs in 4–6 weeks in about 80% of cases. Symptoms may persist and contractures or synkineses may develop. The pathogenesis of Bell's palsy is not clear but may be viral or inflammatory. Associated diseases include diabetes and hypertension [11]. Corticosteroids are effective in Bell's palsy.

Late effects of facial nerve palsy: Synkinesis and residual weakness can be important sequelae [12]. Regeneration can result in involuntary movements and similar conditions, such as blepharospasm, contracture (postparalytic facial dysfunction), facial myokymia, hemifacial spasm, synkinesis and ticks, and crocodile tears. Late effects may be lower with a combination of corticosteroids and antivirals [13].

Permanent loss of taste is rare [7].

Congenital malformation: Arnold Chiari syndrome, Goldenhar syndrome, Möbius syndrome, and syringobulbia.

Genetic conditions: Amyloid (Gelsolin type, Tangier's disease), hereditary myopathies, 3q21–22 and 10q21.3–22.1 mutations.

Granulomatous disease: Sarcoid, Heerfordt syndrome.

Hypertrophic neuropathy of the facial nerve: [14].

Iatrogenic: Oxygen mask used in anesthesia (mandibular branch).

Idiopathic:

Infection: Adenovirus, botulism, CMV, Epstein-Barr virus, haemophilus, HIV, influenzae, mumps, mycoplasma pneumoniae, parotid abscess [15], poliomyelitis, rubella, syphilis, tetanus, tuberculosis.

Leprosy: Zygomatic nerve most frequently affected [16].

Lyme disease: Up to 10% of facial paralyses in endemic areas; often bilateral VII [17, 18].

Combination with other CN in herpes zoster [19].

Ramsay Hunt syndrome (RHS) (Fig. 11.4): Viral, herpes zoster geniculate ganglionitis, caused by reactivation of herpes zoster in the geniculate ganglion. Clinically, a peripheral facial nerve palsy with painful red rash and with fluid-filled blisters in and around one ear. In any peripheral facial nerve paralysis, the inspection of the ear and external acoustic meatus is mandatory. The geniculate ganglion also receives innervation from the glossopharyngeal nerve (CN IX). A prodromal period of otalgia and vesicular eruptions within the external auditory canal as well as the soft palate can appear. Antiviral treatment is warranted.

Bacterial: Acute otitis media can cause dehiscence within the facial canal resulting in nerve paralysis. Additionally, cholesteatomas and necrotizing otitis externa can cause facial nerve palsies.

Neonatal: Abnormal post-birth trauma: Cardiofacial syndrome, congenital dysfunction, hemifacial microsomia, prenatal face compression against mother's sacrum, childbirth forceps, and vaginal births [20].

Neoplastic: Acoustic neurinoma, schwannoma (Figs. 11.5 and 11.6), base of the skull tumors (cholesteatoma dermoids), large meningiomas, parotid tumors, cerebellopontine tumors,

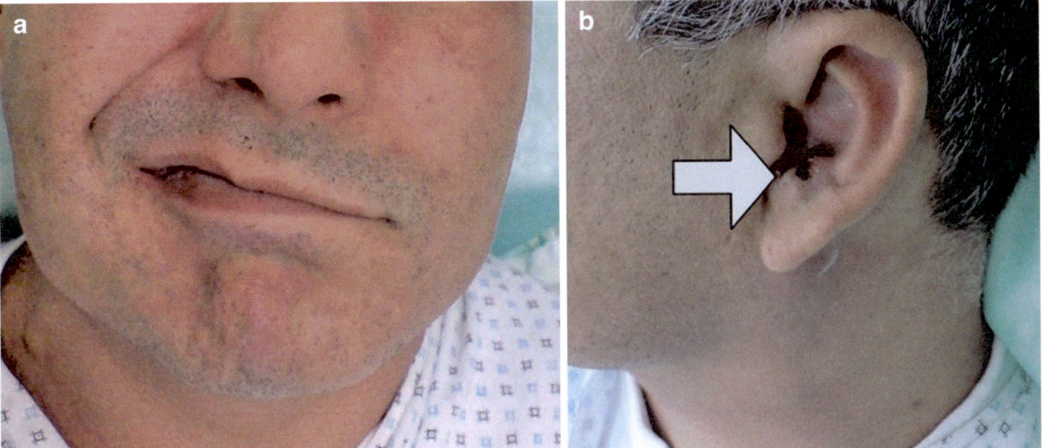

Fig. 11.4 Ramsey Hunt syndrome. (a) This patient suffered from a left-sided peripheral facial nerve palsy. (b) In the ear herpes sores can be seen (*arrow*)

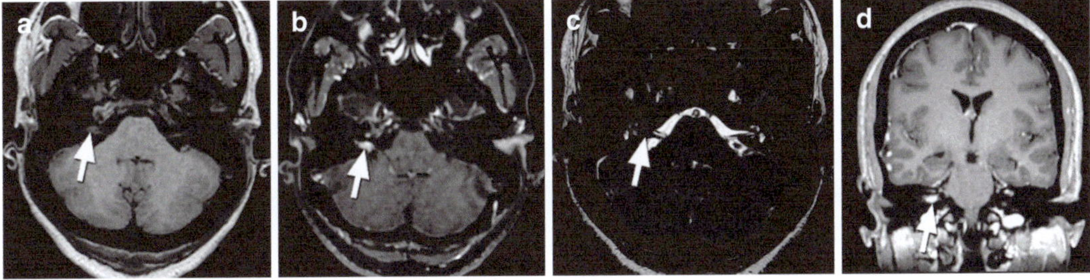

Fig. 11.5 Axial T1-weighted (a) without and (b) with contrast agent administration and axial (c) heavily T2-weighted three-dimensional constructive interference in steady-state (CISS) sequence. (d) Coronal T1-weighted sequence with contrast agent. There is a small vestibular schwannoma of the right vestibular nerve with an almost exclusive intrameatal component (*arrows*)

NF tumors in the parotid gland, leptomeningeal carcinomatosis, metastasis at the base of the skull [21]. Myeloma and metastasis. Tumors of the facial nerve: [22, 23].

Parotid surgery: [24].

Plastic and reconstructive surgery: Cosmetic or restorative surgery can cause lesions of the whole nerve of nerve twigs, *e.g.*, paralysis of the frontalis muscle.

Paraneoplastic: Rare and controversially discussed [25].*Pregnancy and peripartum appearance*: [26, 27].

Toxic: Rare [28].

Trauma: See Chap. 32.

Extracranial: Carotid endarterectomy, gunshot or knife wounds, parotid surgery.

Temporal bone fractures: Motor vehicle accidents, 70–80% from longitudinal fractures.

Facial wounds transecting the branches of the facial nerve can cause total or partial facial nerve palsies. Intracranial damage by surgery, *e.g.*, parotid surgery.

Reconstructive surgery: [29].

Facial war injuries: In association with cranio-maxillofacial injury, such as blunt trauma, falls, gunshot injuries, and blast injuries [30, 31].

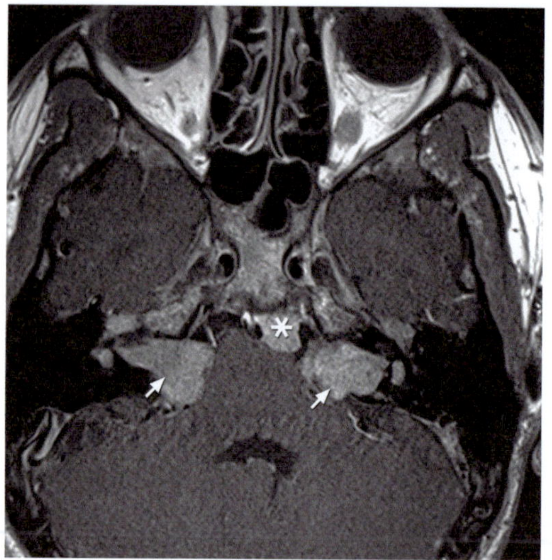

Fig. 11.6 MRI of the skull base, axial plane, T1-weighted contrast medium enhanced in a patient with type 2 neurofibromatosis. Findings include contrast medium enhancing bilateral vestibulocochlear nerve schwannoma (*arrows*) and skull base meningioma (*asterisk*)

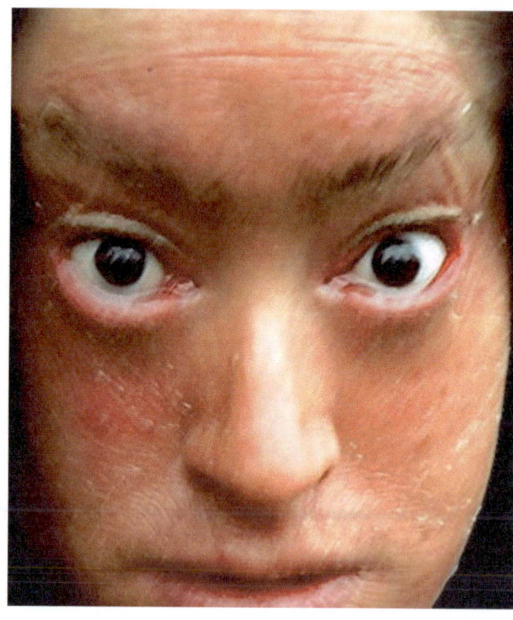

Fig. 11.7 Scleroderma mimicking bilateral "facial" paralysis. Inability to close eyes and masklike face

Otology temporal bone fractures: In about 50% of cases of transverse temporal bone fractures, the facial nerve is damaged within the internal auditory canal. Facial nerve injury occurs in about 50% of cases, and the labyrinth is usually damaged by the fracture. Sixty-five to 80% of fractures are reported to be neither longitudinal nor transverse but oblique. Signs to check are hemotympanum, "Battle's" sign, and nystagmus.

Vascular: Hemifacial spasm is characterized by unilateral, involuntary twitching. Neurovascular contact at the root exit zone of the facial nerve may account for hemifacial spasm (analogous with trigeminal nerve).

Vaccination: Examples: [32, 33].

Other focal conditions:

Myeloma, Paget's disease, porphyria, osteopetrosis [34].

Association of CN VII palsy with other neuropathies: GBS, Lyme disease, polyradiculopathies and sarcoid, Tangiers disease [35].

Periocular weakness, without extraocular movement disturbance: Congenital myopathies, FSHD, muscular dystrophies (myotonic, oculopharyngeal muscle dystrophy), polymyositis. See Muscle chapter. See Chap. 24).

Motor neuron disease/amyotrophic lateral sclerosis (ALS): ALS, bulbospinal muscular atrophy, motor neuron syndromes. Bulbar amyotrophic lateral sclerosis causes perioral facial weakness (weakness in pursing lips).

Facial onset sensory and motor neuronopathy (FOSMN): Early or in the advanced course [36].

Skin diseases: Scleroderma mimics facial nerve weakness (Fig. 11.7).

Hypomimia in extrapyramidal weakness [37].

Bilateral peripheral VII nerve palsy: Rare occurrence compared with isolated facial nerve palsy. Causes include acute intermittent porphyria, GBS, leprosy, Lyme disease, Melkersson-Rosenthal syndrome, Moebius syndrome, myopathies, NF2, neoplastic meningitis, sarcoidosis, and COVID-19 (VII, taste) [38–40].

Main Investigations

Electrophysiology: NCV, EMG.

Imaging: MR and ultrasound.

Classification of paresis: House-Brackmann [41]. Yanagihara grading system, the Sunnybrook facial grading system, and eFACE.

Diagnosis: In addition to the clinical examination, laboratory tests for antinuclear antibody (ANA), angiotensin-converting enzyme (for sarcoidosis), erythrocyte sedimentation rate (ESR), glucose, HIV, rheumatoid arthritis, Lyme serology, microbial tests, serology, and virology. CSF should be examined if an intracranial inflammatory lesion is suspected.

Other tests: Include CT, blink reflex, EMG (facial nerve compound muscle action potential (CMAP), needle EMG), magnetic stimulation, and MRI. Ultrasound can compare the muscle volume between both sides of the face [42].

Nerve ultrasound of the parotid: See Chap. 2.

Electrophysiology: See Chap. 3.

Therapy

The available evidence from randomized controlled trials shows significant benefit from treating Bell's palsy with corticosteroids [43].

Australian study management confirms the use of steroids [44]. Acyclovir, steroids, and surgery were compared, and pooled results from those studies showed better outcomes from steroid-treated vs. nonsteroid-treated patients. The combination of antivirals and corticosteroids may have little or no effect on rates of incomplete recovery in comparison to corticosteroids alone in Bell's palsy of various degrees of severity, or in people with severe Bell's palsy.

Surgical therapies for Bell's palsy are classified into:

Acute surgery: Usually within the first 2–3 weeks to aim for nerve decompression.

Nerve grafting: In later stages up to 2 years (hypoglossal, trigeminal, accessory).

Regional or free muscle transfers: Can be considered in chronic cases after more than 2 years.

Nerve surgery: See also Chap. 29.

A Cochrane review [45] showed no improvement due to acute surgical intervention, and physical therapy was not effective in Bell's palsy. Important additional measures to consider are eye care, eyelid surgery, facial rehabilitation, and botulinum injections for symptomatic synkineses.

Other studies support a role for physiotherapy in Bell's palsy [46], and the use of speech therapy [47] and communicative participation is increasing.

Prognosis: The overall prognosis in Bell palsy is good, with 80–85% of patients recovering.

For NCV prognosis of peripheral facial nerve palsies, the CMAPs of both facial nerves are compared, usually 1 week after onset. Elicitable CMAPs, either normal or reduced, point to a good prognosis. Loss of CMAPs point to axonal loss and bad prognosis.

References

1. Tubbs RS, Steck DT, Mortazavi MM, Cohen-Gadol AA. The nervus intermedius: a review of its anatomy, function, pathology, and role in neurosurgery. World Neurosurg. 2013;79(5–6):763–7.
2. Tang IP, Freeman SR, Kontorinis G, Tang MY, Rutherford SA, King AT, et al. Geniculate neuralgia: a systematic review. J Laryngol Otol. 2014;128(5):394–9.
3. Hopf HC, Muller-Forell W, Hopf NJ. Localization of emotional and volitional facial paresis. Neurology. 1992;42(10):1918–23.
4. Ogawa Y, Sakakibara R. Platysma sign in high cervical lesion. J Neurol Neurosurg Psychiatry. 2005;76(5):735.
5. Salinas NL, Jackson O, Dunham B, Bartlett SP. Anatomical dissection and modified Sihler stain of the lower branches of the facial nerve. Plast Reconstr Surg. 2009;124(6):1905–15.
6. Frunza A, Slavescu D, Lascar I. Perineural invasion in head and neck cancers—a review. J Med Life. 2014;7(2):121–3.
7. Peitersen E. Bell's palsy: the spontaneous course of 2,500 peripheral facial nerve palsies of different etiologies. Acta Otolaryngol Suppl. 2002;549:4–30.
8. Zhang W, Xu L, Luo T, Wu F, Zhao B, Li X. The etiology of Bell's palsy: a review. J Neurol. 2020;267(7):1896–905.
9. Kim SJ, Lee HY. Acute peripheral facial palsy: recent guidelines and a systematic review of the literature. J Korean Med Sci. 2020;35(30):e245.

10. Zandian A, Osiro S, Hudson R, Ali IM, Matusz P, Tubbs SR, et al. The neurologist's dilemma: a comprehensive clinical review of Bell's palsy, with emphasis on current management trends. Med Sci Monit. 2014;20:83–90.
11. Reich SG. Bell's Palsy. Continuum (Minneap Minn). 2017;23(2):447–66. Selected Topics in Outpatient Neurology
12. Yamamoto E, Nishimura H, Hirono Y. Occurrence of sequelae in Bell's palsy. Acta Otolaryngol Suppl. 1988;446:93–6.
13. Gagyor I, Madhok VB, Daly F, Sullivan F. Antiviral treatment for Bell's palsy (idiopathic facial paralysis). Cochrane Database Syst Rev. 2019;9:CD001869.
14. Kania RE, Cazals-Hatem D, Bouccara D, Cyna-Gorse F, Lisovoski F, Henin D, et al. Hypertrophic neuropathy of the facial nerve. Ann Otol Rhinol Laryngol. 2001;110(3):257–62.
15. Chew ZH, Lim EH, Lum SG, Teo D. Facial nerve palsy secondary to parotid abscess: report of a rare case and review of the literature. Cureus. 2022;14(2):e22509.
16. Kumar S, Alexander M, Gnanamuthu C. Cranial nerve involvement in patients with leprous neuropathy. Neurol India. 2006;54(3):283–5.
17. Guez-Barber D, Swami SK, Harrison JB, McGuire JL. Differentiating Bell's Palsy from Lyme-related facial palsy. Pediatrics. 2022;149(6):e2021053992.
18. Figoni J, Chirouze C, Hansmann Y, Lemogne C, Hentgen V, Saunier A, et al. Lyme borreliosis and other tick-borne diseases. Guidelines from the French Scientific Societies (I): prevention, epidemiology, diagnosis. Med Mal Infect. 2019;49(5):318–34.
19. Pandey PK, Chaudhuri Z, Sharma P. Extraocular muscle and facial paresis in herpes zoster ophthalmicus. J Pediatr Ophthalmol Strabismus. 2001;38(6):363–6.
20. Wang B, Kong Q, Li X, Zhao J, Zhang H, Chen W, et al. A high-fat diet increases gut microbiota biodiversity and energy expenditure due to nutrient difference. Nutrients. 2020;12(10):3197.
21. Christopher LH, Slattery WH, Smith EJ, Larian B, Azizzadeh B. Facial nerve management in patients with malignant skull base tumors. J Neuro-Oncol. 2020;150(3):493–500.
22. McRackan TR, Wilkinson EP, Rivas A. Primary tumors of the facial nerve. Otolaryngol Clin N Am. 2015;48(3):491–500.
23. Muhlbauer MS, Clark WC, Robertson JH, Gardner LG, Dohan FC Jr. Malignant nerve sheath tumor of the facial nerve: case report and discussion. Neurosurgery. 1987;21(1):68–73.
24. Marchesi M, Biffoni M, Trinchi S, Turriziani V, Campana FP. Facial nerve function after parotidectomy for neoplasms with deep localization. Surg Today. 2006;36(4):308–11.
25. Kwatra V, Charakidis M, Karanth NV. Bilateral facial nerve palsy associated with amphiphysin antibody in metastatic breast cancer: a case report. J Med Case Rep. 2021;15(1):158.
26. Cohen Y, Lavie O, Granovsky-Grisaru S, Aboulafia Y, Diamant YZ. Bell palsy complicating pregnancy: a review. Obstet Gynecol Surv. 2000;55(3):184–8.
27. Fuzi J, Spencer S, Seckold E, Damiano S, Meller C. Bell's palsy during pregnancy and the post-partum period: A contemporary management approach. Am J Otolaryngol. 2021;42(3):102914.
28. Lee RT, Oster MW, Balmaceda C, Hesdorffer CS, Vahdat LT, Papadopoulos KP. Bilateral facial nerve palsy secondary to the administration of high-dose paclitaxel. Ann Oncol. 1999;10(10):1245–7.
29. Brown S, Isaacson B, Kutz W, Barnett S, Rozen SM. Facial Nerve Trauma: Clinical Evaluation and Management Strategies. Plast Reconstr Surg. 2019;143(5):1498–512.
30. Scott B. Roofe M, Caroline M. Kolb, Jared Seibert. Chapter 18 Cranial nerve injuries. Otolaryngology/head and neck surgery combat casualty care in operation Iraqi freedom and operation enduring freedom 2015. 2016; Textbooks of Military Medicine (ISBN 9780160930348).
31. Abu-Sittah GS, Hoballah JJ, Bakhach J. Reconstructing the war injured patient. Springer. ISBN 978-3-319-56885-0; 2017.
32. Garg RK, Paliwal VK. Spectrum of neurological complications following COVID-19 vaccination. Neurol Sci. 2022;43(1):3–40.
33. Tregoning JS, Russell RF, Kinnear E. Adjuvanted influenza vaccines. Hum Vaccin Immunother. 2018;14(3):550–64.
34. Loke JY, Mohd Ali H, Kamalden TA. Osteopetrosis craniopathy: a rare cause of bilateral compressive optic neuropathy and facial nerve palsy. Postgrad Med J. 2019;95(1127):513.
35. Nagappa M, Taly AB, Mahadevan A, Pooja M, Bindu PS, Chickabasaviah YT, et al. Tangier's disease: an uncommon cause of facial weakness and non-length dependent demyelinating neuropathy. Ann Indian Acad Neurol. 2016;19(1):137–9.
36. Vucic S, Tian D, Chong PS, Cudkowicz ME, Hedley-Whyte ET, Cros D. Facial onset sensory and motor neuronopathy (FOSMN syndrome): a novel syndrome in neurology. Brain. 2006;129(Pt 12):3384–90.
37. Ricciardi L, De Angelis A, Marsili L, Faiman I, Pradhan P, Pereira EA, et al. Hypomimia in Parkinson's disease: an axial sign responsive to levodopa. Eur J Neurol. 2020;27(12):2422–9.
38. Gaudin RA, Jowett N, Banks CA, Knox CJ, Hadlock TA. Bilateral facial paralysis: a 13-year experience. Plast Reconstr Surg. 2016;138(4):879–87.
39. Pothiawala S, Lateef F. Bilateral facial nerve palsy: a diagnostic dilemma. Case Rep Emerg Med. 2012;2012:458371.
40. Hiraga A, Muto M, Kuwabara S. Loss of taste as an initial symptom of a "Facial Diplegia and Paresthesia"

variant of Guillain-Barre Syndrome. Intern Med. 2022;61(19):2957–9.

41. House JW, Brackmann DE. Facial nerve grading system. Otolaryngol Head Neck Surg. 1985;93(2):146–7.

42. Volk GF, Pohlmann M, Sauer M, Finkensieper M, Guntinas-Lichius O. Quantitative ultrasonography of facial muscles in patients with chronic facial palsy. Muscle Nerve. 2014;50(3):358–65.

43. Xiao L, Sonne SB, Feng Q, Chen N, Xia Z, Li X, et al. High-fat feeding rather than obesity drives taxonomical and functional changes in the gut microbiota in mice. Microbiome. 2017;5(1):43.

44. Somasundara D, Sullivan F. Management of Bell's palsy. Aust Prescr. 2017;40(3):94–7.

45. Menchetti I, McAllister K, Walker D, Donnan PT. Surgical interventions for the early management of Bell's palsy. Cochrane Database Syst Rev. 2021;1:CD007468.

46. Beurskens CH, Heymans PG. Physiotherapy in patients with facial nerve paresis: description of outcomes. Am J Otolaryngol. 2004;25(6):394–400.

47. Kim JH, Fisher LM, Reder L, Hapner ER, Pepper JP. Speech and communicative participation in patients with facial paralysis. JAMA Otolaryngol Head Neck Surg. 2018;144(8):686–93.

One sentence: The acoustic nerve has a special sensory function and delivers signals from the cochlea into the brain stem.

Genetic testing	NCV/ EMG	Laboratory	Imaging	Biopsy	Hearing tests
Familial	Auditory test, AEP		+		+

Symptoms

Hearing loss of various degrees. The onset can be acute or chronic, and symptoms can range from mild hearing loss to deafness.

Phenomena such as "tinnitus," which is described as a sensation of a variety of noise qualities that is caused by abnormal excitation of the acoustic apparatus, can appear frequently and be associated with sensorineural hearing loss and at times with dizziness and vertigo. Other auditory phenomena also possible but rare. These can be part of psychiatric diseases (see Chap. 35).

Several auditory phenomena are described, including palinacousis, pareidolia, synesthesia, aura, and acoustic hallucination, among others [1].

Signs

There are no "direct" signs, but absence of acoustic reflexes (e.g., blink reflex) or absent attention to sound can be indicators of hearing loss.

Specific Qualities

Motor:
  Sensory:
  Autonomic:
  Special senses: +, the acoustic nerve has a special sensory function and delivers signals from the cochlea into the brain stem, from where central pathways continue to the cortex.
  Other:

Location of Lesions

Central:
  Cortical: Pure word deafness and sound agnosia.
  The spectrum of cortical hearing loss in stroke is disputed [2].
  Lesions affecting Heschel's gyri result in pure word deafness (auditory verbal agnosia) [3, 4].
  Brain stem lesions: [5, 6].
  Intracranial within the skull:
  Arachnoid space, e.g., cerebellopontine angle tumors (CPA), meningitis.
  Exit of the skull: Temporal bone trauma, fractures, infections, tumors [7].

Combination with Other CNs

At the CPA, or in temporal bone lesions.

© The Author(s), under exclusive license to Springer Nature Switzerland AG 2023
W. Grisold et al., *The Cranial Nerves in Neurology*, https://doi.org/10.1007/978-3-031-43081-7_12

Others: Auditory neuropathy [8] and pure auditory neuropathy [9]. Acute auditory loss in adults [10].

Causes and Frequency

Age: Hearing reduction in elderly is termed presbycusis. The possible contribution of hearing loss to develop dementia is discussed [11, 12]. Common overall cause of sensorineural hearing loss, age-related and mostly affecting high frequencies [13].

Congenital: Congenital anomalies such as cochlear aplasia or dysplasia. Example: Mondini [14] or Michel aplasia and other malformations [15]. Rubeola embryopathy, thalidomide toxicity [16].

Hereditary conditions:

Genetic neuropathies [17].

Other syndromes: Transthyretin (ATTR) amyloidosis, cerebellar ataxia, neuropathy, vestibular areflexia syndrome (CANVAS) [18, 19], Coffin-Lowry syndrome, Connexin 31, Duane's syndrome, Fabry's disease [20], mitochondrial diseases (e.g., mitochondrial encephalopathy, lactic acidosis, and stroke-like episodes (MELAS), myoclonic epilepsy with ragged red fibers (MERFF), DNA polymerase subunit gamma (POLG or POLG1)), neuroaxonal dystrophy (late infantile), neurofibromatosis-2, X-linked dilated cardiomyopathy with sensorineural hearing loss (CMD1J or CMD1K).

Infections: Covid disputed [21], herpes, meningitis, mumps, otitis, sarcoid, suppurative labyrinthitis, syphilis, tuberculosis.

Inflammatory: Acute labyrinthitis. Vestibular neuritis with associated tinnitus and hearing loss. Can follow systemic or middle ear infections or the use of ototoxic drugs (toxic labyrinthitis).

Inflammatory/autoimmune disease: Cogan syndrome [22], Wegener granulomatosis, polyar-

teritis nodosa, temporal arteritis, Buerger disease (thromboangiitis obliterans), systemic lupus erythematodes.

Neuropathies: With neuropathy (several types):

Hereditary neuropathies: [7], transthyretin (TTR) amyloidosis [22].

Acquired: Platinum, glue sniffing [23].

Metabolic: Diabetes, hypothyroidism. Wernicke encephalopathy [24].*Paraneoplastic*: Rare [25].

Radiation therapy (RT): RT of head and neck [26].

Toxic: There are a large number of ototoxic agents; this is an incomplete list:

Antibiotics: Aminoglycosides, chloramphenicol, colistin, erythromycin, ethambutol, isoniazid, streptomycin, sulfonamides, tetracyclines, vancomycin, antibacterial agents [27].

Cancer drugs: Carboplatinum, platinum, vinca alkaloids, thalidomide [28].

Diuretics.

Immune checkpoint inhibitors: Vestibulocochlear damage [29].

Quinine [30].

Salicylates [31].

Other substances: Carbon monoxide, heavy metals such as mercury and lead, pesticides.

Combination of several ototoxicants increases the risk of hearing loss.

Trauma: Temporal bone fractures. Contusion of the cochlea [32]. Noise-induced (prolonged exposure to loud noise causes hair cell loss) [33]. Cochlear hemorrhage [34].

Tumors and compressive lesions: Tumors at the cerebellopontine angle. Neoplastic: Cholesteatoma, meningeal carcinomatosis, metastasis, neurofibromatosis (Fig. 12.1).

Vascular: Hemorrhage, stroke [35]. Labyrinthine hemorrhage or stroke secondary to thrombosis of the labyrinthine (internal auditory) artery. If the cochlear branch is occluded, deafness can occur [36].

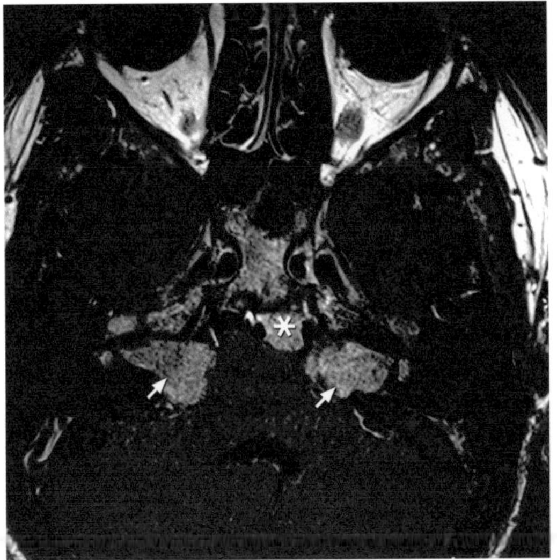

Fig. 12.1 MRI of the skull base, axial plane, T1-weighted contrast medium enhanced in a patient with type 2 neurofibromatosis. Findings include contrast medium enhancing bilateral vestibulocochlear nerve schwannoma (*arrows*) and skull base meningioma (*asterisk*)

Main Investigations

Hearing Tests:
- Weber test. Vibration over midline. Sensorineural loss – louder in normal ear. Conductive loss – louder in affected ear.
- Rinne test. Air conduction (AC) versus bone conduction (BC). Normal: AC > BC (positive Rinne). Sensorineural loss: AC > BC. Conductive loss: BC > AC.
- Schwabach test. Compare the examiner's bone conduction over mastoid with patient. If examiner's is better, sensorineural loss is suspected.

In sensorineural hearing loss, Weber lateralizes to the normal ear, Rinne is positive, and the Schwabach is abnormal.

In conductive hearing loss, Weber lateralizes to the affected ear, Rinne is negative, and the Schwabach is normal.

Therapy

Prognosis depends on cause, usually permanent.

References

1. Marek A. Auditory phenomena as differential diagnostics to tinnitus. Laryngorhinootologie. 2021;100(9):712–9.
2. Bamiou DE. Hearing disorders in stroke. Handb Clin Neurol. 2015;129:633–47.
3. Dieterich M, Brandt T. The bilateral central vestibular system: its pathways, functions, and disorders. Ann N Y Acad Sci. 2015;1343:10–26.
4. Benoudiba F, Toulgoat F, Sarrazin JL. The vestibulocochlear nerve (VIII). Diagn Interv Imaging. 2013;94(10):1043–50.
5. Cohen M, Luxon L, Rudge P. Auditory deficits and hearing loss associated with focal brainstem haemorrhage. Scand Audiol. 1996;25(2):133–41.
6. Chung SH, Jeong SW, Kim LS. A case of auditory neuropathy caused by pontine hemorrhage in an adult. J Audiol Otol. 2017;21(2):107–11.
7. Maillot O, Attye A, Boyer E, Heck O, Kastler A, Grand S, et al. Post traumatic deafness: a pictorial review of CT and MRI findings. Insights Imaging. 2016;7(3):341–50.
8. Loundon N, Marcolla A, Roux I, Rouillon I, Denoyelle F, Feldmann D, et al. Auditory neuropathy or endocochlear hearing loss? Otol Neurotol. 2005;26(4):748–54.
9. Moser T, Starr A. Auditory neuropathy--neural and synaptic mechanisms. Nat Rev Neurol. 2016;12(3):135–49.
10. Pittman CA, Ward BK, Nieman CL. A Review of Adult-Onset Hearing Loss: A Primer for Neurologists. Curr Treat Options Neurol. 2021;23(7).
11. Thomson RS, Auduong P, Miller AT, Gurgel RK. Hearing loss as a risk factor for dementia: a systematic review. Laryngoscope Investig Otolaryngol. 2017;2(2):69–79.
12. Jung J, Bae SH, Han JH, Kwak SH, Nam GS, Lee PH, et al. Relationship between hearing loss and dementia differs according to the underlying mechanism. J Clin Neurol. 2021;17(2):290–9.
13. Michels TC, Duffy MT, Rogers DJ. Hearing loss in adults: differential diagnosis and treatment. Am Fam Physician. 2019;100(2):98–108.
14. Illum P. The Mondini type of cochlear malformation. A survey of the literature. Arch Otolaryngol. 1972;96(4):305–11.
15. Dagkiran M, Dagkiran N, Surmelioglu O, Balli T, Tuncer U, Akgul E, et al. Radiological imaging find-

ings of patients with congenital totally hearing loss. J Int Adv Otol. 2016;12(1):43–8.

16. Takemori S, Tanaka Y, Suzuki JI. Thalidomide anomalies of the ear. Arch Otolaryngol. 1976;102(7):425–7.

17. Lerat J, Magdelaine C, Roux AF, Darnaud L, Beauvais-Dzugan H, Naud S, et al. Hearing loss in inherited peripheral neuropathies: molecular diagnosis by NGS in a French series. Mol Genet Genomic Med. 2019;7(9):e839.

18. Szmulewicz DJ, Roberts L, McLean CA, MacDougall HG, Halmagyi GM, Storey E. Proposed diagnostic criteria for cerebellar ataxia with neuropathy and vestibular areflexia syndrome (CANVAS). Neurol Clin Pract. 2016;6(1):61–8.

19. Ishai R, Seyyedi M, Chancellor AM, McLean CA, Rodriguez ML, Halmagyi GM, et al. The pathology of the vestibular system in CANVAS. Otol Neurotol. 2021;42(3):e332–e40.

20. Yazdanfard PDW, Effraimidis G, Madsen CV, Nielsen LH, Rasmussen AK, Petersen JH, et al. Hearing loss in Fabry disease: a 16 year follow-up study of the Danish nationwide cohort. Mol Genet Metab Rep. 2022;31:100841.

21. Karimi-Galougahi M, Naeini AS, Raad N, Mikaniki N, Ghorbani J. Vertigo and hearing loss during the COVID-19 pandemic - is there an association? Acta Otorhinolaryngol Ital. 2020;40(6):463–5.

22. Haynes BF, Kaiser-Kupfer MI, Mason P, Fauci AS. Cogan syndrome: studies in thirteen patients, long-term follow-up, and a review of the literature. Medicine (Baltimore). 1980;59(6):426–41.

23. Ehyai A, Freemon FR. Progressive optic neuropathy and sensorineural hearing loss due to chronic glue sniffing. J Neurol Neurosurg Psychiatry. 1983;46(4):349–51.

24. Hoistad DL, Hain TC. Central hearing loss with a bilateral inferior colliculus lesion. Audiol Neurootol. 2003;8(2):111–3.

25. Kattah JC, Eggers SD, Bach SE, Dubey D, McKeon AB. Paraneoplastic progressive downbeat nystagmus, ataxia and sensorineural hearing loss due to the ANTI-Kelch-11 protein antibody. J Neuroophthalmol. 2021;41(2):261–5.

26. Azzam P, Mroueh M, Francis M, Daher AA, Zeidan YH. Radiation-induced neuropathies in head and neck cancer: prevention and treatment modalities. Ecancermedicalscience. 2020;14:1133.

27. Snavely SR, Hodges GR. The neurotoxicity of antibacterial agents. Ann Intern Med. 1984;101(1):92–104.

28. Landier W. Ototoxicity and cancer therapy. Cancer. 2016;122(11):1647–58.

29. Vogrig A, Muniz-Castrillo S, Joubert B, Picard G, Rogemond V, Skowron F, et al. Cranial nerve disorders associated with immune checkpoint inhibitors. Neurology. 2021;96(6):e866–e75.

30. Brough H. Acquired auditory neuropathy spectrum disorder after malaria treated with quinine. Trop Dr. 2020;50(3):246–8.

31. Arslan E, Orzan E, Santarelli R. Global problem of drug-induced hearing loss. Ann N Y Acad Sci. 1999;884:1–14.

32. Patel A, Groppo E. Management of temporal bone trauma. Craniomaxillofac Trauma Reconstr. 2010;3(2):105–13.

33. Moore BCJ, Lowe DA, Cox G. Guidelines for diagnosing and quantifying noise-induced hearing loss. Trends Hear. 2022;26:23312165221093156.

34. Chen XH, Zeng CJ, Fang ZM, Zhang R, Cheng JM, Lin C. The natural history of labyrinthine hemorrhage in patients with sudden sensorineural hearing loss. Ear Nose Throat J. 2019;98(5):E13–20.

35. Lingling Neng XS. Vascular pathology and hearing disorders. Curr Opin Physio. 2020;18:79–84.

36. Nam HW, Yoo D, Lee SU, Choi JY, Yu S, Kim JS. Pearls & oy-sters: labyrinthine infarction mimicking vestibular neuritis. Neurology. 2021;97(16):787–90.

One sentence: The vestibular nerve is a special sensory nerve that balances information from the semicircular canals, and its anatomy is best visualized in relation to the temporal bone (Fig. 13.1) and the vestibular organ (Fig. 13.2).

Genetic testing	NCV/ EMG	Laboratory	Imaging	Other	Biopsy
?	+	+	+	Impulse test	

Symptoms

Dizziness, vertigo ("spinning" and tilting), nausea/vomiting, imbalance, and falling.

Signs

Lesions result in abnormal eye movements and balance problems with stance, gait, and equilibrium abnormalities.

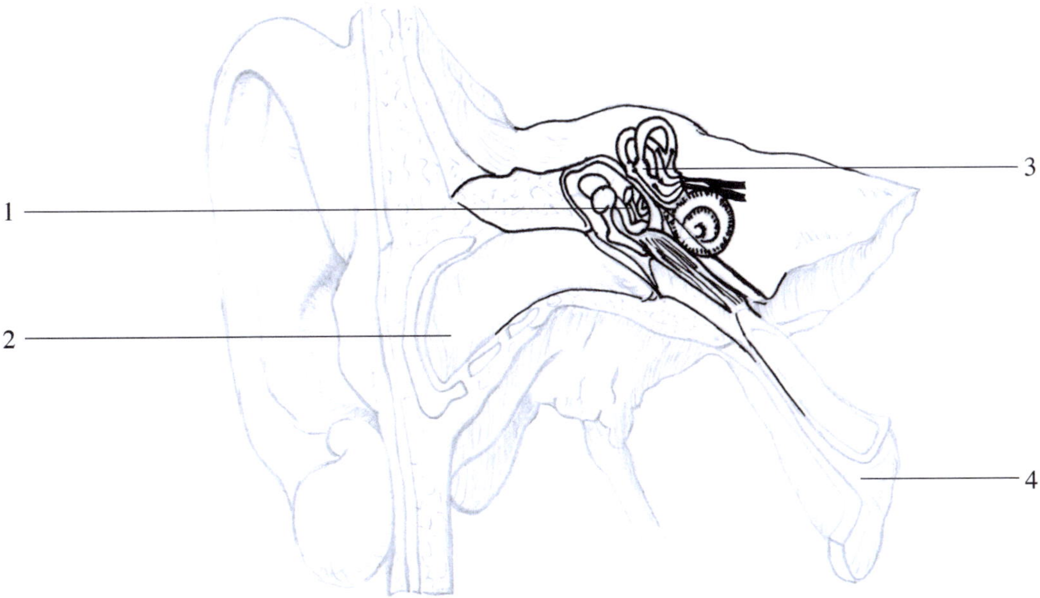

Fig. 13.1 Temporal bone. (*1*) Tympanic cavity, (*2*) external auditory meatus, (*3*) bony labyrinth, (*4*) eustachian tube

W. Grisold et al., *The Cranial Nerves in Neurology*, https://doi.org/10.1007/978-3-031-43081-7_13

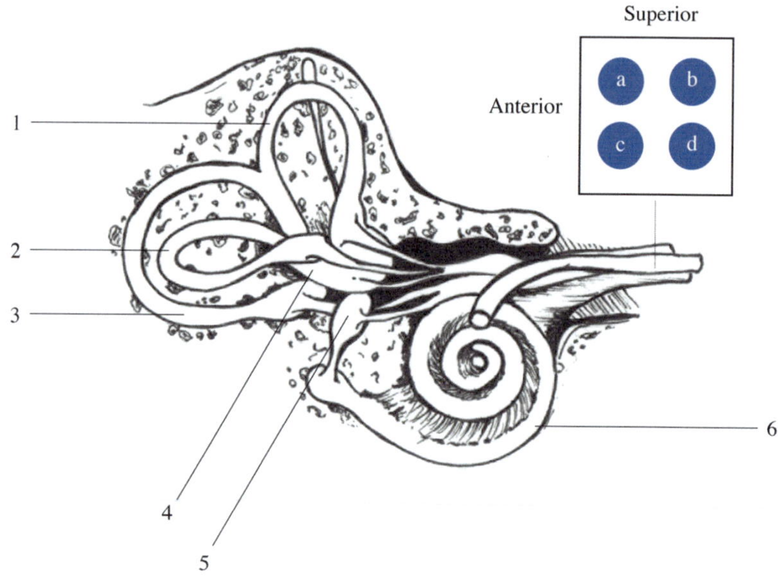

Fig. 13.2 Vestibular nerve. (*1*) Superior semicircular canal, (*2*) lateral semicircular canal, (*3*) posterior semicircular canal, (*4*) utriculus, (*5*) sacculus, (*6*) spiral ganglia. Positions of nerves in the internal auditory meatus: *a* facial nerve, *b* superior vestibular nerve, *c* cochlear nerve, *d* inferior vestibular nerve

Specific symptoms: Vertigo, nystagmus, oscillopsia, and autonomic involvement.

Specific Qualities

Motor:
  Sensory:
  Autonomic:
  Special senses: +.
  Other:

Location of Lesions

Central: The distribution of the cortical vestibular areas is complex [1] and is subject to extensive study. A clearly assigned lesion to a cortical area of vestibular symptoms and signs is clinically difficult, but several paradigms of localization of function have been described [1–3].

Brain stem lesion causes include vascular, inflammatory diseases, infections, and tumors.

Intracranial lesions within the skull: Examples include cerebellopontine angle tumors (CPA) and other intracranial tumors.

Exit of the skull: Temporal bone trauma, fractures. Middle ear damage [4], blast injuries.

Other: Other vestibular syndromes include Menier's disease [5], vestibular neuritis [6], peripheral paroxysmal positional nystagmus [7], positional (central) [8], persistent postural-perceptual dizziness (PPPD) [9], bilateral vestibulopathy ("bilateral vestibular weakness"), vestibular paroyxsmia, and the third mobile window syndromes [10]

Combination with Other CN

In CPA tumors.

Causes and Frequency

Age-related: With increasing age vestibular functions also deteriorate [11]. Presbyastasis is the term coined for aging of sensory systems [12, 13].

Congenital and hereditary: Aplasia; Arnold-Chiari syndrome; atrophy of CN VIII; chromosomal aberrations; Cockayne, Hallgren, and Alström syndrome; hereditary motor and sensory neuropathy (HMSN); Kearns-Sayre; olivoponto-cerebellar atrophy (OPCA); Refsum's disease; retinitis pigmentosa; sensorineural deafness; SMA; thyroid disease.

Cupulolithiasis: Benign paroxysmal positional nystagmus. Several subtypes have been described. Positioning maneuvers: Dix, Hallpike, Semont, or Epley.

Immunologic disorders: Demyelinating neuropathies, Hashimoto, leukodystrophies, MS, periarteritis nodosa, sarcoid.

Infection: Labyrinthitis, specific and unspecific.

Bacterial: Hemophilus, Lyme disease, petrositis, streptococcus pneumoniae, syphilis [14]. Pus reaches the inner ear by either blood or direct invasion (meningoencephalitis).

Viral: AIDS, herpes zoster oticus, Ramsey Hunt syndrome, vestibular neuronitis.

Mycotic: Coccidiomycosis, cryptococcosis, rickettsial infection.

Metabolic: Diabetes, uremia.

Neoplastic: Acoustic nerve neuroma, metastases, neurofibromatosis [15], schwannoma.

Neuropathy: Several associations (polyneuropathy) [16], also several types of CMT.*Perilymphatic fistula*: Communication between the middle ear (air-filled) and inner ear (fluid-filled) following trauma or surgery.

Radiation therapy: Usually as late effects [17].

Toxic: Alcohol, aminoglycosides, chemotherapy (cisplatin, cyclophosphamide, hydroxyurea, platinum [18], vinblastine); heavy metals (lead, mercury); quinine, salicylate [19].

Trauma: Blunt, penetrating, or barotrauma. Transverse fractures are often associated with additional CN VII lesion. The less common transverse fractures damage both facial and vestibulocochlear nerves. These fractures involve the otic capsule, passing through the vestibule of the inner ear, tearing the membranous labyrinth, and lacerating both vestibular and cochlear nerves. Vertigo is the most common neurologic sequel to head injury, and it is a positional vertigo.

Vascular: Anterior inferior cerebellar artery aneurysm, arteria posterior communicans aneurysm, labyrinthine hemorrhage or stroke secondary to thrombosis of the labyrinthine (internal auditory) artery, large vascular loops, vascular lesions of the spiral ganglion, vertebrobasilar circulation disorders (history of diabetes, hypertension).

Vasculitis: Immune mediated, Cogan syndrome.

Vestibular epilepsy: [20].

Vestibular paroxysms.

Others: Hyperviscosity syndromes (hypergammaglobulinemia, polycythemia vera, Waldenström's macroglobulinemia).

Main Investigations

Diagnosis is based on clinical and vestibular testing, laboratory testing (including genetics for hereditary causes), and imaging.

Clinical tests: Romberg, vestibular-ocular reflex test (doll's head test), video head impulse test [21].

Therapy

Depends on the cause of the vestibular nerve damage.

References

1. Dieterich M, Brandt T. Functional brain imaging of peripheral and central vestibular disorders. Brain. 2008;131(Pt 10):2538–52.
2. Nam HW, Yoo D, Lee SU, Choi JY, Yu S, Kim JS. Pearls & Oy-sters: labyrinthine infarction mimicking vestibular neuritis. Neurology. 2021;97(16):787–90.
3. Gam BU, Cho IH, Yeo SS, Kwon JW, Jang SH, Oh S. Comparative study of vestibular projection pathway connectivity in cerebellar injury patients and healthy adults. BMC Neurosci. 2022;23(1):17.
4. Van Hoecke H, Calus L, Dhooge I. Middle ear damages. B-ENT. 2016;12(Suppl. 26):173–83.
5. Christopher LH, Wilkinson EP. Meniere's disease: medical management, rationale for vestibular preservation and suggested protocol in medical failure. Am J Otolaryngol. 2021;42(1):102817.

6. Le TN, Westerberg BD, Lea J. Vestibular neuritis: recent advances in etiology, diagnostic evaluation, and treatment. Adv Otorhinolaryngol. 2019;82:87–92.

7. Imai T, Inohara H. Benign paroxysmal positional vertigo. Auris Nasus Larynx. 2022;49(5):737–47.

8. Macdonald NK, Kaski D, Saman Y, Al-Shaikh Sulaiman A, Anwer A, Bamiou DE. Central positional nystagmus: a systematic literature review. Front Neurol. 2017;8:141.

9. Waterston J, Chen L, Mahony K, Gencarelli J, Stuart G. Persistent postural-perceptual dizziness: precipitating conditions, co-morbidities and treatment with cognitive behavioral therapy. Front Neurol. 2021;12:795516.

10. Strupp M, Dlugaiczyk J, Ertl-Wagner BB, Rujescu D, Westhofen M, Dieterich M. Vestibular disorders. Dtsch Arztebl Int. 2020;117(17):300–10.

11. Balatsouras DG, Koukoutsis G, Fassolis A, Moukos A, Apris A. Benign paroxysmal positional vertigo in the elderly: current insights. Clin Interv Aging. 2018;13:2251–66.

12. Rogers C. Presbyastasis: a multifactorial cause of balance problems in the elderly. South Afr Family Pract. 2010;52(5):431–4.

13. Belal A Jr, Glorig A. Dysequilibrium of ageing (presbyastasis). J Laryngol Otol. 1986;100(9):1037–41.

14. Casas-Limon J, Ordas-Bandera CM, Matias-Guiu JA, Barahona-Hernando R, Abarrategui-Yague B, Garcia-Ramos R, et al. Otosyphilis as the cause of skew deviation and benign paroxysmal positional vertigo. Rev Neurol. 2012;55(1):62–4.

15. Korf BR. Neurofibromatosis. Handb Clin Neurol. 2013;111:333–40.

16. Buetti B, Luxon LM. Vestibular involvement in peripheral neuropathy: a review. Int J Audiol. 2014;53(6):353–9.

17. Kovar M, Waltner JG. Radiation effect on the middle and inner ear. Pract Otorhinolaryngol (Basel). 1971;33(4):233–42.

18. Prayuenyong P, Taylor JA, Pearson SE, Gomez R, Patel PM, Hall DA, et al. Vestibulotoxicity associated with platinum-based chemotherapy in survivors of cancer: a scoping review. Front Oncol. 2018;8:363.

19. Sheppard A, Hayes SH, Chen GD, Ralli M, Salvi R. Review of salicylate-induced hearing loss, neurotoxicity, tinnitus and neuropathophysiology. Acta Otorhinolaryngol Ital. 2014;34(2):79–93.

20. Hewett R, Bartolomei F. Epilepsy and the cortical vestibular system: tales of dizziness and recent concepts. Front Integr Neurosci. 2013;7:73.

21. Halmagyi GM, Chen L, MacDougall HG, Weber KP, McGarvie LA, Curthoys IS. The video head impulse test. Front Neurol. 2017;8:258.

Cranial Nerve IX: Glossopharyngeal Nerve

One sentence: The glossopharyngeal nerve is part of the lower CNs and has motor, sensory, special senses, and autonomic functions, and while it is difficult to investigate in isolation, it is important for swallowing, taste, and autonomic functions (Fig. 14.1).

Genetic testing	NCV/ EMG	Laboratory	Imaging	Biopsy
	+?		+ and endoscopy	

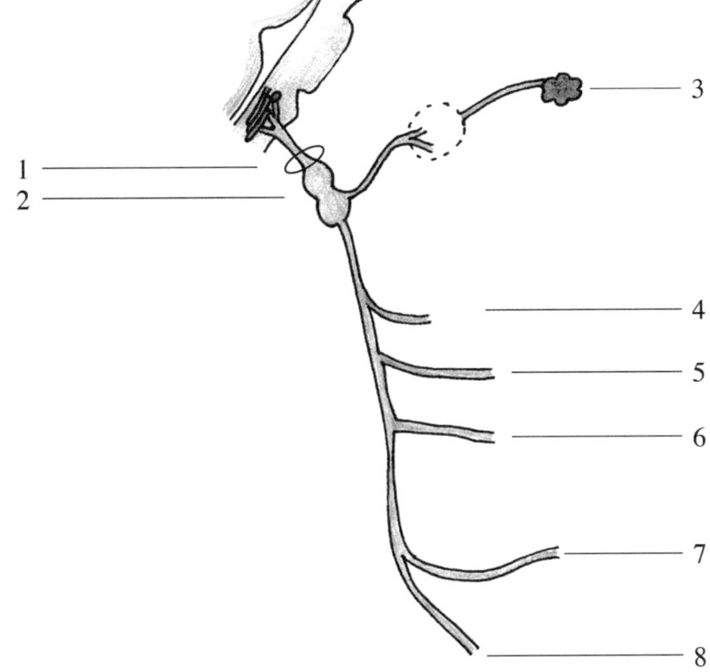

Fig. 14.1 Glossopharyngeal nerve. (*1*) Jugular foramen, (*2*) ganglia, (*3*) otic ganglion, (*4*) nerve to stylopharyngeal muscle, (*5*) pharyngeal branch, (*6*) tonsillar branch, (*7*) lingual nerve, (*8*) carotid body branch

Symptoms

Lesions can cause minor swallowing difficulties, disturbance of taste, glossopharyngeal neuralgia (rare – pain behind the angle of the jaw, deep within the ear, and side of throat), and abnormal lacrimation ("crocodile tears" and "Bogorad" syndrome), but these symptoms may also be a complication of Bell's palsy with lesions proximal to the geniculate ganglion.

Signs

Taste on the soft palate, pharynx, and posterior third of the tongue is abnormal with decreased saliva production. The gag reflex is reduced or absent, which may result in swallowing and aspiration problems.

Specific Qualities

Motor: Stylopharyngeus muscle.

Sensory: Posterior third of the tongue, skin of the external ear, and the internal surface of the tympanic membrane.

Autonomic: Fibers to stimulate the parotid gland. Visceral sensory sensation, carotid body, and sinus.

Special senses: Taste from the posterior third of the tongue [1].

Other: Branchial. Visceral motor: Otic ganglion, general sensory, special sensory.

Location

Central:

Supranuclear lesion:

Unilateral: No deficit.
Bilateral: Corticobulbar innervation results in "pseudobulbar palsy."
Usually vascular causes.

Brain stem: Swallowing difficulties, bulbar symptoms combined with long tract signs, vascular brain stem lesions (*e.g.*, Bonnier's syndrome); medulla oblongata, pons, and pontine tumors; Wallenberg's syndrome.

Intracranial within the skull:

Inflammatory: GBS, meningitis, "polyneuritis cranialis."

Tumors: Neurinoma; cerebellopontine angle tumors, meningeal carcinomatosis, and schwannomas are rare [2], as is neurofibromatosis and malignant peripheral nerve sheath tumor (MPNST) [3].

Venous thrombosis.

Exit of the skull:

Jugular foramen syndrome (with CN X, XI; Vernet's syndrome), fracture of the base of the skull, metastasis, neurinoma, and other local tumors.

Outside of the skull: *i.e.*, neck.

Iatrogenic: Carotid operations, neck dissection (ENT and neurosurgical procedures), resection of aneurysms. Tonsillectomy is rarely a cause (0.1%). Lesions of the lateral pharyngeal wall.

Embolization of the ascending pharyngeal artery (tumor embolization in base of the skull tumors).

Lesions are rarely isolated and often associated with vagus nerve lesions.

Specific syndromes: Bonnier syndrome, Collet-Sicard syndrome, Villaret syndrome, Eagle's syndrome [4], Drummond syndrome, Frey syndrome.

Combination with Other CNs

Lesion of the jugular foramen.
Base of skull lesions.

Causes and Frequency

Amyloidosis of the pharynx: [5].*Eagle's syndrome*: [4, 6].

Iatrogenic: Anesthesia [7], carotid operations, embolization of the ascending pharyngeal artery (tumor embolization of base of the skull tumors), neck dissection (ENT and neurosurgical procedures), lesions of the lateral pharynx wall, resection of aneurysms; tonsillectomy is rarely a cause (0.1%) [8].

Immune dysphagia: [9].

Infectious: Diphtheria, herpes zoster, poliomyelitis.

Inflammatory/immune-mediated: Cryoglobulinemia, GBS, Miller Fisher syndrome, panarteritis nodosa, sarcoid, serum sickness, systemic lupus erythematodes (SLE).

Metabolic: Amyloid deposition, porphyria.

Motor neuron disease.

Myopathies: dermatomyositis, inclusion body myositis (IBM).

Neoplastic: Leptomeningeal carcinomatosis, leukemia, myeloma, vagal rootlet neuroma [10].

Neuromuscular transmission disorders: Myasthenia gravis, others.

Neuropathies: Diphtheria, GBS, paraneoplastic.*Radiotherapy*: [11].

Surgery: Tonsillectomy [12].

Tardive dyskinesia: Can involve swallowing function.

Tonsillectomy: Post tonsillectomy [12, 13].

Toxic: Tetanus toxin, nitrofurantoin, salvarsan intoxication.

Trauma: Basal fracture of the skull.

Vascular: Brain stem lesions; see topographical lesions.*Other syndromes*:

Baroreceptors can be affected in syphilis and diabetes and autonomic disorders [14, 15].

Baroreflex failure after carotid surgery [14].

Glossopharyngeal neuralgia is a rare occurrence and is much less frequent than trigeminal neuralgia but with several trigger points. The pain radiates into the ear, pharynx, neck, and the base of the tongue. The attacks are brief but can be associated with excruciating pain. Glossopharyngeal neuralgia can be associated with fainting (reflex associated with the vagus nerve, which can cause syncope and bradycardia) [16].

Main Investigations

ENT, US, muscle myofascial release therapy (MRT); swallowing, endoscopy; EMG; baroreceptor testing.

Differential diagnosis: Bulbar muscular disorders, motor neuron disorders, myasthenia gravis, pain, trigeminal neuralgia.

Therapy

Depending on the symptoms:

Specific: *E.g.,* "swallowing," logopedic interventions.

Neuralgia: Pain therapy, *e.g.*, amitriptyline, carbamazepine, gabapentin.

Surgery: See Eagle's syndrome.

Interventions for specific conditions:

Eagle's syndrome: Surgery, various approaches [6].

Glossopharyngeal neuralgia: Decompression [17–19].

Prognosis: Depends on the cause.

References

1. Heckmann JG, Lang CJG. Neurological causes of taste disorders. Adv Otorhinolaryngol. 2006;63:255–64.
2. Sweasey TA, Edelstein SR, Hoff JT. Glossopharyngeal schwannoma: review of five cases and the literature. Surg Neurol. 1991;35(2):127–30.
3. Guerra-Mora JR, Del Castillo-Calcaneo JD, Cordoba-Mosqueda ME, Yanez-Castro J, Garcia-Gonzalez U, Soriano-Navarro E, et al. Malignant nerve sheath tumor involving glossopharyngeal, vagus and spinal nerve with intracranial-extracranial extension and systemic metastases in a patient with type 1 neurofibromatosis: a case report. Int J Surg Case Rep. 2016;29:196–200.
4. Badhey A, Jategaonkar A, Anglin Kovacs AJ, Kadakia S, De Deyn PP, Ducic Y, et al. Eagle syndrome: a comprehensive review. Clin Neurol Neurosurg. 2017;159:34–8.

5. Pietruszewska W, Wagrowska-Danilewicz M, Klatka J. Amyloidosis of the head and neck: a clinicopathological study of cases with long-term follow-up. Arch Med Sci. 2014;10(4):846–52.
6. Soh KB. The glossopharyngeal nerve, glossopharyngeal neuralgia and the Eagle's syndrome—current concepts and management. Singap Med J. 1999;40(10):659–65.
7. Hickman N, Mathews A. Cranial nerve injuries with supraglottic airway devices—more common than we think? Anaesthesia. 2015;70(9):1095–6.
8. Uzun C, Adali MK, Karasalihoglu AR. Unusual complication of tonsillectomy: taste disturbance and the lingual branch of the glossopharyngeal nerve. J Laryngol Otol. 2003;117(4):314–7.
9. Stathopoulos P, Dalakas MC. Autoimmune neurogenic dysphagia. Dysphagia. 2022;37(3):473–87.
10. Pomfrett CJ, Glover DG, Pollard BJ. The vagus nerve as a conduit for neuroinvasion, a diagnostic tool, and a therapeutic pathway for transmissible spongiform encephalopathies, including variant Creutzfeldt-Jacob disease. Med Hypotheses. 2007;68(6):1252–7.
11. Heir GM, Masterson M. Bilateral glossopharyngeal neuropathy following chemo and radiation therapy for a primitive neuroectodermal tumour. J Oral Rehabil. 2016;43(2):154–8.
12. Erdogan BA, Batum K. A rare complication of tonsillectomy: glossopharyngeal neuralgia. J Craniofac Surg. 2021;32(1):e100–e1.
13. Goins MR, Pitovski DZ. Posttonsillectomy taste distortion: a significant complication. Laryngoscope. 2004;114(7):1206–13.
14. Shah-Becker S, Pennock M, Sinoway L, Goldenberg D, Goyal N. Baroreceptor reflex failure: review of the literature and the potential impact on patients with head and neck cancer. Head Neck. 2017;39(10):2135–41
15. Iturriaga R, Alcayaga J, Chapleau MW, Somers VK. Carotid body chemoreceptors: physiology, pathology, and implications for health and disease. Physiol Rev. 2021;101(3):1177–235.
16. ICHD-3 IC. https://ichd-3org/13-painful-cranial-neuropathies-and-other-facial-pains/13-2-glossopharyngeal-neuralgia/13-2-1-glossopharyngeal-neuralgia/13-2-1-1-classical-glossopharyngeal-neuralgia/.
17. Jarrahy R, Cha ST, Eby JB, Berci G, Shahinian HK. Fully endoscopic vascular decompression of the glossopharyngeal nerve. J Craniofac Surg. 2002;13(1):90–5.
18. Zhu J, Sun J, Li R, Yu Y, Zhang L. Fully endoscopic versus microscopic vascular decompression for hemifacial spasm: a retrospective cohort study. Acta Neurochir. 2021;163(9):2417–23.
19. Pearce JM. Glossopharyngeal neuralgia. Eur Neurol. 2006;55(1):49–52.

One sentence: The vagus nerve is the longest CN, with the widest anatomical distribution, and it is important for swallowing and autonomic function (Figs. 15.1 and 15.2).

Genetic testing	NCV/EMG Autonomic testing	Laboratory	Imaging	Biopsy
	+		+	

Symptoms

Patients with vagus nerve damage experience swallowing difficulty and hoarseness of voice. "High" vagus nerve lesions are rare and are associated with ear and occipital pain.

Signs

Vagus nerve damage can cause paralysis of the palate, pharynx, and larynx according to the site of the lesion and cause dysphagia. Bilateral lesions can lead to a nasal voice and regurgitation through the nose. The gag reflex can be absent, and the uvula deviates away from the side of the lesion as a failure of palatal elevation occurs.

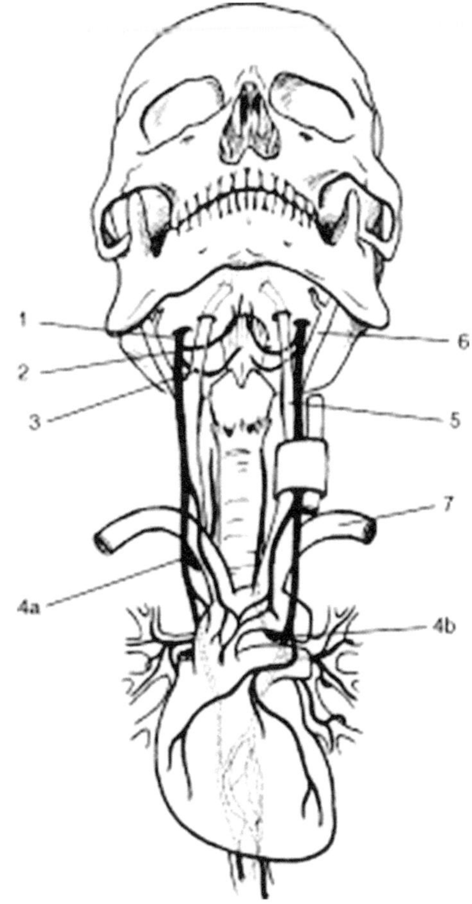

Fig. 15.1 *1* Vagus nerve, *2* pharyngeal branch, *3* internal laryngeal branch, *4a* right recurrent laryngeal nerve (across the subclavian artery), *4b* left recurrent laryngeal nerve (across the arch of the aorta), *5* internal carotid artery, *6* external carotid artery, *7* left subclavian artery

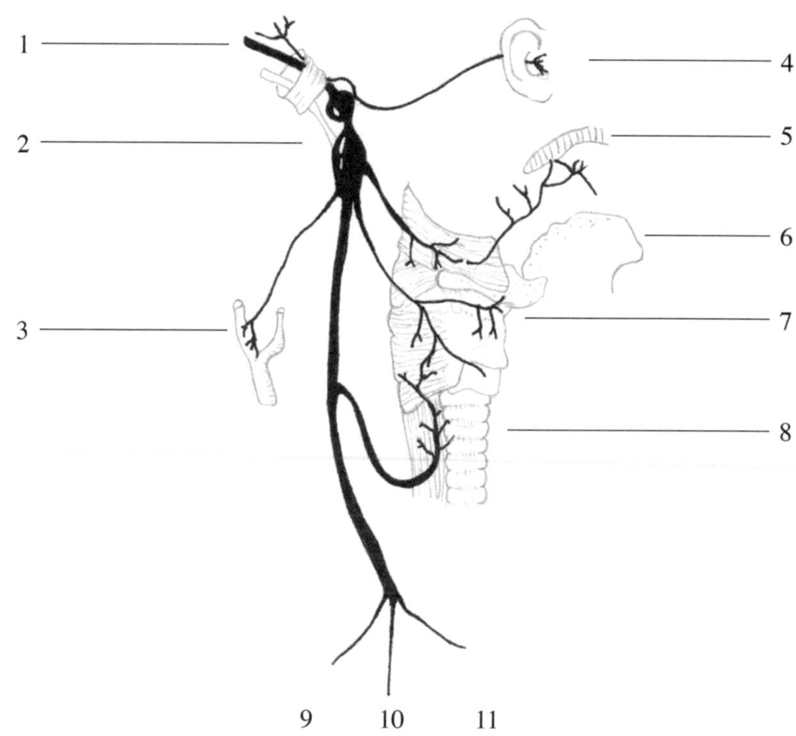

Fig. 15.2 Vagus nerve. *1* Vagus nerve, *2* ganglia, *3* branch to sinus, *4* auricular branch, *5* pharyngeal branch, *6* superior laryngeal nerve, *7* internal laryngeal nerve, *8* recurrent laryngeal nerve, and branches to *9* lung, *10* gastrointestinal tract, and *11* heart

Specific Qualities

Motor: +.

Branchial motor: Pharynx (except stylopharyngeus and tensor veli palatini), larynx, tongue. Striated muscle of soft palate.

Visceral motor: Smooth muscle and glands of pharynx, larynx, thoracic and abdominal viscera.

Sensory: +.

General sensory: Auditory meatus, skin on the back of the ear, external tympanic membrane, pharynx.

Visceral sensory: Larynx, trachea, esophagus, thoracic and abdominal viscera, stretch receptors in the wall of the aortic arch, chemoreceptors in the aortic body.

Autonomic: +.

Special senses: + (taste pharyngeal).

Other:

Location of Lesions

Central:

Supranuclear: Brain motor fibers for the ambiguous nucleus travel from the precentral gyrus via corticobulbar fibers. Impairment jointly with CN IX, XI, and XII.

Only mild symptoms occur in unilateral lesions. Bilateral lesions cause supranuclear palsy.

The dorsal motor nucleus (parasympathetic) receives input from the hypothalamus, olfactory nucleus, and reticular formation.

Brain stem and nuclear: Vascular syndromes, e.g., Avellis and Wallenberg syndrome.

Tumor: Brain stem glioma. Gross total surgical removal of malignant glioma [1].

Infection: diphtheria, herpes zoster encephalitis [2], poliomyelitis.

Intracranial Within the Skull:

The vagus nerve emerges from the medulla oblongata with several rootlets and exits through the jugular foramen, within the same dural sleeve as the accessory nerve.

Two external ganglia, the superior and inferior vagal ganglia, are found along the nerve's course within the jugular fossa of the petrous temporal bone.

Exit of the Skull:

The jugular foramen can be subdivided into three compartments (anterior, anteromedial, and posterolateral). CN IX, CN X, and CN XI are contained in the intermediate compartment. In the anteromedial portion of the jugular foramen, the tympanic branch of the glossopharyngeal nerve (Jacobsen's nerve) is located. The foramen is located behind the carotid canal.

CN X has two ganglia, the superior and the inferior.

The jugular foramen syndrome is well described in metastatic disease.

Vernet syndrome (jugular foramen syndrome): Describes lesions below the jugular foramen, also including CN XII.

Outside of the Skull:

Extracranial pathway: In the neck region, the nerve branches into the meningeal and auricular ramus, the pharyngeal rami, and the superior laryngeal nerve (internal and external rami). The pharyngeal rami innervate all the muscles of the pharynx, except the stylopharyngeus and the tensor veli palatini muscles. The superior laryngeal nerve divides into the internal and external laryngeal nerves. The external laryngeal branch supplies the inferior constrictor muscles. The vocal cords are innervated by the superior laryngeal nerve and the external and internal rami of the inferior laryngeal nerve. The esophageal ramus innervates the striated muscles of the esophagus.

The cervical branches can be asymmetric and are important in vagus nerve stimulation [3]. More distal branches are divided into thoracal and abdominal branches and carry autonomic fibers.

Thoracic branches: Inferior cardiac branches, anterior bronchial branches, posterior bronchial nerve.

Abdominal branches: Gastric, celiac, hepatic nerve.

Combination with Other CNs

Jugular foramen and base of the skull.

Causes and Frequency

Iatrogenic: Surgery of thyroid, neck, and mediastinal tumors, mediastinoscopy, surgery of the trachea and esophagus, thoracotomy, thyroid surgery (recurrent nerve), gastric surgery.

Infectious: Botulism, diphtheria, herpes, meningitis, poliomyelitis, tetanus [4].

Inflammatory/immune-mediated: Dermato- and polymyositis and sarcoid [5].

Neoplastic: Jugular foramen tumor, meningeal carcinomatosis, metastasis (with CN IX involvement), lymphoma [6].

Metabolic: Hyperpotassemia and hypophosphatemia.

Motor neuron disease.

Neuromuscular transmission disorders: Myasthenia gravis, others.

Side effects of vagus nerve stimulation: Voice alterations, vocal cord palsy, throat pain [7].

Surgery: Lung, mediastinum, esophageal cancer, and recurrent nerve in thyroid surgery [8].

Trauma: Fractures that affect the jugular foramen (uncommon). Hyperextension neck injuries are also sometimes associated with injury to these nerves at the cranio-cervical junction [9].

Combat and war: Recurrent laryngeal nerve, unilateral or bilateral, base of the skull injuries.

Toxic: Alcoholic polyneuropathy and thallium.

Tumor (rare): Glomus tumors [10], lymphoma [11], neurofibroma, neurogenic tumors [12], neurilemmoma [13], schwannoma.

Vascular: Medullary infarction, pharyngeal artery embolization (damage of vasa nervorum).

Others: Familial hypertrophic polyneuropathy, myopathies (chronic progressive external ophthalmoplegia, oculopharyngeal muscular dystrophy), polyneuropathies (amyloid – some types, diphtheria, alcohol). Tardive dyskinesia can involve laryngeal muscles.

Special nerve segments:

"High vagus lesions" involving the meningeal and occipital branch: Swallowing difficulties, hoarseness, local occipital pain, hypersensitivity of the ear [14].

Vagus recurrent nerve:

Focal superior and recurrent laryngeal neuropathies: Peripheral lesions affecting the recurrent laryngeal nerve, with or without involvement of the superior laryngeal nerve, are most common from trauma, surgery, thyroidectomies, carotid endarterectomies, or idiopathic causes.

The laryngeal neuropathy causes inability to forcefully cough, and hoarseness appears. Causes of focal damage of the recurrent laryngeal nerve include diseases of the lungs, tumors in the thoracic cavity (*e.g.*, lung cancer), and heart and lung transplant: [15] Aneurysm of the aortic arch, enlarged lymph nodes, and thyroid surgery. Cervical disc surgery by anterior approach [16]. About 25% of cases are idiopathic [17].

Recurrent laryngeal nerve lesions: Hoarseness is observed in local anesthetic procedures, presumably due to excessive local anesthetic spread.

Multiple CN: [18].

Other entities:

Focal laryngeal dystonia.

The gag reflex can be diminished in patients with schizophrenia, obesity treatment, sexual dysfunction in women after spinal cord injury, and spastic dystonia.

Neuralgia of the laryngeal nerve (rare) [19].

Main Investigations

Diagnosis can be facilitated with ENT examination and vocal cord inspection (with endoscopy), imaging, and video swallowing studies. EMG of the cricothyroid muscle (superior laryngeal nerve) or thyroarytenoid muscle (recurrent nerve) can be done but is uncommon.

Differential diagnosis: Bulbar disorders. Motor neuron diseases, neuromuscular transmission disorders.

Therapy

Treatment depends upon the etiology:

Surgical reinnervation techniques after trauma [20].

Monitoring: Thyroid surgery [21].

Vagus nerve stimulation for intractable hiccup treatment [22].

Prognosis: Prognosis depends upon the etiology.

References

1. Kyoshima K, Sakai K, Goto T, Tanabe A, Sato A, Nagashima H, et al. Gross total surgical removal of malignant glioma from the medulla oblongata: report of two adult cases with reference to surgical anatomy. J Clin Neurosci. 2004;11(1):75–80.
2. Cao DH, Xie YN, Ji Y, Han JZ, Zhu JG. A case of varicella zoster encephalitis with glossopharyngeal and vagus nerve injury as primary manifestation combined with medulla lesion. J Int Med Res. 2019;47(5):2256–61.
3. Hammer N, Glatzner J, Feja C, Kuhne C, Meixensberger J, Planitzer U, et al. Human vagus nerve branching in the cervical region. PLoS One. 2015;10(2):e0118006.
4. Amin MR, Koufman JA. Vagal neuropathy after upper respiratory infection: a viral etiology? Am J Otolaryngol. 2001;22(4):251–6.
5. Vaile JH, Davis P. Isolated unilateral vagus nerve palsy in systemic lupus erythematosus. J Rheumatol. 1998;25(11):2287–8.
6. Mustafa R, Neth BJ, Stitt D. Bilateral Vagus nerve enhancement in a patient with leptomeningeal lymphoplasmacytic lymphoma presenting with intractable hiccups. JAMA Neurol. 2021;78(4):493–4.
7. Verlinden TJ, Rijkers K, Hoogland G, Herrler A. Morphology of the human cervical vagus nerve: implications for vagus nerve stimulation treatment. Acta Neurol Scand. 2016;133(3):173–82.

8. Gunn A, Oyekunle T, Stang M, Kazaure H, Scheri R. Recurrent laryngeal nerve injury after thyroid surgery: an analysis of 11,370 patients. J Surg Res. 2020;255:42–9.

9. Aygun D, Acar E. Isolated unilateral vagus nerve palsy secondary to trauma. Ulus Travma Acil Cerrahi Derg. 2013;19(2):180–2.

10. Netterville JL, Jackson CG, Miller FR, Wanamaker JR, Glasscock ME. Vagal paraganglioma: a review of 46 patients treated during a 20-year period. Arch Otolaryngol Head Neck Surg. 1998;124(10):1133–40.

11. Boasquevisque GS, Guidoni J, Moreira de Souza LA, Gonçalves PG, Andrade CV, Pedras FV, Boasquevisque EM, Boasquevisque ET. Bilateral vagus nerve neurolymphomatosis diagnosed using PET/CT and diffusion-weighted MRI. Clin Nucl Med. 2012;37(9):e225–8.

12. Sugio K, Inoue T, Inoue K, Tateishi M, Ishida T, Sugimachi K. Neurogenic tumors of the mediastinum originated from the vagus nerve. Eur J Surg Oncol. 1995;21(2):214–6.

13. Yumoto E, Nakamura K, Mori T, Yanagihara N. Parapharyngeal vagal neurilemmoma extending to the jugular foramen. J Laryngol Otol. 1996;110(5):485–9.

14. Grisold W, Schwarzmeier J, Frei K, Neumuller G, Breier F. Ti.: "High" vagus nerve lesions in varicella zoster infection. eNeurologicalSci 2021;23:100337

15. Murty GE, Smith MC. Recurrent laryngeal nerve palsy following heart-lung transplantation: three cases of vocal cord augmentation in the acute phase. J Laryngol Otol. 1989;103(10):968–9.

16. Bertalanffy H, Eggert HR. Complications of anterior cervical discectomy without fusion in 450 consecutive patients. Acta Neurochir. 1989;99(1-2):41–50.

17. Reiter R, Hoffmann TK, Rotter N, Pickhard A, Scheithauer MO, Brosch S. Etiology, diagnosis, differential diagnosis and therapy of vocal fold paralysis. Laryngorhinootologie. 2014;93(3):161–73.

18. Erman AB, Kejner AE, Hogikyan ND, Feldman EL. Disorders of cranial nerves IX and X. Semin Neurol. 2009;29(1):85–92.

19. Kandan SR, Khan S, Jeyaretna DS, Lhatoo S, Patel NK, Coakham HB. Neuralgia of the glossopharyngeal and vagal nerves: long-term outcome following surgical treatment and literature review. Br J Neurosurg. 2010;24(4):441–6.

20. Aynehchi BB, McCoul ED, Sundaram K. Systematic review of laryngeal reinnervation techniques. Otolaryngol Head Neck Surg. 2010;143(6):749–59.

21. Abt NB, Puram SV, Kamani D, Modi R, Randolph GW. Neuromonitored thyroid surgery: optimal stimulation based on intraoperative EMG response features. Laryngoscope. 2020;130(12):E970–E5.

22. De Vloo P, Dallapiazza RF, Lee DJ, Zurowski M, Peng PW, Chen R, et al. Long-term relief of intractable hiccups with vagal nerve stimulation. Brain Stimul. 2018;11(6):1385–7.

One sentence: The accessory nerve, or CN XI, is a motor nerve that stems from the brainstem and cervical cord, and it is involved in complex eye tracking movements.

Genetic testing	NCV/ EMG	Laboratory	Imaging	Biopsy
	+		+	

Symptoms

Weakness of the shoulder and shoulder drop. Damage to the accessory nerve can cause shoulder pain of variable severity over the shoulder and scapula.

Signs

Trapezius muscle weakness causes shoulder drop, atrophy of trapezius muscle. Inability to lift the shoulder and raise the arm above the horizontal plane. If affected, atrophy and weakness of the sternocleidomastoid muscle and impaired head rotation to the opposite side. Scapular winging (medial margin).

Specific Qualities

Motor: Most of the motor supply to the trapezius muscle is derived from the accessory nerve, with contribution from the cervical plexus [1].

Sensory:

Autonomic:

Special senses:

Other: The accessory nerve is the only cranial nerve which enters and exits the skull. Anatomically, a distinction between the brainstem and spinal fibers is made. The "transitional nerve" is involved in laryngopharyngeal innervation. The sternocleidomastoid muscles have a prominent role in oculomotor tracking (Fig. 16.1).

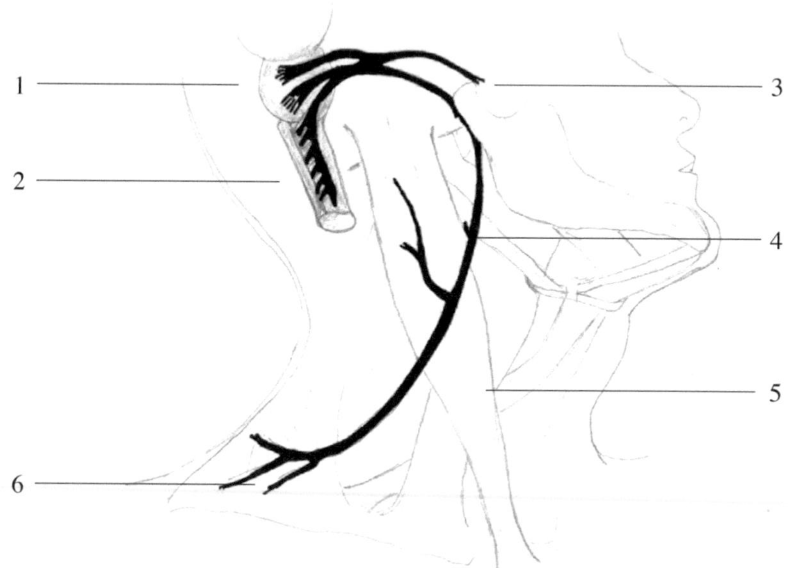

Fig. 16.1 Accessory nerve. *1* cranial roots, *2* spinal roots, *3* branch to soft palate, *4* accessory nerve, *5* sternocleidomastoid muscle, *6* trapezius muscle

Location of Lesion

Central: The "central" unilateral supranuclear lesions tend to cause mild and transient weakness, as the accessory nerve nuclei receive bilateral cortical input. Hemispheric lesions rarely cause a clinically relevant CN XI paresis.

"Dissociated weakness" of the sternocleidomastoid and trapezius muscles have been reported in brainstem lesions.

Intracranial within the skull: Infections; tumors, e.g., schwannoma.

Exit of the skull: At the jugular foramen: Lesions occur in association with the glossopharyngeal and vagus nerves, e.g., Vernet's syndrome, local tumors, schwannomas, metastasis, sarcoidosis, and Collet–Sicard syndrome.

A lesion at the cervicomedullary junction produces a weakness of the ipsilateral sternocleidomastoid and weakness of the *contralateral* trapezius.

Outside of the skull: Injury to the neck: Biting, blunt trauma, carotid endarterectomy, coronary bypass surgery, radiation, shoulder blows, shoulder dislocation, stretch/hyperextension injury, strangulation, variants of neuralgic amyotrophy.

Combination with Other CN

CN IX, X in base of the skull lesions or tumors.

Causes and Frequency

Dystonia: A cervical lesion of the CN XI can result in cervical dystonia or torticollis (in addition to the more common cause of centrally caused dystonia).

Iatrogenic: Surgery in the neck (posterior cervical triangle), deep cervical lymph node removal, "neck dissection procedures," shunt implantation (Fig. 16.2), fibrosis following radiotherapy, shoulder support in the Trendelenburg position.

Neoplastic: Collet–Sicard syndrome, ENT tumors, base of skull metastases (all tumors, in particular multiple myeloma, prostate, ENT, and

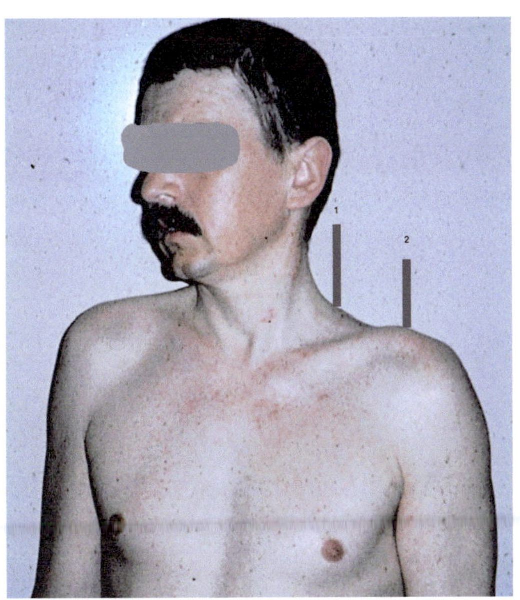

Fig. 16.2 Accessory lesion below the left sternocleido-mastoid muscle (after a shunt procedure). *1* atrophy of the trapezius muscle, *2* prominent difference in shoulder rounding, lower position of clavicula

Hodgkin's disease). Neurolemmoma, nerve sheath tumors. Spinal tumors, retrograde infiltration from adjacent tumors [2].

Torticollis: [3].

Trauma: [4], strangulation [5]. War and combat: Blunt and penetrating injuries to the neck, fractures of the jugular foramen.

Others: Motor neuron disorders, neck surgery (Fig. 16.3); spinal tumors and syringomyelia.

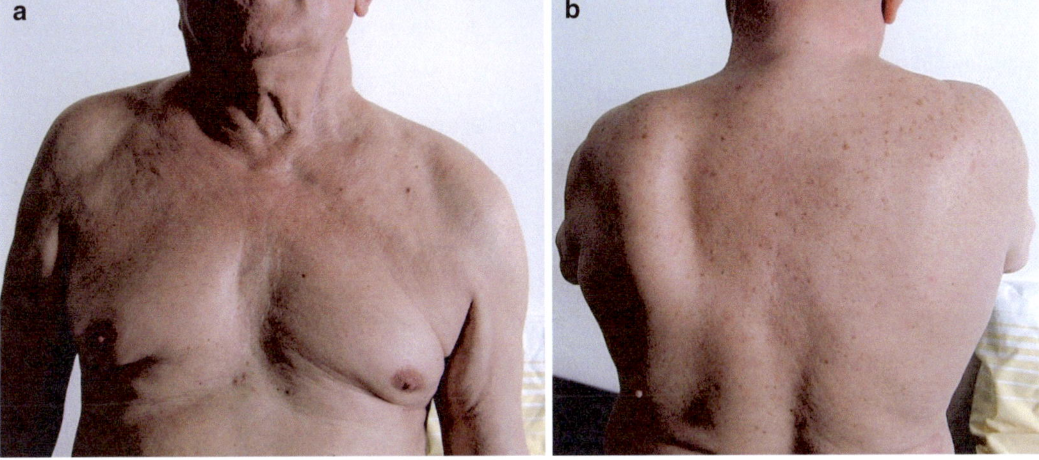

Fig. 16.3 Left accessory nerve palsy, following carotid resection: (**a**) note the unilateral atrophy of the trapezoid muscle and (**b**) the winging of the scapula with the abduction of the medial scapular border

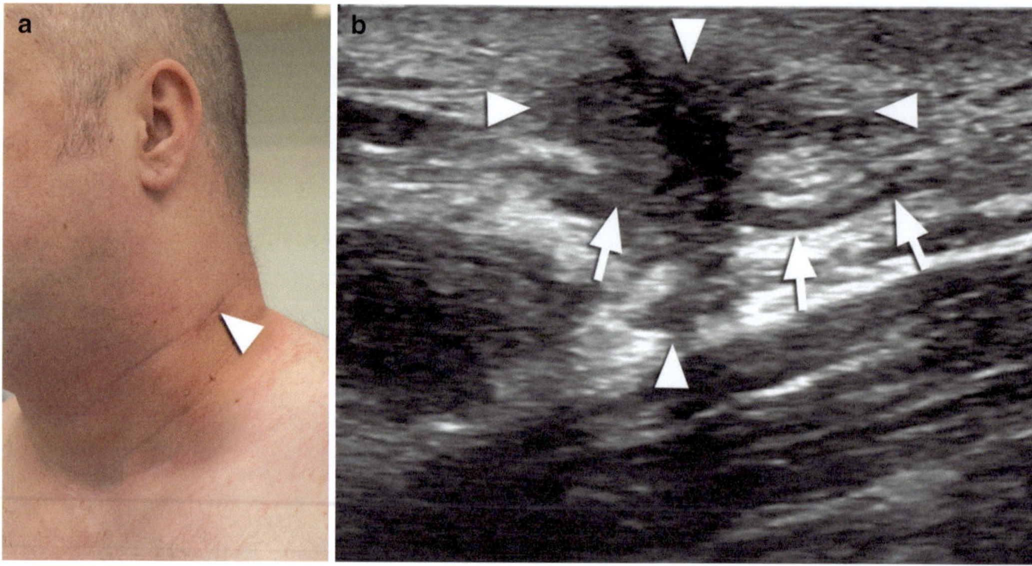

Fig. 16.4 Ultrasound of the accessory nerve. (**a**) A complete loss of function of the trapezius muscle occurred after diagnostic surgical lymph node removal. (**b**) Ultrasound examination revealed a scar tissue formation (arrowheads) surrounding the accessory nerve (arrows), which is intact

Main investigations

Clinical and electrophysiology diagnosis.

Sternocleidomastoid muscle: Impaired head rotation.

Trapezius muscle: Upper, middle, and lower parts of the trapezius muscle must be examined separately. Upper and middle part lesions may produce winging of the scapula.

NCV: Stimulation of the nerve at the posterior aspect of the sternocleidomastoid muscle.

EMG: Sternocleidomastoid, trapezoid upper, middle, and lower part.

Imaging: MR of neck and shoulder muscles.

Ultrasound: The sternocleidomastoid muscle can be visualized in ultrasound (Fig. 16.4).

Therapy

Nerve grafting (bridge): Reconstruction of the spinal accessory nerve with [6]; operations are not effective in long-standing scars; orthotic devices are not effective. The nerve is also used as a transferable nerve in neurotization and reinnervation [7].

Prognosis: Uncertain; recovery is slow and often incomplete. Further exploration is warranted if no improvement occurs after closed trauma.

References

1. Johal J, Iwanaga J, Tubbs K, Loukas M, Oskouian RJ, Tubbs RS. The accessory nerve: a comprehensive review of its anatomy, development, variations, landmarks and clinical considerations. Anat Rec (Hoboken). 2019;302(4):620–9.
2. Fabrizi AP, Poppi M, Giuliani G, Gambari PI, Gaist G. Benign solitary nerve sheath tumors of the spinal accessory nerve in the posterior triangle of the neck. Report of two cases. J Neurosurg Sci. 1992;36(4):247–50.
3. Tomczak KK, Rosman NP. Torticollis. J Child Neurol. 2013;28(3):365–78.
4. Tekin T, Ege T. Late-onset spinal accessory nerve palsy after traffic accident: case report. Ulus Travma Acil Cerrahi Derg. 2012;18(4):364–6.
5. Iserson KV. Strangulation: a review of ligature, manual, and postural neck compression injuries. Ann Emerg Med. 1984;13(3):179–85.
6. Mayer JA, Hruby LA, Salminger S, Bodner G, Aszmann OC. Reconstruction of the spinal accessory nerve with selective fascicular nerve transfer of the upper trunk. J Neurosurg Spine. 2019;31(1):133–8.
7. Rohde RS, Wolfe SW. Nerve transfers for adult traumatic brachial plexus palsy (brachial plexus nerve transfer). HSS J. 2007;3(1):77–82.

One sentence: The hypoglossal nerve controls the somatic motor intrinsic and extrinsic muscles of the tongue, except for the palatoglossus muscle (Fig. 17.1).

Genetic testing	NCV/ EMG	Laboratory	Imaging	Biopsy
	+		+	+

Symptoms

Unilateral loss of hypoglossal function causes mild difficulties with speaking, but swallowing is not impaired. Bilateral impairment leads to speech difficulties and severe difficulty with bolus transport due to reduced oral transport. Headache may occur in hypoglossal lesions due to its anastomosis with the ansa cervicalis.

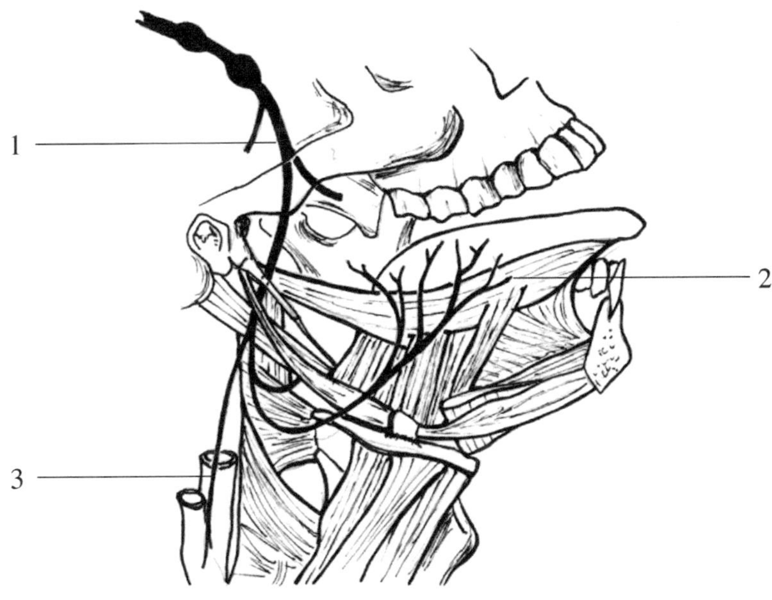

Fig. 17.1 Hypoglossal nerve. *1* hypoglossal nerve, *2* branches to the tongue, *3* branches to carotid body

Signs

Central lesions with weakness cause a deviation to the side of the weakness upon protrusion of the tongue. Spasticity can reduce tongue movements. Brainstem bulbar lesions are rare.

Peripheral lesions cause wasting of the tongue on the affected side, with deviation of the tongue towards the side of weakness. Bilateral wasting occurs in motor neuron disease (MND) and bilateral peripheral lesions. Fasciculations are characteristic. Difficulty with food transport occurs within the oral cavity.

Specific Qualities

Motor: + Somatic motor intrinsic and extrinsic muscles of the tongue except the palatoglossus muscle.

Sensory:

Autonomic:

Special senses:

Other: The hypoglossal nerve has several types of anastomoses with the cervical plexus [1].

Location: [2]

Central:

Unilateral supranuclear lesions have small effects and are usually associated with other associated neurologic findings, such as in stroke [3].

Bilateral supranuclear lesions (e.g., pseudobulbar palsy from bilateral or repeated infarctions) cause bilateral tongue paralysis and dysarthria.

Brainstem nuclear lesions: Vascular, demyelinating diseases, tumors, infections (poliomyelitis), and syringobulbia.

Intracranial within the skull:

Lesions in the subarachnoid space.

Infections: Meningitis, osteomyelitis.

Tumors: Meningioma, metastases, paraglioma, schwannoma. Nasopharyngeal as well as head and neck malignancies can extend posteriorly to the clivus and reach the hypoglossal canal.

Other causes: Trauma, skull fracture, and vertebral artery dissection.

Exit of the skull:

Lesion of the canalis nervi hypoglossi: Metastasis and tumors.

Infections, osteomyelitis, and trauma, e.g., occipital fractures.

Outside of the skull:

Lesions within the carotid space: Aneurysm, dissection [4, 5], carotid artery interventions. Close contact with the cervical plexus [6].

Infections: Teeth conditions and dentistry [7].

Iatrogenic: Carotid endarterectomy, post radiotherapy, local puncture or interventions.

Movement disorders: Tongue tremor is rarely seen in Parkinson disease [8]. The tongue can be involved in dystonic movements, such as in oromandibular dystonia (cranial dystonia).

Neoplastic: Schwannoma, metastasis, and other tumors.

Trauma: [9].

Others: Tongue atrophy indicates a peripheral lesion. Macroglossia can occur in several conditions; see "tongue," e.g., amyloid deposition (Fig. 17.2c).

Lesions in the sublingual space and tongue: Iatrogenic (floor of mouth surgery), infection (e.g., odontogenic abscess), neoplasms (squamous cell cancer from base of the tongue), tongue tumor [10], tongue necrosis.

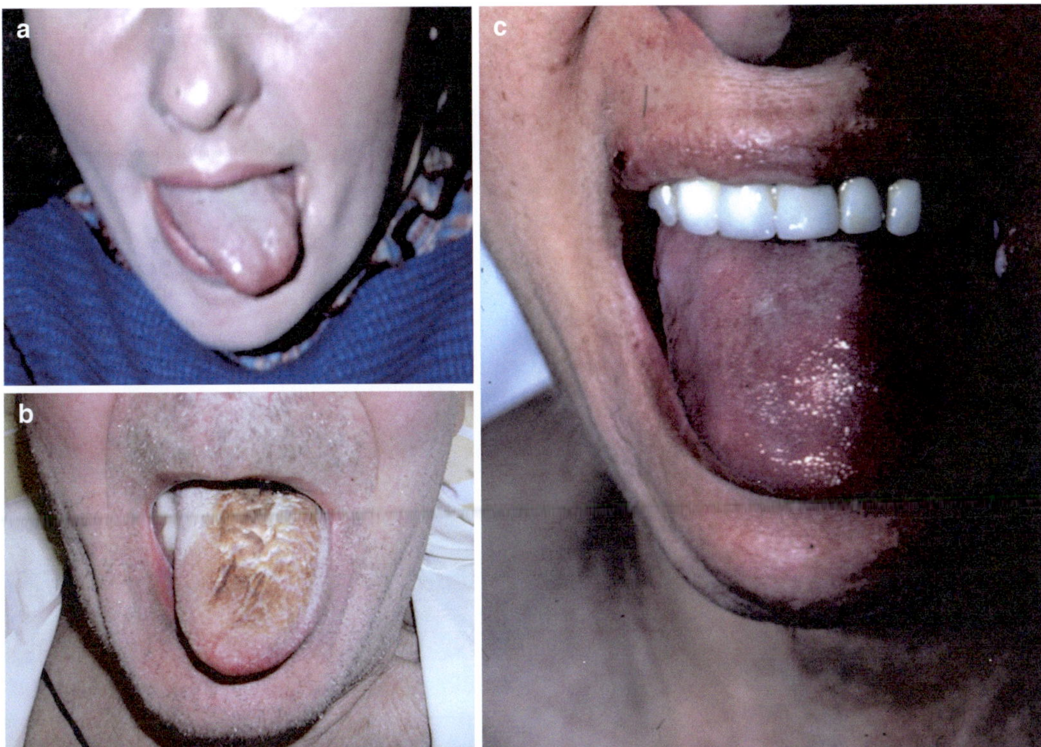

Fig. 17.2 (**a**) Left hypoglossal peripheral paresis. Note deviation of the tongue to the left. (**b**) Right-sided hypoglossal paresis, in a patient with meningeal carcinomatosis. Midline of the tongue is shifted to the right. (**c**) Amyloid tongue in a patient with multiple myeloma. Patient's subjective impression was that the tongue was "too big"

Combination with Other CN

Multiple CN (IX, X, XI) lesions: Collet–Sicard syndrome and base of the skull tumors.

Causes and Frequency

This CN is rarely affected in isolation, except in disorders of the base of the skull and neck.

Genetic: Chiari malformation, cerebral, ocular, auricular, dental, skeletal (CODAS), hemiatrophy tongue [11], hereditary liability to pressure palsies (HNPP) [12].

Iatrogenic: Surgery of the oral cavity and neck and dentistry [13].

Carotid endarterectomy, radiotherapy, in association with other CNs, compression of the lateral part of the tongue (with lingual nerve following laryngoscopy, intubation, neck extension, tooth extraction) [14].

Idiopathic: Isolated unexplained pathogenesis, usually reversible (Fig. 17.2a).

Immune-mediated: Myasthenia gravis, triple furrowed tongue (Fig. 17.3).

Infection: Basal meningitis, mononucleosis, granulomatous meningitis, postvaccination mononeuropathy, toxoplasmosis.

Inflammatory/immune-mediated: Rheumatoid arthritis (subluxation of odontoid process in rheumatoid arthritis), Paget's disease, giant cell arteritis, and tongue necrosis.

Neoplastic: Schwannoma, primary nerve tumors (neurinoma, neurofibroma) (Fig. 17.4), metastasis to the base of the skull, meningeal carcinomatosis (Fig. 17.2b), clivus metastasis (can be bilateral as nerves are close to the midline), lesion of the hypoglossal canal by glomus jugulare tumors, meningioma, and chordoma (sometimes in association with other CNs). Tongue carcinoma can infiltrate the nerve and lymph nodes, as with Hodgkin's disease and Burkitt's lymphoma, amyloid nerve deposition in myeloma, and post radiation of neck tumors. Hemangioma [15].

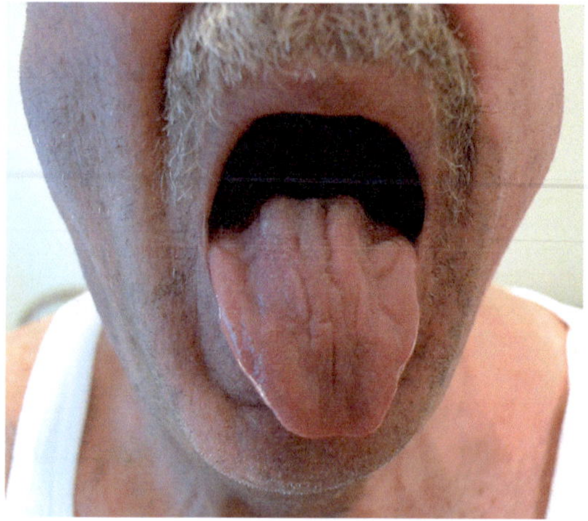

Fig. 17.3 Triple furrowed tongue: this patient suffered about 20 years from myasthenia gravis. Despite modern and intensive treatment, the bulbar symptoms were never completely controlled. The tongue shows "tripled furrowed tongue" atrophy

Paraneoplastic: Rare [16].

Tongue necrosis: Giant cell arteritis, endotracheal tubes, overinflated cuff or an oversized endotracheal tube.

Variety of conditions, most frequently from vasculitides, hypercoagulable states, or arterial emboli and thrombi [17]. Hematoma and anticoagulation [18].

Rarely bilateral [19].

Trauma: Head injury, penetrating head wound (often with other CN injuries), or dental extraction. Hyperextension of the neck.

Gunshot wound [20, 21] and knife lesions. Rare.

Anesthesiology airway mask [22].

Vascular: Vertebral basilar aneurysm, dissection of internal carotid artery [4].

Vasculitis: Giant cell arteritis and tongue necrosis [23].

Brainstem lesion: Medial medulla oblongata.

Blood supply of the lower CNs: The neuromeningeal trunk of the ascending pharyngeal artery supplies CN IX–XII. Embolization or ligation of this vessel in selective tumor therapy can cause CN damage. See Angiosomal supply of the lower CN.

Other causes:

Bilateral CN XII lesions: Motor neuron disorders, especially ALS, appear as bilateral hypo-

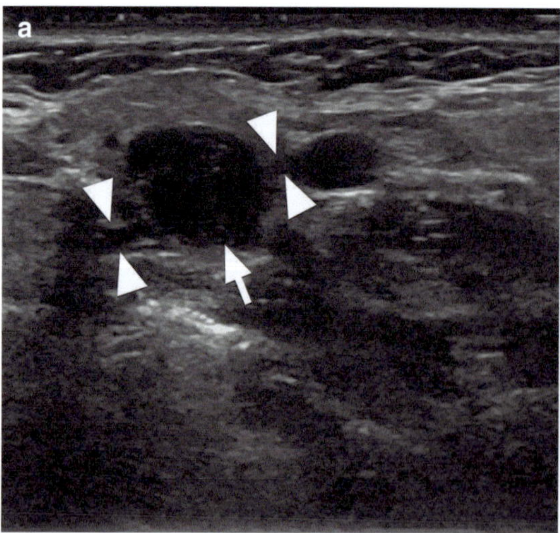
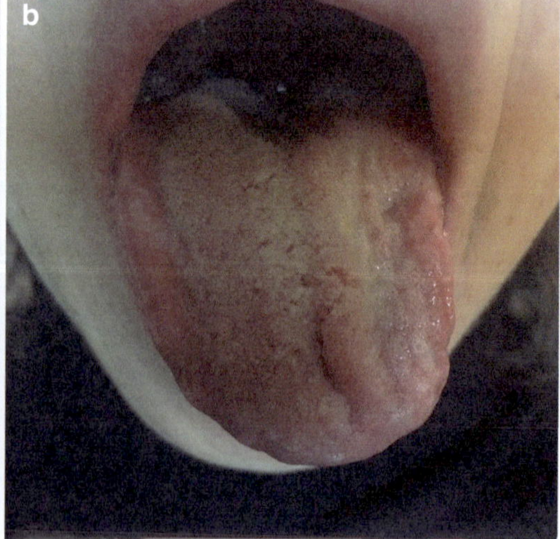

Fig. 17.4 Tumor in the hypoglossal nerve. (**a**) High-resolution ultrasound scan of the hypoglossal nerve (*arrowheads*) which is infiltrated by a tumor (*arrow*) causing (**b**) the hemiatrophy of the tongue

glossal nerve lesions. Intubation, MS, neoplasm, tongue necrosis. Facial onset sensory and motor neuropathy (*FOSMN*) and hereditary motor–sensory neuropathy type 4D (CMT 4D) causing tongue atrophy.

Reconstructive surgery: Use of CN XII in facial nerve palsy (anastomosis) [24] and motor relearning in rehabilitation [25].

Other tongue-related syndromes: See Chap. 18.

Glossodynia: Burning pain in the tongue and also oral mucosa, usually occurring in middle-aged or elderly persons.

"Burning" tongue: Vitamin B12 deficiency and several systemic diseases.

Eagle syndrome: Unilateral or bilateral [26].

Movement disorders: Orolingual tremor, Parkinson's disease [27], essential tongue tremor [8], myokymia (post RT) [28], glossopharyngeal spasm (neuroleptics).

Main Investigations

Clinical examination: Ultrasound (Fig. 17.5), CT, MR.

Electrophysiology: EMG of the tongue, magnetic brain stimulation.

Magnetic resonance tomography (MRT): Dynamic MRT swallowing, muscle tissue (muscle denervation: acute edema, T2 hyperintense, contrasts enhancement, minimal fatty replacement.)

Differential diagnosis: Motor neuron disease (ALS), pseudobulbar involvement, local tumors affecting the tongue, tongue necrosis.

Therapy

Treatment is based on the underlying cause.

References

1. Caliot P, Dumont D, Bousquet V, Midy D. A note on the anastomoses between the hypoglossal nerve and the cervical plexus. Surg Radiol Anat. 1986;8(1):75–9.
2. Manoli A, Ploumidou K, Georgopapadakos N, Stratzias P, Skandalakis PN, Angelis S, et al. Hypoglossal nerve: anatomy, anatomical variations comorbidities and clinical significance. J Long Term Eff Med Implants. 2019;29(3):197–203.
3. Brown DL, Chervin RD, Wolfe J, Hughes R, Concannon M, Lisabeth LD, et al. Hypoglossal nerve dysfunction and sleep-disordered breathing after stroke. Neurology. 2014;82(13):1149–52.
4. Lindsay FW, Mullin D, Keefe MA. Subacute hypoglossal nerve paresis with internal carotid artery dissection. Laryngoscope. 2003;113(9):1530–3.
5. Allingham W, Devakumar V, Herwadkar A, Punter M. Hypoglossal nerve palsy due to internal carotid artery dissection. Neurohospitalist. 2018;8(4):199.
6. Kariuki BN, Butt F, Mandela P, Odula P. Surgical anatomy of the cervical part of the hypoglossal nerve. Craniomaxillofac Trauma Reconstr. 2018;11(1):21–7.
7. Durrani F, Singh R. Isolated hypoglossal nerve palsy due to infected impacted tooth. Case Rep Med. 2009;2009:231947.
8. Kusanale A, Wilson A, Brennan P. Tongue tremor: a rare initial presentation of essential tremor. Br J Oral Maxillofac Surg. 2011;49(8):e82–3.
9. Muthukumar N. Delayed hypoglossal palsy following occipital condyle fracture—case report. J Clin Neurosci. 2002;9(5):580–2.
10. Nestola DF, Lombardi M, Brucoli M, Pia F, Aluffi P. Isolated hypoglossal nerve palsy mimicking a base of tongue tumor. J Craniofac Surg. 2017;28(1):e78–80.
11. Strauss KA, Jinks RN, Puffenberger EG, Venkatesh S, Singh K, Cheng I, et al. CODAS syndrome is associated with mutations of LONP1, encoding mitochondrial AAA+ Lon protease. Am J Hum Genet. 2015;96(1):121–35.
12. Winter WC, Juel VC. Hypoglossal neuropathy in hereditary neuropathy with liability to pressure palsy. Neurology. 2003;61(8):1154–5.

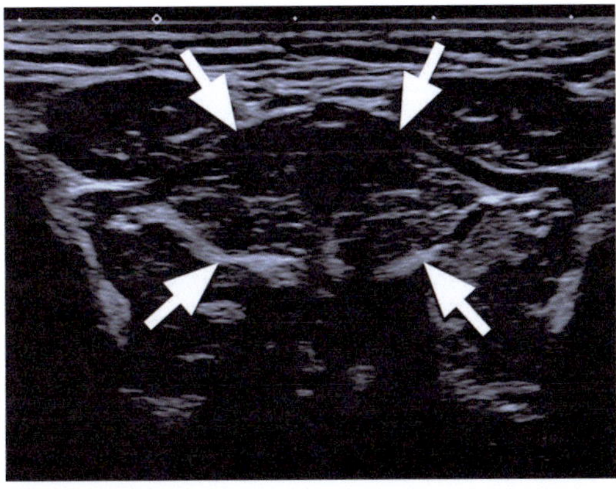

Fig. 17.5 Ultrasound of tongue. This technique allows a painless investigation of the tongue tissue and can detect movements as fasciculations. Arrows indicate circumference of the tongue

13. De Santis F, Martini G, Thuringen P, Thaler M, Mani G, Steckholzer K. Internal carotid artery dissection after inferior alveolar nerve block for third molar dental care presented as hypoglossal nerve palsy. Vasc Endovasc Surg. 2012;46(7):591–5.
14. Fritz MA, Kang BJ, Fox TP, Bhatia N, Mandel SM. Iatrogenic hypoglossal nerve palsy. Expert opinion. 2014:13–6. https://practicalneurology.com/pdfs/PN0214_ExpertOpinion_IHNP.pdf.
15. Kamala KA, Ashok L, Sujatha GP. Cavernous hemangioma of the tongue: a rare case report. Contemp Clin Dent. 2014;5(1):95–8.
16. Ohta Y, Kawahara Y, Tadokoro K, Sato K, Sasaki R, Takahashi Y, et al. Asymmetrical and isolated hypoglossal nerve palsy accompanied by a new subset of anti-ganglioside antibodies in a patient with diffuse large B cell lymphoma. Intern Med. 2019;58(2):283–6.
17. Braun V, Mayer M, Antoniadis G, Richter HP, Schroder JM. Reconstruction of the spinal accessory nerve with an anastomosis to the dorsal C3 branch: technical note. Neurosurgery. 1996;38(1):208–10.
18. Nogueira J, Parente AR, Mendes A, Lavadinho I. Tongue hematoma with necrosis. Cureus. 2021;13(1):e12741.
19. Sainuddin S, Saeed NR. Acute bilateral tongue necrosis—a case report. Br J Oral Maxillofac Surg. 2008;46(8):671–2.
20. Roofe SB, Kolb CM, Seibert J. Chapter 18. Cranial nerve injuries. In: Otolaryngology/head and neck surgery combat casualty care in operation Iraqi freedom and operation enduring freedom 2015. 2016. Textbooks of military medicine. isbn:9780160930348.
21. Shahzadi S, Abouzari M, Rashidi A. Bilateral traumatic hypoglossal nerve transection in a blast injury. Surg Neurol. 2007;68(4):464–5.
22. Stewart A, Lindsay WA. Bilateral hypoglossal nerve injury following the use of the laryngeal mask airway. Anaesthesia. 2002;57(3):264–5.
23. Payen C, Kucharczak F, Favier V. Giant cell arteritis presenting with progressive dysphagia and tongue necrosis. CMAJ. 2022;194(11):E420.
24. Ozsoy U, Hizay A, Demirel BM, Ozsoy O, Bilmen Sarikcioglu S, Turhan M, et al. The hypoglossal-facial nerve repair as a method to improve recovery of motor function after facial nerve injury. Ann Anat. 2011;193(4):304–13.
25. Negley KJ, Rasool A, Byrne PJ. Motor relearning after hypoglossal-facial nerve anastomosis. Am J Phys Med Rehabil. 2021;100(6):e85–8.
26. Altun D, Camci E. Bilateral hypoglossal nerve paralysis following elongated styloid process resection: case report. J Anesth. 2016;30(6):1082–6.
27. Fabbri M, Abreu L, Santos T, Ferreira JJ. Resting and reemergent tongue tremor as presenting symptoms of Parkinson's disease. Mov Disord Clin Pract. 2017;4(2):273–4.
28. Leupold D, Schilg L, Felbecker A, Kim OC, Tettenborn B, Hundsberger T. Unilateral tongue myokymia—a rare topodiagnostic sign of different clinical conditions. J Clin Neurosci. 2017;45:132–3.

The term "side topics" refers to CN functions which are often not confined to an isolated CN, but are within the control of several CNs or other local structures.

An example is the pupil, which is regulated by the function of several CNs with different functions (special, sensory, and autonomic). Another example is the eyelids, where function also depends on the mechanical aspects of the lid, fibers and fascia, and other tissues and mechanical components.

It is helpful to have a detailed description of some of the different functions. This information will be structured in a compendial way and will limit the anatomy to essentials, as anatomy is mentioned in a previous respective chapter.

Herein, we include short clinical comments on:

- The pupil
- Horner's syndrome
- The eyelids
- Ptosis
- The oral cavity and dysphagia
- The tongue
- Multiple CN lesions
- CNs in coma
- Anastomosis of CNs
- The concept of angiosoma

Pain in CNs is covered in Chap. 34.

The Pupil

Sympathetic innervation	Parasympathetic innervation	Optic nerve (reflex)
Dilatator pupillae	Sphincter pupillae	Afferent for light perception

The pupil is innervated by two antagonistic muscles. The circular muscle of the iris, the dilatator, is innervated by the sympathetic nerve (cervical sympathetic), and the pupillary sphincter is innervated by parasympathetic fibers from CN III.

The pupil reacts to light, depending on the function of the optic nerve, and convergence, which also needs the function of the optic nerve and additionally an intact complex reflex mechanism, which may be impaired in the elderly [1]. Convergence paresis is rarely unilateral [2].

Usually the pupils are symmetric, have the same size (isocoria), and react directly and indirectly to light as well as constrict with convergence. They are usually round and, at constant light exposure, maintain their size. A difference in size is termed anisocoria. About 20% of the population has a slight anisocoria [3]. Dyscoria is the term for an abnormal shape of the pupil.

Mechanical anisocoria can be caused by trauma, inflammation, angle closure glaucoma leading to iris occlusion, and local tumors. In addition to pupillary changes due to light and convergence, spontaneous movements of the pupils occur rarely (e.g., hippus) [4].

Congenital anomalies include aniridia, coloboma, and ectopic pupil.

Aged persons have often smaller and mildly unrounded pupils.

Conditions Associated with Pupillary Dysfunction

Paralysis of sphincter pupillae: Lesion between the Edinger–Westphal nucleus and the eye. The pupil widens due to the unantagonized action of the sympathetic iris dilatator muscle.

Paralysis of dilatator pupillae: Ocular sympathetic paralysis, as in Horner's syndrome.

Paralysis of accommodation: Drugs such as antidepressants, atropine, eserine, homatropine, pilocarpine, and psychotropics. Cocaine causes dilatation by stimulating sympathetic nerve endings.

Pharmacological effects: Cocaine, apraclonidine, hydroxyamphetamine, and pilocarpine are used in testing various dysfunctions of the pupil to distinguish between central (first order), preganglionic (second order), or postganglionic (third order) lesion.

Mydriasis: Can be caused by anticholinergics (atropine, homatropine, tropicamide, scopolamine, and cyclopentolate) and sympathomimetics (adrenaline, clonidine, and phenylephrine). Scopolamine patches, glycopyrrolate antiperspirants, nasal vasoconstrictors, blue nightshade, and Angel's trumpet can also dilate the pupils.

Miosis: Pilocarpine is a nonselective muscarinic receptor agonist in the parasympathetic nervous system that may cause a small and poorly reactive pupil. Prostaglandins, opioids, and organophosphate insecticides can constrict pupils.

Anisocoria: Adie's tonic pupil or Adie syndrome (tonically dilated pupil with poor reactivity to light); most cases are unilateral and associated with a loss of deep tendon reflexes in the lower extremities [5], Argyle–Robertson pupil, cataract surgery [6], chronic anterior uveitis, diabetes [7], pupillary sphincter tear, unilateral use of miotics or mydriatics, third nerve palsy (can also appear as "pupil sparing"), trigeminal autonomic cephalalgias.

Symptoms and Signs

Pain, headache, ptosis, diplopia, blurred vision, numbness, weakness, or ataxia indicates imminent evaluation for conditions, such as traumatic injury, intracranial hemorrhage or mass, aneurysm, or carotid dissection.

Horner's Syndrome

Horner's syndrome is an oculosympathetic palsy described by the triad of (partial) ptosis, miosis, and rarely enophthalmos and facultatively anhidrosis [8]. It indicates a lesion of the ipsilateral sympathetic nerve trunk. The sympathetic nerve trunk innervates the iris dilator muscle, the superior tarsal muscle, and the sweat glands. The elevation of the lower lid is termed "upside-down ptosis."

Horner's syndrome is usually acquired, but manifestations in childhood also occur (congenital Horner's syndrome).

Signs (Fig. 18.1)

Mild ptosis of the upper lid.

The lower lid is often at a slightly higher level than normal, decreased palpebral aperture compared to the unaffected eye.

Pupil: Miosis of the affected eye, more visible in the dark. Dilation lag when a bright light source is removed.

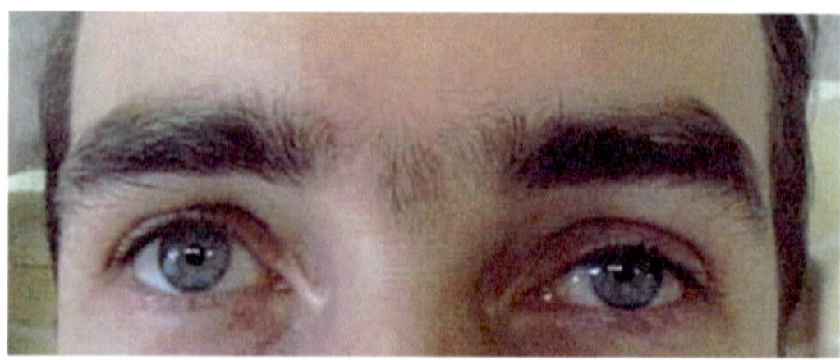

Fig. 18.1 Horner's syndrome. Left Horner's syndrome with mild ptosis and miosis

Anhidrosis and sympathetic denervation is variable. Preganglionic lesions produce more noticeable anhidrosis. Anhidrosis is often not noticeable in postganglionic lesions. Ipsilateral conjunctival injection, changes in accommodation, and lower intraocular pressure can occur.

Extraocular eye movements are only involved in lesions of the brainstem or the cavernous sinus which affect additional fibers of the optomotor system.

Congenital Horner's syndrome: Iris heterochromia (different colored irides) in children.

Transient Horner's syndrome: Cluster headache [9, 10], migraine (some types) [11], trigeminal autonomic cephalalgia [12].

Other types: "Reverse Horner's syndrome," e.g., Pourfour du Petit syndrome [13, 14]; tonic pupil [15]; Harlequin syndrome [16].

Causes: See Table 18.1

Carotid artery dissection, manipulation of cervical spine and neck, myelopathy, neck trauma, nerve blocks, sympathectomy.

In combination with other signs of the trigeminal or oculomotor nerves: Cavernous sinus (associated with CN VI and CN V lesion) or superior orbital fissure syndrome.

Main Investigations

Carotid ultrasound, chest X-rays, CT, MRA, MR, eye exam.

Pharmacological testing:

Topical cocaine causes dilation of the pupil with intact sympathetic innervation.

Topical apraclonidine is an alpha adrenergic agonist and causes pupillary dilation of the Horner's pupil due to denervation supersensitivity. In the normal pupil it produces a mild pupillary constriction.

Topical hydroxyamphetamine is used to differentiate pre- and postganglionic HS. Hydroxyamphetamine causes a release of norepinephrine from intact adrenergic nerve endings causing pupillary dilation.

Table 18.1 Sites of lesions causing Horner's syndrome

First order	Second order (preganglionic)	Third order (postganglionic)
The hypothalamus to the first synapse in the cervical spinal cord (Level C8–T2) *Lesions*: Stroke, tumors, lateral medullary syndrome, neck trauma. or demyelinating disease (e.g., MS)	Axons from neurons destined for the head and neck exit the spinal cord and travel in the cervical sympathetic chain through the brachial plexus, over the pulmonary apex and synapse in the superior cervical ganglion *Lesions*: Pancoast tumor, mediastinal or thyroid mass, cervical rib, neck and brachial plexus trauma, or surgery	Neurons for the orbit enter the cranium within the adventitia of the internal carotid artery into the cavernous sinus The oculosympathetic fibers exit the internal carotid artery in close proximity to the trigeminal ganglion and CN VI and join the first division of the trigeminal nerve (CN V) to enter the orbit *Lesions*: Carotid artery dissection, cavernous sinus lesion, otitis media, head or neck trauma

New (acute) onset Horner's syndrome requires radiologic evaluation of the brain, cervical spinal cord, cerebral vessels, head, neck, and thorax.

The Eyelids

The eyelids have several important ocular functions, including protection of the eye from injury and providing an ocular tear film [17]. The nictitating membrane occurs rarely in humans [18].

Individual nerves serving the eyelids (Table 18.2):

- V1, the ophthalmic nerve: The ophthalmic nerve has three major branches—the frontal, lacrimal, and nasociliary nerves.

Table 18.2 Eyelid innervation

Function	Nerve
Motor	CN III, CN VII, and sympathetic innervation (tarsalis Mueller muscle)
Sensory	Trigeminal nerve V1, V2 Anastomosis with CN VII
Autonomic	CN III and sympathetic fibers

- V2, the maxillary nerve: The maxillary nerve has three branches—the infraorbital, zygomatic, and pterygopalatinal nerves.
- Sensory innervation of the eyelid is via the ophthalmic nerve (V1) and maxillary (V2) divisions. V1 innervates the upper eyelid (lacrimal, supraorbital, supratrochlear nerves) and the medial part of both lower and upper lids. The lower lid receives fibers from V2 via the zygomaticofacial and infraorbital nerves (Fig. 18.2).

Eyelid functions: Blinking (spontaneous, voluntary, and reflexive), voluntary eye closure (gentle or forced), partial lid lowering during squinting, lid retraction in emotional states (fear or surprise).

Abnormal lid function: Apraxia of lid opening, blepharospasm, excessive lid closure (cerebral ptosis), excessive lid opening (peripheral facial nerve palsy and midbrain lid retraction [19]), Horner's syndrome, mechanical (fibrosis), neuromuscular transmission disorders (e.g., myasthenia gravis), oculomotor palsy, pseudo-Graefe synkinesia (a sign of mis-regeneration), supranuclear lid retraction (e.g., progressive supranuclear palsy), abnormal lid movements (myokymia

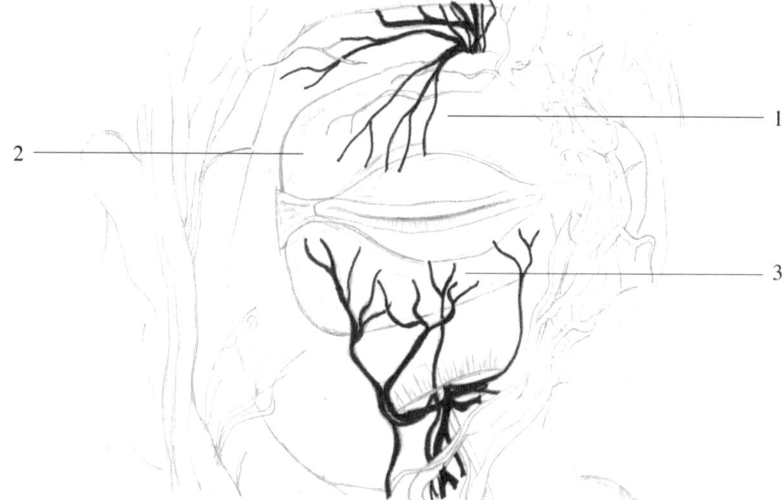

Fig. 18.2 Eyelid innervation. *1* orbicularis oculi muscle (VII), *2* ophthalmic nerve, *3* maxillary nerve; in addition, levator palpebrae (III) and superior and inferior tarsal muscle (sympathetic nerve)

[20–23]; lid tremor, blepharospasm), topiramate-induced [24].

Neoplastic changes: Eyelid tumors [25], metastasis [26].

Ptosis

Appearance

Unilateral and bilateral, permanent and transient, complete and incomplete ptosis.

Classification

According to cause.

Neurogenic ptosis: Damage or dysfunction of specific parts of the central nervous system (e.g., midbrain lesion) and of CNs within the skull, exiting the skull, or in the orbit (e.g., oculomotor nerve).

Myogenic ptosis: Myogenic ptosis can be caused by myopathies, such as congenital myopathies, chronic external ophthalmoplegia (CPEO), facioscapulohumeral muscular dystrophy, mitochondriopathy, myotonic dystrophy, and oculopharyngeal muscular dystrophy (OPMD). See Chap. 24.

Neuromuscular transmission (NMT) disorders: Includes MG, LEMS, and botulism.

Drug induced: Use of high doses of opioid drugs such as morphine, oxycodone, heroin, or hydrocodone can cause ptosis. Pregabalin, an anticonvulsant drug, has also been known to cause mild ptosis. Snake venoms [27].

Causes

Aponeurotic ptosis.

Oculomotor nerve lesion.

Senile ptosis.

Transient: Migraine [28, 29], cluster headache [30], NMT disorders (Fig. 18.3).

Incomplete ptosis: Horner's syndrome, senile ptosis.

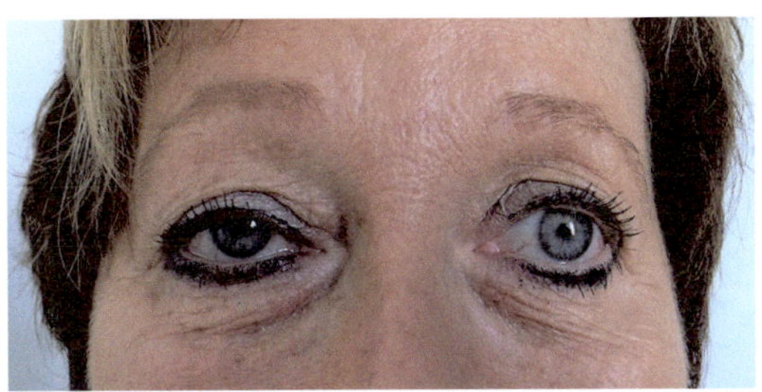

Fig. 18.3 Bilateral incomplete ptosis in a patient with myasthenia gravis. Also note the deviation of bulbi

Other: Blepharospasm and eyelid apraxia [31]; aponeurotic ptosis in elderly patients; mechanical ptosis associated with increased eyelid weight (mass, lesion, heavy skin tissues); traumatic ptosis; traumatic levator muscle weakness; pseudoptosis associated with contralateral retracted eyelid, brow ptosis, upper eyelid swelling, or decreased orbital volume. Psychogenic pseudoptosis [32] or psychogenic unilateral pseudoptosis [33].

The Oral Cavity and Dysphagia

The oral cavity, as one of the most important entry gates, is innervated by several CNs and muscles and sustains important functions, such as swallowing, taste perceptions, and speaking, among others (Fig. 18.4).

In addition to neurological causes, mechanical aspects, such as local infections, tumors, trauma, fibrosis, and amyloidosis, can cause dysfunction.

In adults, there is an age-related deterioration of swallowing, termed presbyphagia, that is also accentuated in sarcopenia.

Oral Cavity Functions

Oral sensations: Taste, oral somatosensation, and retronasal olfaction are mediated via several CNs.

Other oral sensations include phantom taste, touch, or pain sensations (e.g., glossodynia or burning mouth syndrome [34]); these can be associated with neuropsychiatric conditions [35].

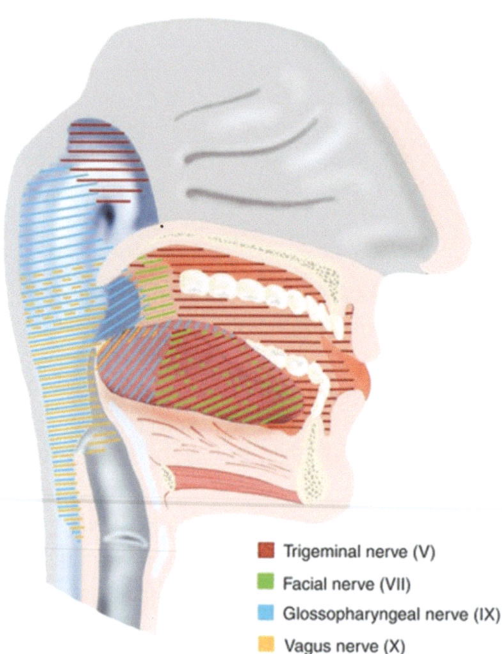

Fig. 18.4 Oral cavity. The image illustrates the innervation of the oral cavity and tongue. The taste perception of the anterior two-thirds of the tongue is transmitted by the facial nerve, the posterior third by the glossopharyngeal nerve. The sensory innervation by the trigeminal nerve V3 overlapping in the buccal area with V2. The buccinator muscle, which innervates the cheeks, is innervated by the facial nerve

Main Investigations

The "BTG pronunciation examination test" is a simple and useful bedside examination to assess oral function.

- "B"—Entrance to the oral cavity: Mouth and lips
- "T"—The oral cavity:
  Within: Tongue, gums, mucous membranes, glands
  Sensory motor innervation and feedback: Chewing.
- "G"—Posterior part: Gag and swallowing

"B" ventral part and mouth closure: The muscles of the entrance of the oral cavity are innervated by the facial nerve, and sensory innervation is via the trigeminal nerve. The lips are innervated in particular by the orbicularis oris muscle, while the sensory innervation stems from the mental and infraorbital nerve. The closure of the oral cavity is an important first step in feeding; lip closure is as important in drinking and eating. Both motor dysfunction of the facial nerve and trigeminal sensory dysfunction reduce lip function. The causes can be central or peripheral and muscular or mechanical.

"T" middle of the oral cavity and tongue: The boundaries of the oral cavity are the cheeks and lips, the hard palate, and posteriorly the oropharynx. The sensory innervation of the cheeks comes from the mental and maxillary nerves; the muscles are predominantly innervated by the buccinator muscle (facial nerve). Both the tongue and the cheeks act as a functional unit during sucking, blowing, and chewing.

The tongue fills the oral cavity. It consists of a root, body, and tip and is divided into an oral and a pharyngeal part. Its functions are taste (lingual papillae and taste buds), participation in mastication, deglutition (swallowing), articulation (speech), and cleansing of the oral cavity. The tongue's main functions are squeezing food into the pharynx when swallowing and forming words during speech. The muscle is innervated by the hypoglossal nerve. It has several intrinsic muscles. The tongue is also linked with extrinsic muscles, such as the genioglossus, hypoglossus, styloglossus, and palatoglossus muscles.

"G" posterior part, gag and swallowing: The food is propelled by the tongue to the oropharynx. In the pharyngeal stage, two events occur: (1) the passage of the food bolus through the pharynx and (2) then airway protection.

The soft palate elevates and closes the nasopharynx. The base of the tongue pushes the bolus against the pharyngeal walls. The pharyngeal wall muscles contract sequentially to press the bolus downward.

Dysphagia: Swallowing difficulty, also known as dysphagia, is a frequent and severely incapacitating problem that can have many causes. Associated neurological conditions can be central or peripheral, and dysphagia is frequent in neurological diseases, including stroke, motor neuron diseases, and neuromuscular transmission disorders such as myasthenia gravis, as well as in CN lesions. It also occurs in autoimmune diseases, such as myositis [36].

Causes of Dysphagia

Age: Presbyphagia describes age-related changes in the swallowing mechanisms and concern both formation, passage, tongue pressure, and loss of teeth, which are of heterogenous causes. These changes can cause difficulties in forming and propelling the bolus, decreased pressure of the tongue, obstruction of the passage of the bolus, stoppage of the bolus when swallowing, a decrease in the sensation of smell and taste (which makes swallowing more difficult), and also the loss of teeth which can be an important factor. All these conditions can also make mastication difficult [37].

Brainstem lesions: Vascular brainstem lesions, e.g., Wallenberg's syndrome

Cancer: Cachexia and dysphagia are considered [38, 39].

Central:

Cerebral: Vascular, usually bilateral causing "pseudobulbar" palsy.

Dementia.

Advanced Parkinson's disease.

CN dysfunction:

Facial nerve dysfunction (lip closure).

Sensory trigeminal nerve (numbness affecting facial nerve innervation).

Lower cranial nerve lesions (individual or multiple).

High vagus nerve lesions.

Dementia: Dysphagia in dementia [40].

Infections: Botulism, mononucleosis, local infections (candida and other oral cavity infections)

Local pathology: Head and neck tumors, infections, trauma, mechanical causes, tumor, embolization [41].

Muscle diseases: [42]; see Chap. 24.

Neuromuscular transmission disorders: Myasthenia gravis, botulism.

Neuropathies: Diphtheria.

Oral sensory damage: [43].

Pharmacologic: Dry mouth is caused by several drugs [44].

Radiation therapy: Radiogenic dysphagia, radiation fibrosis.

Sarcopenic dysphagia: [45, 46].

Salivation disorders:

Hyposalivation: Sjögren's syndrome, drugs, sicca syndrome [47].

Hypersalivation: Psychoactive drugs.

Inability to swallow: Motor neuron disease.

The Tongue

The tongue is a central part of the oral cavity. In addition to being essential for food transport, the swallowing process, and speech production, the tongue is an important component of the sensory innervation of the oral cavity and the receptors for the special senses for taste. The muscular parts of the tongue are innervated by the hypoglossal nerve and several other CNs, including V, VII, IX, and X [48]. See also the hypoglossal neve, Chap. 17.

Tongue Dysfunction

Impairment of motor function results in tongue weakness and atrophy, either unilaterally or bilaterally (see hypoglossal nerve or motor neuron disease).

Central innervation deficits in hemiparesis, pseudobulbar palsy, and spasticity can produce mild or severe weakness. Spasticity in motor neuron disease can also cause tongue movement dysfunction.

Rarely, the tongue can be enlarged. Macroglossia can heave several causes, including amyloid deposition (Fig. 18.5), muscle disease, hypothyroidism, primary lateral sclerosis (PLS) [49], and several other conditions, e.g., Beckwith–Wiedemann syndrome. Focal enlargement can be the sign of a tumor, or rarely tongue infraction or tongue necrosis [50, 51].

Unilateral atrophy is usually caused by a CN XII lesion. Bilateral tongue atrophy is characteristic of motor neuron disease, but may also occur in other conditions (tongue atrophy [52], Sjögren syndrome [53], TTR tongue [54], bilateral CN XII in Hodgkin's disease).

Sensory innervation: the tongue is innervated by the trigeminal nerve (anterior two-thirds) and glossopharyngeal nerve (posterior third). Numbness of the tongue can be produced by dental procedures and also dental surgery. Lingual nerve damage can result in persistent numbness and may need intervention [55].

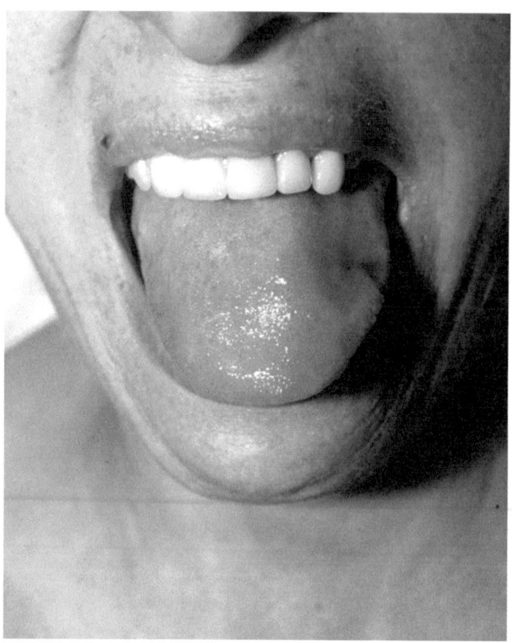

Fig. 18.5 Amyloid tongue. Enlarged tongue in a patient with amyloidosis in paraproteinemia. Subjectively, the tongue was perceived to be too large

Several symptoms of tongue sensation include:

Burning tongue
Glossodynia
Oral dysesthesia, often associated with diabetic neuropathies [56].
Oral phantom sensations, such as the "burning mouth."

Tongue changes and burning mouth occur also in hematological disorders, e.g., anemia [57].

There are also various mouth sensations in depression and functional disorders. See Chap. 35.

Special Senses

The special senses of taste are the facial nerve (CN VII) for the anterior two-thirds of the tongue and the greater petrosal nerve, supplying the taste buds of the soft palate, and the glossopharyngeal nerve (cranial nerve IX) for the posterior third of the tongue. The vagus nerve (CN X) provides fibers to the epiglottic region.

Movement Disorders

Several tongue movements occur in movement disorders, such as essential tremor [58], orolingual tremor [59], and rarely Parkinson's tremor [60].

The tongue can also be involved in movement disorders, such as dystonia, tardive dyskinesia [61], tongue and throat spasm, the posttraumatic galloping tongue [62], tongue cramps [63], and neck tongue syndrome [64].

Main Investigations

Inspection or examination for specific appearance of the tongue:

Black and hairy tongue [65–67].
Tripple furrow tongue [68].
The tone in common oral lesions [69].

The assessment of tongue function is also gaining importance and can be assessed by:

Evaluating tongue protrusion, tongue pressure [70], and tongue strength [71].
Electrophysiology: EMG of the tongue, various approaches.
Ultrasound of the tongue: Shows morphology as well as movements.
Magnetic resonance tomography (MRT): MRT "bright tongue sign" [72] in denervation.

Other Specific Conditions

Tongue hematoma [73].
Infection [74], COVID-19 dysphagia [75].
Lingual sarcopenia [76].
Muscle specific tyrosine kinase (MuSK), myasthenia gravis: Triple furrowed tongue [77].
Sarcopenic dysphagia [78].
Seizures: Epilepsy—tongue biting [79].

Tongue tumors: Accessory tongue [80], lymphoma [81, 82], MRT [83], schwannoma [84, 85], hemangioma [38], other tumors [39].

Tongue infarcts: Infarction [51, 78, 86, 87], e.g., in Wegener's disease [88, 89].

Trauma: Laceration, self-bites.

Vascular lesions or malformations.

CNs in Coma

Genetic testing	NCV/ EMG	Laboratory	Imaging	Biopsy	Other
	+	+	++		Thermic test, Ice water

CN examination in coma (Table 18.3): The examination of the comatose patient is a highly specific and clinically important task. The types and causes of coma vary, and usually deep coma is characterized by absent cranial functions, which may be indistinguishable from brain death. Practically, persons with this condition are investigated by imaging techniques, such as CT, laboratory tests, toxicology, and CSF examinations.

The clinical examination can give clues to the coma stage, laterality, and also preserved CN functions. Careful monitoring of the patient in intensive care enables following improvement or progression. Deep sedation or intoxications can hamper the function of CNs and suggest severe and progressed brain damage. Care must be taken to consider the extent of sedation when judging CN functions.

Table 18.3 CN examination in coma

Pupil	Metabolic and toxic causes often spare the light reflex. Nonreacting "pinpoint pupils" point to either structural damage (pontine) or opiate intoxication. Midbrain lesions can produce large, fixed unresponsive pupils. Lids must be passively held open: anisocoria, consensual light reaction. Early manifestation of herniation syndrome—decline of pupillary reaction, usually on the side of the mass, followed by an ipsilateral mydriatic pupil. Differential diagnosis: eye drops, organophosphates
Perception within the visual field	Can be tested by examining if the patient "blinks to threat"

Table 18.3 (continued)

Oculovestibular reflexes are dependent on the functions of VIII, III, IV, and VI	Extraocular movements are more sensitive to toxic and metabolic influences. Quick and saccadic eye movements are absent. Clinical test: oculocephalic maneuver, caloric testing. Doll's head reflex. Deviation of eyes to one side. Eye movements in resting position: conjugate, dysconjugate, roving, bobbing, inverse ocular bobbing (dipping), retractory nystagmus, convergence nystagmus. Lesions of the MLF with internuclear ophthalmoplegia
Palatal and gag reflex	Relatively well-preserved reflex: absent gag is a severe sign. Imminent danger of aspiration
Corneal reflex	Needs localizing, if unilaterally absent. Bilateral absence not particularly a sign of structural lesion but could also be caused by metabolic or toxic encephalopathy
Pain	Pain can be elicited in the trigeminal nerve distribution. The "ciliospinal" reflex evokes a dilatation of the pupil by noxious cutaneous stimulation. Pain in the limbs and body may induce mimic changes and ipsilateral dilatation of the pupil
Trismus	Lesion above midpons
Acoustic startle reflex	The acoustic startle reflex is usually present in superficial coma. Exaggerated acoustic startle reflex can be a sign of disinhibition, as observed in hypoxic brain damage. The startle reflex can be elicited by acoustic or optic stimuli

Multiple CN Lesions

Sites of multiple CN lesions are noted in Table 18.4.

Table 18.4 Site of multiple CN lesions

Site of lesion	Cause	Associated findings
Brainstem	Infarction, hemorrhage	Brainstem signs
	Encephalitis, infections, abscess (e.g., listeria)	
	Leigh syndrome	
	Metabolic: Wernicke's encephalopathy	
	Paraneoplastic brainstem encephalitis	
	Tumor (e.g., glioma)	
Subarachnoid space	Aneurysm	Often multiple CNs involved
	Clivus tumor	
	Cerebellopontine angle tumors	
	Meningeal carcinomatosis	
	Infections, Meningitis	e.g., TBC, mucormycosis
	Trauma	
Base of the skull	Base of the skull syndromes, e.g., trauma, local destruction: metastasis	Several locations
	Retrograde nerve infiltration from outside of the cranial vault, e.g., neck, sinus, anastomosis between CN and cervical plexus	
	Infections: tuberculous meningitis, granulomatous diseases	
Cavernous sinus	Aneurysm	Often V1, V2 involved
	Carotico-cavernous fistula	Orbital swelling
	Infection: herpes zoster, mucormycosis	
	Mucocele	
	Pituitary apoplexy	
	Tolosa–HHunt syndrome	
	Tumor: llymphoma, meningioma, nasopharyngeal carcinoma	
Fissura orbitalis superior (apex of the orbit)	Metastasis, trauma, tumors	
Orbit	Orbital cellulitis	Proptosis (particularly in advanced age)
	Orbital dysthyroid eye disease	
	Pain and vision loss: consider anterior optic pathways	
	Pseudotumor	
	Trauma	
Uncertain	Cranial arteritis	Pain, polymyalgia
	Miller Fisher syndrome	Associated ataxia
	Oculomotor nerve palsies, toxic	Vincristine
Specific causes	Site of lesion	Associated finings
War and combat injury	CN IX, X, XII Penetrating neck injury Base of skull injuries	Dysphagia, velopharyngeal insufficiency, dysarthria High mortality
Neoplastic	Leptomeningeal carcinomatosis, dural infiltration, base of the skull tutors	
Ophthalmoplegia: various causes	Heterogenous examples for ophthalmoplegia: CIDP, herpes [90], migraine [28], myositis [91], tumors [92], venoms [27]	
Radiotherapy		Late effects
Surgical interventions	Base of skull surgery, shunt placement	
Infections	Botulinum toxin, diphtheria, leprosy, venoms (animal bites and toxins)	

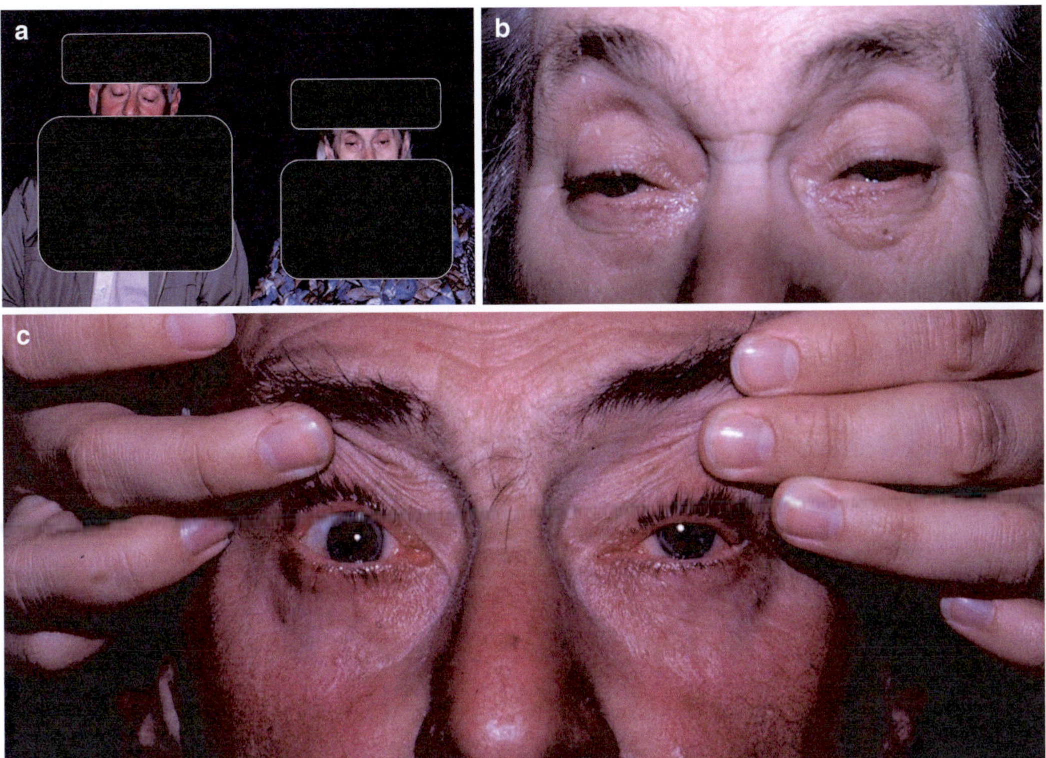

Fig. 18.6 Family with chronic progressive external ophthalmoplegia (CPEO). (**a**) Sister and brother, (**b**) bilateral incomplete ptosis, and (**c**) static optomotor system, with no voluntary eye movements

Differential Diagnosis

Multiple CN lesions can indicate focal disease as base of the skull lesions [93], cavernous sinus lesions, cerebellopontine angle (CPA), and diseases affecting the cavernous sinus and the superior orbital fissure. In these circumstances, focal lesions such as infections, tumors, and trauma can be suspected.

Multiple CN lesions can also be caused by systemic neuropathies, such as GBS, medial longitudinal fascicle (MLF) lesions, and others, including toxic conditions, and they are usually but not necessarily symmetric.

A third type of lesion can be caused by direct involvement of CNs, such as in leptomeningeal carcinomatosis, infections like tuberculosis, and others, such as inflammatory, autoimmune, and granulomatose diseases.

Neuromuscular transmission (NMT) disorders, such as myasthenia gravis (MG) and botulism, can appear with multiple CN lesions. Depending on the cause of NMT, fluctuations are typical, e.g., for MG and LEMS, whereas they are static in botulinum toxin intoxications.

Muscle involvement is usually symmetric, e.g., orbital muscle disease, including thyroid disease and rare ocular myopathies (Fig. 18.6). See Chap. 33.

Anastomosis of CNs

The role of nerve anastomosis is underestimated and is important in several circumstances, particularly for anastomotic connections of autonomic fibers. Figure 18.7 illustrates the connections between parasympathetic fibers and the oculomotor nerve and sympathetic fibers in regard to pupillary functions. The CNs are interconnected with a variety of anastomosis, particularly autonomic, sympathetic, and parasympathetic. The

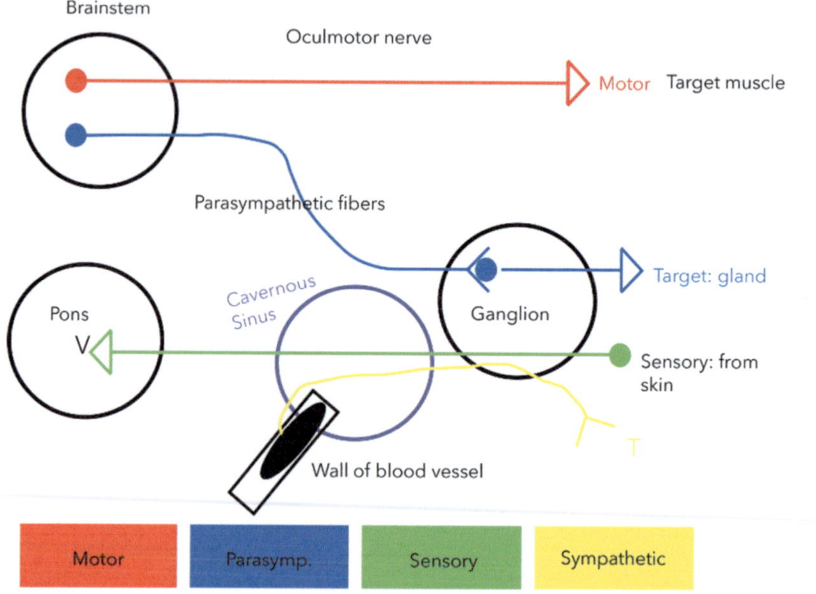

Fig. 18.7 Autonomic fibers traveling with different CNs is also termed "hitchhiking." As an example, the oculomotor nerve (CN III) and the trigeminal nerve (CN V) travel through the cavernous sinus. The parasympathetic fibers from the oculomotor nerve travel with the oculomotor nerve; then change to the trigeminal nerve to reach the ganglion, where they synapse; and then travel to the target (gland). The sympathetic fibers leave the vessel wall and travel as postsynaptic fibers to their target. Sensory fibers travel from the periphery to the brainstem

examples of autonomic nerves travelling over various structures are also termed "hitchhiking."

In the chapter on CN V, several anastomoses and functions of the trigeminal nerve are mentioned (see Chap. 9).

The Concept of Angiosoma

The concept of angiosoma [94] explains the vascular supply of all tissues of the body. For the CNs, the regions of vascular supply differ considerably from the concept of innervation of the skull, skin, and the CNs [95] which is based on dermatomes and myotomes. For practical purposes, this concept is used for head and skull surgery, and following these vascular patterns surgery is performed [94].

For the function of CNs, it has several important aspects, with three of them being mentioned as examples:

1. The vasa nervorum from the lower CN come from the external carotid and ascending pharyngeal artery. Lesion of these vessels, such as by interventions or embolization, can cause damage to the lower CN.
2. Another example is the angiosomic and vascular system of the tongue, which is characterized by a strict unilateral supply without anastomosis [96].
3. In surgery of the skull, the territory of the CN in regard to motor and sensory distribution does not correspond with the angiosomic distribution.

It is also noteworthy that the CNs exiting the skull pass through several angiosomatic areas in the neck, which can influence their function via alterations of the blood supply of the vasa nervorum.

References

1. Hashemi H, Nabovati P, Yekta A, Aghamirsalim M, Rafati S, Ostadimoghaddam H, et al. Convergence insufficiency in the geriatric population. Optom Vis Sci. 2021;98(6):613–9.

2. Lindner K, Hitzenberger P, Drlicek M, Grisold W. Dissociated unilateral convergence paralysis in a patient with thalamotectal haemorrhage. J Neurol Neurosurg Psychiatry. 1992;55(8):731–3.

3. Lam BL, Thompson HS, Corbett JJ. The prevalence of simple anisocoria. Am J Ophthalmol. 1987;104(1):69–73.

4. Turnbull PR, Irani N, Lim N, Phillips JR. Origins of pupillary hippus in the autonomic nervous system. Invest Ophthalmol Vis Sci. 2017;58(1):197–203.

5. Sarao MS, Elnahry AG, Sharma S. Adie syndrome. Treasure Island: StatPearls; 2022.

6. Ba-Ali S, Lund-Andersen H, Brondsted AE. Cataract surgery affects the pupil size and pupil constrictions, but not the late post-illumination pupil response. Acta Ophthalmol. 2017;95(3):e252–e3.

7. Jacobson DM. Pupil involvement in patients with diabetes-associated oculomotor nerve palsy. Arch Ophthalmol. 1998;116(6):723–7.

8. Kanagalingam S, Miller NR. Horner syndrome: clinical perspectives. Eye Brain. 2015;7:35–46.

9. Havelius U. A Horner-like syndrome and cluster headache. What comes first? Acta Ophthalmol Scand. 2001;79(4):374–5.

10. Gupta VK. Painless Horner's syndrome in cluster headache. J Neurol Neurosurg Psychiatry. 1996;60(4):462–3.

11. Khan Z, Bollu PC. Horner Syndrome. Treasure Island: StatPearls; 2022.

12. Rozen TD, Kline MT. Chronic persistent Horner's syndrome in trigeminal autonomic cephalalgia subtypes and alleviation with treatment: two case reports. J Med Case Rep. 2019;13(1):60.

13. Villalba Martinez G, Navalpotro Gomez I, Serrano Perez L, Gonzalez Ortiz S, Fernandez-Candil JL, Steinhauer EG. Surgical position, cause of extracranial internal carotid artery dissection, presenting as Pourfour Du Petit syndrome: case report and literature review. Turk Neurosurg. 2015;25(4):666–9.

14. Aouba A, Der Agopian P, Genty-Le Goff I, Mutschler C, Janin N, Patri B. [Pourfour du Petit syndrome: a rare aetiology of unilateral exophthalmos with mydriasis and lid retraction]. Rev Med Interne. 2003;24(4):261–265.

15. Ahmad R, Saurabh K. Two cases of tonic pupil: Ross and Ross syndrome plus. Cureus. 2022;14(2):e22305.

16. Tascilar N, Tekin NS, Erdem Z, Alpay A, Emre U. Unnoticed dysautonomic syndrome of the face: Harlequin syndrome. Auton Neurosci. 2007;137(1–2):1–9.

17. Helmchen C, Rambold H. The eyelid and its contribution to eye movements. Dev Ophthalmol. 2007;40:110–31.

18. Heralgi M, Thallangady A, Venkatachalam K, Vokuda H. Persistent unilateral nictitating membrane in a 9-year-old girl: a rare case report. Indian J Ophthalmol. 2017;65(3):253–5.

19. Rucker JC. Normal and abnormal lid function. Handb Clin Neurol. 2011;102:403–24.

20. Banik R, Miller NR. Chronic myokymia limited to the eyelid is a benign condition. J Neuroophthalmol. 2004;24(4):290–2.

21. Medrano-Martinez V, Perez-Sempere A, Molto-Jorda JM, Fernandez-Izquierdo S, Frances-Pont I, Mallada-Frechin J, et al. Eyelid myokymia in patients with migraine taking topiramate. Acta Neurol Scand. 2015;132(2):143–6.

22. Wessel M, Zimerman M, Timmermann JE, Hummel FC. Eyelid myokymia in an older subject after repetitive sessions of anodal transcranial direct current stimulation. Brain Stimul. 2013;6(3):463–5.

23. Vuppala AD, Griepentrog GJ, Walsh RD. Swallow-induced eyelid myokymia: a novel Synkinesis syndrome. Neuroophthalmology. 2020;44(2):108–10.

24. Khalkhali M. Topiramate-induced persistent eyelid myokymia. Case Rep Psychiatry. 2016;2016:7901085.

25. Squamous carcinoma of the eyelid. American Academy of Opthalmology; 2022. https://eyewiki org/Squamous_Carcinoma_of_the_Eyelid.

26. Bianciotto C, Demirci H, Shields CL, Eagle RC Jr, Shields JA. Metastatic tumors to the eyelid: report of 20 cases and review of the literature. Arch Ophthalmol. 2009;127(8):999–1005.

27. Praveen Kumar KV, Praveen Kumar S, Kasturi N, Ahuja S. Ocular manifestations of venomous Snake bite over a one-year period in a tertiary care hospital. Korean J Ophthalmol. 2015;29(4):256–62.

28. Gelfand AA, Gelfand JM, Prabakhar P, Goadsby PJ. Ophthalmoplegic "migraine" or recurrent ophthalmoplegic cranial neuropathy: new cases and a systematic review. J Child Neurol. 2012;27(6):759–66.

29. Gulkilik G, Cagatay HH, Oba EM, Uslu C. Ophthalmoplegic migraine associated with recurrent isolated ptosis. Ann Ophthalmol (Skokie). 2009;41(3–4):206–7.

30. Nesbitt AD, Goadsby PJ. Cluster headache. BMJ. 2012;344:e2407.

31. Verghese J, Milling C, Rosenbaum DM. Ptosis, blepharospasm, and apraxia of eyelid opening secondary to putaminal hemorrhage. Neurology. 1999;53(3):652.

32. Hop JW, Frijns CJ, van Gijn J. Psychogenic pseudoptosis. J Neurol. 1997;244(10):623–4.

33. Bagheri A, Abbasnia E, Pakravan M, Roshani M, Tavakoli M. Psychogenic unilateral pseudoptosis. Ophthalmic Plast Reconstr Surg. 2015;31(3):e55–7.

34. Klein B, Thoppay JR, De Rossi SS, Ciarrocca K. Burning mouth syndrome. Dermatol Clin. 2020;38(4):477–83.

35. Yu JRT, Yu XX, Rajaram R, Fernandez HH, Siddiqui J. Burning mouth syndrome to oral cenesthopathy: a spectrum of neuropsychiatric and sensory complications in neurodegenerative parkinsonism? Parkinsonism Relat Disord. 2022;104:1–2.

36. Labeit B, Pawlitzki M, Ruck T, Muhle P, Claus I, Suntrup-Krueger S, et al. The impact of dysphagia in myositis: a systematic review and meta-analysis. J Clin Med. 2020;9(7)

37. Yigman ZA, Umay E, Cankurtaran D, Guzel S. Swallowing difficulty in the older adults: presby-

phagia or dysphagia with sarcopenia? Int J Rehabil Res. 2021;44(4):336–42.

38. Wakabayashi H, Matsushima M, Uwano R, Watanabe N, Oritsu H, Shimizu Y. Skeletal muscle mass is associated with severe dysphagia in cancer patients. J Cachexia Sarcopenia Muscle. 2015;6(4):351–7.

39. Okuni I, Otsubo Y, Ebihara S. Molecular and neural mechanism of dysphagia due to cancer. Int J Mol Sci. 2021;22(13):7033.

40. Wijsmuller AR, Giraudeau C, Leroy J, Kleinrensink GJ, Rociu E, Romagnolo LG, Melani AGF, Agnus V, Diana M, Soler L, Dallemagne B, Marescaux J, Mutter D. A step towards stereotactic navigation during pelvic surgery: 3D nerve topography. Surg Endosc. 2018;32:3582–91. https://doi.org/10.1007/s00464-018-6086-3.

41. Gartrell BC, Hansen MR, Gantz BJ, Gluth MB, Mowry SE, Aagaard-Kienitz BL, et al. Facial and lower cranial neuropathies after preoperative embolization of jugular foramen lesions with ethylene vinyl alcohol. Otol Neurotol. 2012;33(7):1270–5.

42. Argov Z, de Visser M. Dysphagia in adult myopathies. Neuromuscul Disord. 2021;31(1):5–20.

43. Snyder DJ, Bartoshuk LM. Oral sensory nerve damage: causes and consequences. Rev Endocr Metab Disord. 2016;17(2):149–58.

44. Sroussi HY, Epstein JB, Bensadoun RJ, Saunders DP, Lalla RV, Migliorati CA, et al. Common oral complications of head and neck cancer radiation therapy: mucositis, infections, saliva change, fibrosis, sensory dysfunctions, dental caries, periodontal disease, and osteoradionecrosis. Cancer Med. 2017;6(12):2918–31.

45. Maeda K, Akagi J. Treatment of Sarcopenic dysphagia with rehabilitation and nutritional support: a comprehensive approach. J Acad Nutr Diet. 2016;116(4):573–7.

46. Hashida N, Shamoto H, Maeda K, Wakabayashi H, Suzuki M, Fujii T. Rehabilitation and nutritional support for sarcopenic dysphagia and tongue atrophy after glossectomy: a case report. Nutrition. 2017;35:128–31.

47. Kramer E, Seeliger T, Skripuletz T, Godecke V, Beider S, Jablonka A, et al. Multimodal assessment and characterization of Sicca syndrome. Front Med (Lausanne). 2021;8:777599.

48. Chauhan S, Chavre S, Chandrashekar NH, B SN. Perforator peroneal artery flap for tongue reconstruction. J Maxillofac Oral Surg. 2017;16(1):123–6.

49. Chang MC, Kwak S. Macroglossia in primary lateral sclerosis: a case report. Int J Neurosci. 2019;129(12):1189–91.

50. Renehan A, Morton M. Acute enlargement of the tongue. Br J Oral Maxillofac Surg. 1993;31(5):321–4.

51. Kagami H, Inaba M, Ichimura S, Hara K, Inamasu J. Endovascular revascularization of external carotid artery occlusion causing tongue infarction: case report. Neurol Med Chir (Tokyo). 2012;52(12):910–3.

52. Yamanaka G, Goto K, Matsumura T, Funakoshi M, Komori T, Hayashi YK, et al. Tongue atrophy in facioscapulohumeral muscular dystrophy. Neurology. 2001;57(4):733–5.

53. Zampeli E, Kalogirou EM, Piperi E, Mavragani CP, Moutsopoulos HM. Tongue atrophy in Sjogren syndrome patients with mucosa-associated lymphoid tissue lymphoma: autoimmune epithelitis beyond the epithelial cells of salivary glands? J Rheumatol. 2018;45(11):1565–71.

54. Goyal NA, Mozaffar T. Tongue atrophy and fasciculations in transthyretin familial amyloid neuropathy: an ALS mimicker. Neurol Genet. 2015;1(2):e18.

55. Biglioli F, Allevi F, Colletti G, Lozza A. Cross-tongue procedure: a new treatment for long-standing numbness of the tongue. Br J Oral Maxillofac Surg. 2015;53(9):880–2.

56. Moore PA, Guggenheimer J, Orchard T. Burning mouth syndrome and peripheral neuropathy in patients with type 1 diabetes mellitus. J Diabetes Complicat. 2007;21(6):397–402.

57. Adeyemo TA, Adeyemo WL, Adediran A, Akinbami AJ, Akanmu AS. Orofacial manifestations of hematological disorders: anemia and hemostatic disorders. Indian J Dent Res. 2011;22(3):454–61.

58. Teive HA. Essential tremor: phenotypes. Parkinsonism Relat Disord. 2012;18(Suppl 1):S140–2.

59. Silverdale MA, Schneider SA, Bhatia KP, Lang AE. The spectrum of orolingual tremor—a proposed classification system. Mov Disord. 2008;23(2):159–67.

60. Toda H, Asanuma K, Kondo T, Terada Y, Saiki H. Tongue tremor as a manifestation of atypical Parkinsonism treated with coaxial deep brain stimulation of thalamus and subthalamic area. Parkinsonism Relat Disord. 2017;44:154–6.

61. Pi EH, Simpson GM. Tardive dyskinesia and abnormal tongue movements. Br J Psychiatry. 1981;139:526–8.

62. Keane JR. Galloping tongue: post-traumatic, episodic, rhythmic movements. Neurology. 1984;34(2):251–2.

63. Torbergsen T, Jurkat-Rott K, Stalberg EV, Loseth S, Hodneo A, Lehmann-Horn F. Painful cramps and giant myotonic discharges in a family with the Nav1.4-G1306A mutation. Muscle Nerve. 2015;52(4):680–3.

64. Gelfand AA, Johnson H, Lenaerts ME, Litwin JR, De Mesa C, Bogduk N, et al. Neck-tongue syndrome: a systematic review. Cephalalgia. 2018;38(2):374–82.

65. Lawoyin D, Brown RS. Drug-induced black hairy tongue: diagnosis and management challenges. Dent Today. 2008;27(1):60, 62–3; quiz 93, 58.

66. Thompson DF, Kessler TL. Drug-induced black hairy tongue. Pharmacotherapy. 2010;30(6):585–93.

67. Gurvits GE, Tan A. Black hairy tongue syndrome. World J Gastroenterol. 2014;20(31):10845–50.

68. Young NP, Sorenson EJ, Milone M, Harper CM. Triple furrowed atrophic tongue of myasthenia gravis. J Clin Neuromuscul Dis. 2017;19(1):47–8.

69. Randall DA, Wilson Westmark NL, Neville BW. Common oral lesions. Am Fam Physician. 2022;105(4):369–76.

70. Mano T, Katsuno M, Banno H, Suzuki K, Suga N, Hashizume A, et al. Tongue pressure as a novel

biomarker of spinal and bulbar muscular atrophy. Neurology. 2014;82(3):255–62.

71. Chen KC, Lee TM, Wu WT, Wang TG, Han DS, Chang KV. Assessment of tongue strength in sarcopenia and sarcopenic dysphagia: a systematic review and meta-analysis. Front Nutr. 2021;8:684840.

72. Karam C, Dimitrova D, Yutan E, Chahin N. Bright tongue sign in patients with late-onset Pompe disease. J Neurol. 2019;266(10):2518–23.

73. Lo BM, Campbell BH. A traumatic swollen tongue. Resuscitation. 2010;81(3):267.

74. Chong GM, Ong DSY, de Mendonca MM, van Hellemond JJ. Painful and swollen tongue: mucosal leishmaniasis due to Leishmania infantum. Int J Infect Dis. 2021;113:109–12.

75. Can B, Ismagulova N, Enver N, Tufan A, Cinel I. Sarcopenic dysphagia following COVID-19 infection: a new danger. Nutr Clin Pract. 2021;36(4):828–32.

76. Machida N, Tohara H, Hara K, Kumakura A, Wakasugi Y, Nakane A, et al. Effects of aging and sarcopenia on tongue pressure and jaw-opening force. Geriatr Gerontol Int. 2017;17(2):295–301.

77. Takahashi H, Kawaguchi N, Ito S, Nemoto Y, Hattori T, Kuwabara S. Is tongue atrophy reversible in anti-MuSK myasthenia gravis? Six-year observation. J Neurol Neurosurg Psychiatry. 2010;81(6):701–2.

78. Moncayo-Hernandez BA, Herrera-Guerrero JA, Vinazco S, Ocampo-Chaparro JM, Reyes-Ortiz CA. Sarcopenic dysphagia in institutionalised older adults. Endocrinol Diabetes Nutr (Engl Ed). 2021;68(9):602–11.

79. Brigo F, Nardone R, Bongiovanni LG. Value of tongue biting in the differential diagnosis between epileptic seizures and syncope. Seizure. 2012;21(8):568–72.

80. Ohara K, Kanaya T, Harabuchi Y. An accessory tongue in a child: a clinical case. Auris Nasus Larynx. 2021;48(6):1214–6.

81. Baik J, Baek HJ, Ryu KH, An HJ, Song S, Lee HJ, et al. MALT lymphoma of the tongue in a patient with Sjogren's syndrome: a case report and literature review. Diagnostics (Basel). 2021;11(9):1715.

82. Goteri G, Ascani G, Filosa A, Rubini C, Olay S, Balercia P. Primary malt lymphoma of the tongue. Med Oral Patol Oral Cir Bucal. 2004;9(5):461–3; 59–61.

83. Liu X, Cheng D, Wang W. MRI in differentiation of benign and malignant tongue tumors. Front Biosci (Landmark Ed). 2015;20(4):614–20.

84. Haider MY, Rahim M, Bashar NMK, Hossain MZ, Islam SMJ. Schwannoma of the base of the tongue: a case report of a rare disease and review of literatures. Case Rep Surg. 2020;2020:7942062.

85. Kavcic J, Bozic M. Schwannoma of the tongue. BMJ Case Rep. 2016;2016:bcr2016215799.

86. Kagami H, Inaba M, Ichimura S, Hara K, Inamasu J. Endovascular revascularization of external carotid artery occlusion causing tongue infarction. Neurol Med Chir (Tokyo). 2012;52:910–3.

87. Daniela Patino-Hernandez M, Borda MG, Sanabria LCV, Diego Andrés Chavarro-Carvajal M, Cano-Gutiérrez CA. Sarcopenic dysphagia. Rev Col Gastroenterol. 2016;31(4):412–7.

88. Carter LM, Brizman E. Lingual infarction in Wegener's granulomatosis: a case report and review of the literature. Head Face Med. 2008;4:19.

89. Souviron Encabo R, Garcia de Pedro F, Encinas A, Rodriguez A, Scola Yurrita B. [Necrosis of the tongue secondary to bilateral carotid thrombosis after radiotherapy]. Acta Otorrinolaringol Esp 2007;58(7):331–332.

90. Archambault P, Wise JS, Rosen J, Polomeno RC, Auger N. Herpes zoster ophthalmoplegia. Report of six cases. J Clin Neuroophthalmol. 1988;8(3):185–93.

91. Tatsumi F, Fushimi Y, Sanada J, Shimoda M, Kohara K, Kimura T, et al. Idiopathic bilateral extraocular myositis in a subject with poorly controlled type 2 diabetes mellitus: case report. Front Med (Lausanne). 2021;8:700307.

92. Greenberg HS, Deck MD, Vikram B, Chu FC, Posner JB. Metastasis to the base of the skull: clinical findings in 43 patients. Neurology. 1981;31(5):530–7.

93. Greenberg HS, Deck MD, Vikram B. Metastasis to the base of the skull: clinical findings in 43 patients. Neurology. 1981;31:530–7.

94. Taylor GI, Palmer JH. The vascular territories (angiosomes) of the body: experimental study and clinical applications. Br J Plast Surg. 1987;40(2):113–41.

95. Houseman ND, Taylor GI, Pan WR. The angiosomes of the head and neck: anatomic study and clinical applications. Plast Reconstr Surg. 2000;105(7):2287–313.

96. Lopez R, Lauwers F, Paoli JR, Boutault F, Guitard J. Vascular territories of the tongue: anatomical study and clinical applications. Surg Radiol Anat. 2007;29(3):239–44.

Part III

The Cranial Nerves in Specific Conditions (diseases)

This series of chapters describes the involvement of Cranial nerves in several conditions, ranging from infections towards neoplastic involvement towards misperception in cranial nerves. in psychiatric conditions.

Central Innervation of Motor Cranial Nerves

Bullet Points

- The unique neuroanatomical pattern of central innervation for each motor cranial nerve (CN) nucleus has important clinical and functional implications.
- Given the anatomy of hemispheric control of lateral gaze in regard to CNs III and VI, destructive lesions of one hemisphere affecting the frontal eye field will cause conjugate lateral eye deviation towards the side of the lesion.
- Given the anatomy of brainstem (pontine) control of lateral gaze in regard to CNs III and VI, a destructive lesion of one side of the brainstem affecting the pontine lateral gaze center will cause conjugate lateral eye deviation away from the side of the lesion.
- As a consequence of the mechanisms of voluntary control of gaze and the yoking of movement of one eye with movement of the contralateral eye, it is difficult for individuals to voluntarily move one eye independently.
- Given the pattern of central innervation in regard to CN VII, muscles of the forehead receive input from both the right and the left motor cortex and therefore typically do not become weak in the setting of most central lesions, such as stroke.
- As a consequence of the central innervation pattern to the muscles of the upper face, voluntary control of the upper facial muscles on one side of the face (winking) is more difficult than voluntary control of movement of one side of the lower part of the face
- Given the pattern of bilateral upper motor neuron supply to motor nuclei of CNs IX and X, there is less likelihood of palatal or swallowing dysfunction after a unilateral hemispheric stroke than bilateral hemispheric lesion or after brainstem stroke.
- As a consequence of the bilateral upper motor neuron innervation to CN IX and X motor nuclei via the corticobulbar tracts to the nucleus ambiguus, voluntary unilateral palatal or laryngeal movement is not generally possible.
- In regard to the 12th cranial nerve, due to bilateral motor cortex input to the hypoglossal nucleus, injury to the primary motor cortex or internal capsule will not typically result in significant tongue weakness and therefore will not cause deviation of the tongue to either side.

Authors of this chapter: Carrie Katherine Grouse and Steven L. Lewis.

W. Grisold et al., *The Cranial Nerves in Neurology*, https://doi.org/10.1007/978-3-031-43081-7_19

Introduction

Each motor CN emanates from a CN nucleus with axons that exit the brainstem and innervates unilateral muscles of the head and neck. Each CN nucleus has central innervation; knowledge of the functional anatomy of this central innervation can inform neurologists about neuroanatomical localization, with important clinical implications. The classic case is that of the CN VII nucleus, which receives unilateral innervation to the part of the nucleus that is responsible for movement of the lower part of the face and bilateral innervation to the part of the nucleus that is responsible for movement of the upper part of the face. Knowing this information helps the neurologist immediately understand that their patient with new-onset unilateral weakness of the lower part of the face likely has a central localization (e.g., a stroke), whereas their patient with unilateral full facial weakness likely has a peripheral lesion (e.g., Bell's palsy). In addition to assistance in localization, however, concepts underlying the central innervation of the CN nuclei has lesser known, but clinically relevant, functional implications regarding the voluntary control of CN function, such as the ability to unilaterally wink one eye voluntarily.

This chapter details what is known of the central innervation of the most clinically relevant motor CNs (III, IV, VI, VII, IX, X, and XII) and describes anatomic features, clinical implications (e.g., regarding localization), and functional implications (e.g., regarding voluntary and independent control of CN-innervated muscles) related to their unique patterns of central innervation.

Central Innervation of CNs III, IV, and VI

This section details the anatomy, clinical implications, and functional implications of the central innervation of the third, fourth, and sixth CNs, the ocular motor nerves.

Anatomy of the Central Innervation of the Third, Fourth, and Sixth CNs

Voluntary control of horizontal eye movements begins in the frontal eye fields which occupy the caudal part of the middle frontal gyrus (Brodmann area 8) [1, 2]. Axons project from the frontal eye fields of each cerebral hemisphere to the contralateral pons [3]. The fibers from the frontal eye fields do not project directly to the cranial nerve nuclei, but rather to the center for lateral gaze in the contralateral pons consisting of the pontine paramedian reticular formation (PPRF) and adjacent abducens nucleus [1].

The lateral gaze mechanisms in the pons are linked with medial movement of the contralateral eye by the medial longitudinal fasciculus (MLF), which projects to the medial rectus subnucleus of CN III. For example, when voluntarily looking to the right, the signal from the frontal eye fields of the left hemisphere projects to the PPRF in the right pons and then activates the right abducens nucleus for right eye abduction; subsequently, fibers projecting from the right lateral pons cross and ascend via the MLF to the medial rectus subnucleus of the left CN III, causing left eye adduction.

Clinical Implications of Central Innervation of the Third, Fourth, and Sixth CNs

Given the anatomy of hemispheric control of lateral gaze described above, destructive lesions of one hemisphere affecting the frontal eye field will cause conjugate lateral eye deviation towards the side of the lesion as a result of the unopposed action of the contralateral, intact, frontal eye field. As an example, a stroke of the left hemisphere affecting the left frontal eye field will result in conjugate horizontal gaze deviation to the left. Conversely, as opposed to a destructive lesion, a process that causes increased stimulation of the frontal eye field of one hemisphere will cause conjugate lateral eye deviation away from the side of the lesion. As an example, a seizure emanating from the left hemisphere affecting the left frontal eye field will result in conjugate horizontal gaze deviation to the right [3].

Also, given the anatomy of brainstem (pontine) control of lateral gaze described in the section above, a destructive lesion of one side of the brainstem affecting the pontine lateral gaze center will cause conjugate lateral eye deviation away from the side of the lesion as a result of the unopposed action of the contralateral, intact pontine lateral gaze mechanisms. As an example, a stroke affecting the left pons involving the left lateral gaze center will result in conjugate horizontal gaze deviation to the right [3].

Conjugate horizontal movement of the eyes occurs due to the interconnection between the pons and the midbrain via the MLF, linking abduction of one eye with adduction of the contralateral eye. A lesion of the MLF on one side of the brainstem will therefore cause impaired adduction of the eye on the side that the MLF is ascending towards. As an example, a lesion of the left pons affecting the MLF on the left will cause impaired adduction of the left eye on rightward gaze, despite full abduction of the right eye (a left internuclear ophthalmoplegia) [3].

Functional Implications of Central Innervation of the Third, Fourth, and Sixth CNs

As a consequence of the mechanisms of voluntary control of gaze and the yoking of movement of one eye with movement of the contralateral eye, it is difficult for individuals to voluntarily move one eye independently, or, in other words, to decouple voluntary movement of one eye from the movement of the contralateral eye. This is in contrast to certain animals, such as ectotherms and birds, which have eye movements that are frequently independent of each other [4].

Summary

The neuroanatomy of central innervation of CNs III, IV, and VI has significant implications with regard to the localization (cerebral hemisphere versus brainstem) and consequences of destructive versus stimulating processes affecting the frontal eye fields of the cerebral hemispheres, as well as functional implications regarding difficulty in independent control of either eye.

Central Innervation of CN VII

This section details the anatomy, clinical implications, and functional implications of the central innervation of the seventh cranial nerve, the facial nerve.

Anatomy of the Central Innervation of CN VII

The central innervation of CN VII starts with motor neurons in the primary motor cortex, in the region representing the facial area in the precentral gyrus. These project as part of the corticobulbar tract through the genu of the internal capsule and then descend and cross to lower motor neurons in the contralateral facial nucleus of the pons, while some fibers also descend without crossing the ipsilateral facial nucleus of the pons. The portion of the facial nucleus subserving movement of the upper part of the face receives innervation from bilateral motor cortices, whereas the portion of the facial nucleus subserving movement of the lower part of the face receives only innervation from the contralateral motor cortex. The seventh CN projects from the facial nucleus in the pons to the ipsilateral muscles of the face [2].

Using control of movement of the right side of the forehead as an example, muscles that raise the right eyebrow and close the right eye have input from the motor cortex from both the right and left hemisphere. Muscles that move the right side of the cheek and lips have input from only the motor cortex from the left hemisphere.

Clinical Implications of Central Innervation of CN VII

Given this pattern of central innervation, the muscles of the forehead receive input from both the right and left motor cortex and therefore typically do not become weak in the setting of most central lesions, such as stroke. The muscles of the lower part of the face, which primarily have input from the contralateral motor cortex, will become weak with hemispheric lesions. Pathology of the facial nucleus or CN VII (Bell's palsy being a classic example of the latter) can cause weakness of both the upper and lower part of the ipsilateral face. Upper facial weakness can be subtle, manifesting in reduced eyebrow lift, reduced forehead wrinkling, or *signe des cils de Souqes*, a sign of orbicularis oculi muscle weakness seen when the patient closes their eyes forcefully: The eyelashes on the affected side appear longer due to less coverage by the eyelid [5].

Cases exist, however, where upper facial muscles can also become weak with central lesions [6–9]. Kojima et al. [6] reported two patients who suffered strokes affecting the left anterior central gyrus, resulting in clinical weakness of the lower part of the right face, and EMG studies revealed relative weakness of the right orbicular muscles of both the eye and mouth compared to those of the left side. Willoughby et al. [7] noted that in 76 patients with facial weakness from a unilateral cerebral vascular lesion, 25% had weakness of the forehead, though usually mild and less striking than weakness of the lower part of the face. Lin et al. [8] noted that 6.6% of patients with unilateral stroke and central facial paralysis had weakness of eye closure. This was noted more frequently in right hemispheric lesions (12 of 16, 75%). While the cause of these findings is not yet clear, Lin et al. [8] proposed various possible mechanisms and suggested that the right hemisphere could potentially be dominant in the control of upper face motility.

Functional Implications of Bilateral Innervation of CN VII

Voluntary control of the upper facial muscles on one side of the face is more difficult than voluntary control of movements of one side of the lower part of the face. For example, most people have no difficulty raising one side of the mouth; however, it is not uncommon for people to have difficulty raising one eyelid or closing only one eye (unilateral winking). This is likely a consequence of bilateral cortical innervation to muscle movements of the upper part of the face. However, unilateral winking can be learned.

Regarding the ability to wink, Lin et al. [10] studied 63 subjects, 22 who could wink bilaterally and 41 who could wink unilaterally and who were asked to blink and wink while being monitored by functional magnetic resonance imaging. Those who could only wink unilaterally were then trained to wink on the other side. It was found that left eye winking results in activation of the left frontal lobe, while right eye winking activated bilateral frontal lobes with right-sided predominance. For subjects who could only wink unilaterally, learning to wink on the other side activated similar cortical areas in subjects capable of bilateral winking without training.

Regarding emotional versus voluntary facial movements, Willoughby et al. [7] studied voluntary and emotional facial movements in patients with unilateral cerebral vascular lesions causing hemiparesis and noted that in 21%, facial weakness was less noticeable during an emotional response than during voluntary facial movement.

Summary

The neuroanatomy of central innervation of CN VII has significant implications with regard to localization (hemispheric versus brainstem/peripheral) of the cause of facial weakness, as well as functional implications regarding voluntary control of movements of the upper or lower part of the face.

Central Innervation of CNs IX and X

This section details the anatomy, clinical implications, and functional implications of the central innervation of the ninth and tenth CNs, the glossopharyngeal and vagus nerves.

Anatomy of the Central Innervation of CNs IX and X

This section groups the ninth (glossopharyngeal) and tenth (vagus) CNs together, as the voluntary (special visceral efferent) motor components of these CNs are functionally indistinguishable [2]. The central innervation of the motor nuclei of CNs IX and X starts with motor neurons in the primary motor cortex, in the region representing palatal and laryngeal function. These project as part of the corticobulbar tract to innervate the contralateral and ipsilateral nucleus ambiguus of both the glossopharyngeal and the vagus nerves, each nerve innervating the muscles of the palate and larynx ipsilateral to each nucleus ambiguus [2].

Clinical Implications of the Central Innervation of CNs IX and X

The bilateral upper motor neuron supply to motor nuclei of CNs IX and X has significant implications regarding the presence or absence of dysphagia after stroke. Although dysphagia can occur as a consequence of a variety of central and peripheral insults [11], there is less likelihood of significant palatal or swallowing dysfunction after unilateral hemispheric stroke (or other causes of unilateral hemispheric lesions) than bilateral hemispheric lesions [12] or after brainstem stroke. Lesions of the brainstem cause dysphagia because of involvement of either the bilateral corticobulbar tracts or the motor nuclei of CNs IX and X. In a systematic review, Martino et al. [13] noted that studies have shown that hemispheric lesions have been associated with an approximately 40% incidence of dysphagia, whereas brainstem lesions were associated with a 40–80% incidence of dysphagia.

Bilateral hemispheric strokes are a well-known cause of bilateral corticobulbar tract dysfunction, causing pseudobulbar palsy [3], with spastic dysarthria and dysphagia and pseudobulbar affect (uncontrollable laughing and crying). As noted above, dysphagia can occur, however, from unilateral hemispheric strokes [12]. As described by Singh and Hamdy [14], upper motor neuron innervation of swallowing is asymmetrically represented in the two hemispheres, so that dysphagia is more likely to occur in unilateral hemispheric stroke affecting the hemisphere that is dominant for swallowing, with recovery of swallowing occurring over time. In a study of 16 consecutive patients with unilateral ischemic infarcts and dysphagia, Daniels et al. [15] noted that despite the right hemispheric lesions in their study patients being smaller than the left-sided lesions, dysphagia seemed more significant in patients with right hemispheric strokes, particularly when affecting the insular cortex.

Regarding vocal cord involvement, Venketasubramanian et al. [16] performed endoscopic vocal cord examinations in 54 patients with acute ischemic stroke involving various locations. They found vocal cord paralysis not only in all 5 of their patients with lateral medullary strokes (typically affecting the ipsilateral vocal cord), but also found vocal cord paralysis in 2 of their patients with cortical or large subcortical hemisphere strokes. The authors questioned the common assumption that the nucleus ambiguus is invariably bilaterally innervated and suggested that in patients with vocal cord paralysis from hemispheric lesions, the nucleus ambiguus was predominantly supplied by crossed upper motor neuron fibers [16].

Functional Implications of Bilateral Innervation of CNs IX and X

As a consequence of the bilateral upper motor neuron innervation to the ninth and tenth CN motor nuclei via the corticobulbar tracts to the nucleus ambiguus, voluntary unilateral palatal or laryngeal movement is not generally possible.

Summary

The neuroanatomy of central innervation of CNs IX and X has significant implications with regard to localization (cortex versus brainstem) of the cause of dysphagia or palatal weakness, as well as functional implications regarding inability to unilaterally control palatal or laryngeal movement.

Central Innervation of CN XII

This section details the anatomy, clinical implications, and functional implications of the central innervation of CN XII, the hypoglossal nerve.

Anatomy of the Central Innervation of CN XII

The central innervation of the twelfth CN starts with motor neurons in the primary motor cortex, in the region representing the tongue in the peri-Sylvian area. These project as part of the corticobulbar tract (cortico-hypoglossal fibers) which passes through the corona radiata and the internal capsule and then descend to lower motor neurons in the hypoglossal nuclei in the medulla. Input from the motor cortex to the hypoglossal nuclei is bilateral; generally, fibers that descend to the contralateral hypoglossal nucleus pass through the medial part of the ventral pons prior to crossing at the pontomedullary junction, while fibers that descend to the ipsilateral hypoglossal nucleus pass through the lateral part of the ventral pons without crossing [2, 17–19]. CN XII emerges from the medulla between the pyramid and the inferior olive and projects to ipsilateral muscles of the tongue. The genioglossus muscle causes the tongue to protrude to the opposite side, so paralysis of this muscle results in the tongue deviating towards the weak side [7].

Clinical Implications of the Central Innervation of CN XII

Due to bilateral motor cortex input to the hypoglossal nucleus, injury to the primary motor cortex or internal capsule will not typically result in significant tongue weakness and therefore will not cause deviation of the tongue to either side [17]. In contrast, the genioglossus muscle

becomes weak on the ipsilateral side (tongue deviating to the side of the lesion) in the setting of injury to the hypoglossal nucleus or hypoglossal nerve, seen in medial medullary strokes, for example.

However, it has been demonstrated in a prior study that tongue deviation can occur in the setting of cerebral hemisphere lesions. Willoughby et al. [7] studied 100 patients hospitalized with hemiparesis and a diagnosis of unilateral cerebral hemisphere vascular lesion and noted that in 97 patients who were asked to protrude their tongue as far as possible, 12 patients were noted to have tongue deviation towards the side of the hemiparesis. In an unblinded study of 300 patients with acute unilateral ischemic stroke (not including the lower brainstem), Umapathi et al. [20] found that 29% of patients, compared to 5% of healthy controls, had tongue deviation, always towards the side of the limb weakness. The authors attributed this finding to asymmetric supranuclear control of the hypoglossal nucleus [20].

Functional Implications of Central Innervation of CN XII

Unlike the other motor CNs with bilateral supranuclear input, humans have the ability to voluntarily control tongue movement to either side. Other motor CNs with bilateral supranuclear input, such as CN VII (eyebrow raise) or CNs IX or X (palate elevation), are not easily voluntarily controlled in this way. The anatomic reason for this retained ability for unilateral control is unclear, but has significant implications with regard to the importance of tongue movement for communication and eating, both important to human survival.

Summary

The neuroanatomy of central innervation of CN XII has implications with regard to localization in that significant tongue weakness is more likely to occur due to brainstem disorders than from hemispheric lesions.

Conclusion

Each CN nucleus has central innervation. As described above, knowledge of the anatomy of this central innervation has important implications with regard to function (e.g., voluntary control of certain muscles of the head and neck), neurologic localization (e.g., upper versus lower motor neuron, brainstem versus hemisphere), and, in some cases, whether a lesion is destructive versus excitatory (e.g., direction of deviation of the eyes with pathology of the frontal eye fields).

References

1. Waxman SG. Clinical neuroanatomy. 29th ed. McGraw Hill; 2020.
2. Carpenter MB. Core text of neuoroanatomy. 4th ed. Williams & Wilkins; 1991.
3. Lewis SL. Field guide to the neurologic examination. Lippincott Williams & Wilkins; 2005.
4. Katz H, Lustig A, Lev-Ari T, Nov Y, Rivlin Y, Katzir G. Eye movements in chameleons are not truly independent—evidence from simultaneous monocular tracking of two targets. J Exp Biol. 2015;218:2097–105.
5. Broussolle E, Loiraud C, Thobois S. Achille Alexandre Soques (1860-1944). J Neurol. 2010;257(6):1047–8.
6. Kojima Y, Kaga K, Shindo M, Hirose A. Electromyographic examination of patients with unilateral cortical facial paralysis. Otolaryngol Head Neck Surg. 1997;117(6):S121–4.
7. Willoughby EW, Anderson NE. Lower cranial nerve motor function in unilateral vascular lesions of the cerebral hemisphere. Br Med J. 1984;289:791–4.
8. Lin J, Chen Y, Wen H, Yang Z, Zeng J. Weakness of eye closure with central facial paralysis after hemispheric stroke predicts a worse outcome. J Stroke Cerebrovasc Dis. 2017;26(4):834–41.
9. Onder H, Albayrak L, Polat H. Frontal lobe ischemic stroke presenting with peripheral type facial palsy: a crucial diagnostic challenge in emergency practice. Turk J Emerg Med. 2017;17:112–4.
10. Lin CCK, Lee KJ, Huang CH, Sun YN. Cerebral control of winking before and after learning: an event-related fMRI study. Brain Behav. 2019;9(12):e01483.
11. Zald DH, Pardo JV. The functional neuroanatomy of voluntary swallowing. Ann Neurol. 46:281–6.
12. Meadows JC. Dysphagia in unilateral cerebral lesions. J Neurol Neurosurg Psychiatry. 1973;36:853–60.
13. Martino R, Foley N, Bhogal S, Diamant N, Speechley M, Teasell R. Dysphagia after stroke: incidence, diagnosis, and pulmonary complications. Stroke. 2005;36:2756–63.
14. Singh S, Hamdy S. Dysphagia in stroke patients. Postgrad Med J. 2006;82:383–91.
15. Daniels SK, Foundas AL, Iglesia GC, Sullivan MA. Lesion site in unilateral stroke patients with dysphagia. J Stroke Cerebrovasc Dis. 1996;6(1):30–4.
16. Venketasubramanian N, Seshadri R, Chee N. Vocal cord paresis in acute ischemic stroke. Cerebrovasc Dis. 1999;9:157–62.
17. Zhou C, Cheng M. Contralateral tongue deviation due to paramedian pontine infarction: a brief review of cortico-hypoglossal projections. Am J Case Rep. 2022;23:e936511.
18. Urban P, Hopf H, Connemann B, Hundemer H, Koehler J. The course of cortico-hypoglossal projections in the human brainstem. Brain. 1996;119:1031–8.
19. Blumenfeld H. Neuroanatomy through clinical cases. 2nd ed. Sinauer Associates; 2010.
20. Umapathi T, Venketasubramanian N, Leck K, Tan C, Lee W, Tjia H. Tongue deviation in acute ischaemic stroke: a study of supranuclear twelfth cranial nerve palsy in 300 stroke patients. Cerebrovasc Dis. 2000;10:462–5.

Bullet Points

- Cranial neuropathies are relatively infrequent in diabetes, unlike other forms of neuropathy, but the association is definite.
- The most commonly involved CNs are CNs III, VI, VII, and X.
- The clinical characteristics of cranial neuropathies are often distinct, but evaluation has to be done to rule out alternate causes.
- In general, the prognosis is favorable and patients tend to have good recovery.
- Cranial neuropathies affect less than 1% of patients with diabetes, but there is a four to sevenfold increased risk of having cranial neuropathy in those with diabetes compared to those without.

Introduction

Neuropathy in diabetes mellitus is broadly classified on the basis of clinical presentation into generalized and focal neuropathies [1]. Diabetic cranial neuropathies belong to the group of focal neuropathies, are acute in onset and sometimes painful, and have a favorable prognosis with spontaneous recovery by 3–6 months in most cases [2]. In many aspects, they constitute a distinctive subset with regards to the clinical presentation, association with diabetes, and pathophysiology. Also, unlike other forms of diabetic neuropathy, electrodiagnostic studies have a limited role in their identification, but other diagnostic evaluations help exclude more sinister differential diagnoses. While other forms of diabetic neuropathy, such as diabetic sensorimotor polyneuropathy (DSP), are much more common and have received wider attention, the literature regarding diabetic cranial neuropathies is not extensive. In this chapter, we discuss various aspects of diabetic cranial neuropathies, as summarized in Table 20.1.

Authors of this chapter: Deepak Menon and Vera Bril.

Table 20.1 Summary of the diabetic cranial neuropathies and their relevant features

Cranial neuropathy	Presentation	Relative frequency among cranial neuropathies	Unique clinical feature	Differential diagnoses
Olfactory	Olfactory dysfunction	+	–	Upper respiratory infections Neurodegenerative diseases
Optic	NA-ION Diabetic papillopathy Optic atrophy secondary to diabetic retinopathy	+	Characteristic retinal telangiectasias	Arteritic ION Papilledema Optic neuritis?
Oculomotor	Medial rectus, superior and inferior rectus, inferior oblique weakness with ptosis	++++	Painful, pupillary sparing, though a mild anisocoria can be seen	Evolving lesions in anterior cavernous sinus, orbital apex, or superior orbital fissure Compressive lesions, such as pCOM Aneurysm
Trochlear	Superior oblique palsy	++		More common etiologies include congenital and trauma
Trigeminal	Trigeminal neuralgia	+	Ophthalmic and maxillary segments more commonly involved, resistance to carbamazepine	Multiple sclerosis Vascular compression
Abducens	Lateral rectus palsy	++++		
Facial	LMN facial palsy	+++	Taste is spared	Bell's palsy Ramsay Hunt syndrome Middle ear infections
Acoustic nerve	Sensorineural hearing loss	+	High-frequency hearing loss	Presbycusis, noise-induced hearing loss, idiopathic
Glossopharyngeal		Rare reports	Bilateral orofacial pain	Other causes of glossopharyngeal neuralgia, but only rarely bilateral
Vagus	Cardiac autonomic symptoms Resting tachycardia Exercise intolerance Hoarseness of voice	+++[a]	–	Other acquired and inherited autonomic neuropathies
Spinal accessory		Association not reported		
Hypoglossal		Single case report		–

LMN lower motor neuron, *NA-ION* non-arteritic ischemic optic neuropathy, *pCOM* posterior communicating artery, *PGE1* prostaglandin E1, *VEGG* vascular endothelial growth factor

[a] Most frequent among cranial neuropathies if the prevalence of diabetic cardiac autonomic neuropathy (CAN), which ranges from 16 to 22%, is considered [3]. CAN also presents with hoarseness of voice and dysphagia

Epidemiology

Compared to the other forms of diabetic neuropathy, the incidence and prevalence of clinical cranial neuropathies (excepting CAN) are rare in diabetes [2]. In hospital- and population-based studies, the frequency of diabetic cranial neuropathies ranged from 0 to 0.1%, while other forms of diabetic neuropathy were found in 23–66% of the same cohorts [4, 5]. Nevertheless, there is an unambiguous association between diabetes and cranial neuropathies. One of the earliest studies that compared ocular abnormalities among diabetics and nondiabetics noted external ophthalmoplegia in 0.4% of 2002 cases of diabetes compared to 1 in 457 of nondiabetics (0.1%) [6]. Watanabe found cranial neuropathies in 0.97% of diabetes patients, while cranial neuropathies were present in only 0.13% of those without diabetes [7]. In the 19 of 1961 diabetes patients having cranial neuropathies, the most common affected nerve was the facial nerve in 9, followed by the oculomotor nerve in 6, abducens nerve in 2, and combined CN III and VI in 2 [7]. Subsequent studies in larger cohorts revealed the frequency of ophthalmoplegia to be 0.32% and that of cranial neuropathies to be 0.75% in diabetes patients [8, 9]. Conversely, most large cohort studies examining cranial neuropathies have noted diabetes to be one of the rarer associations, though one report showed an association in 13.7% of cases [10–12]. In another series of 979 patients with multiple cranial neuropathies, only 2% of the cases were ascribed to diabetes [13].

Overall, cranial neuropathies affect less than 1% of patients with diabetes, but there is a four to sevenfold increased risk of having cranial neuropathies in diabetics compared to nondiabetics. The third, sixth, and seventh CN palsies account for the overwhelming majority of diabetic cranial neuropathies, excluding consideration of CAN [2, 9, 14, 15].

Risk Factors

Unlike DSP, the risk factors for diabetic cranial neuropathies are not well understood. Meta-analysis shows that the risk factors associated with DSP in type 2 diabetes include duration of diabetes, age, HbA1c, and diabetic retinopathy [16]. In diabetic cranial neuropathies, age, duration of diabetes, male gender, and the presence of retinopathy and nephropathy may be risk factors [8] In patients with diabetes, the frequency of CN III cranial neuropathy was 0.8% in those less than 45 years of age compared with 2.1% in those older than 45 years of age [17]. The basic mechanisms underlying DSP appear to be metabolic and microvascular alterations. Increased glucose levels, excessive free radical generation, and advanced glycosylation end products interfere with neuronal function directly and trigger an inflammatory cascade leading to microvasculitis and ischemic neuropathy [1, 18]. The same pathophysiologic mechanisms might lead to cranial neuropathies, but some contradictory evidence suggests that this is not the case.

Several studies have noted that the prevalence of diabetic complications, including DSP, are significantly lower in patients with cranial neuropathies compared to matched controls, which would not be expected if the same mechanisms were operative [10, 19–21]. CN IV has the longest course and would therefore be expected to be most prone for a vascular injury, but CN IV cranial neuropathies are the least reported among diabetic cranial neuropathies. There also are conflicting reports on the association of diabetes control, cardiac function, and renal function with diabetic ocular cranial neuropathies [15, 20]. A difference in cranial neuropathies was found in some studies with CN VI cranial neuropathy, which was found to be associated with more severe diabetes and its complications, compared to CN III or VII cranial neuropathies [9, 22]. Patients with diabetic ocular cranial neuropathies have a higher prevalence of metabolic syndrome and other vascular risk factors, such as hypertension, hyperlipidemia, and fibrinogen levels, compared to patients with facial cranial neuropathies [9, 22]. Thus, the conventional pathophysiological mechanisms of diabetic complications do not appear to explain cranial neuropathy lesions.

Overall, there is no difference in association between CN and the type of diabetes although some studies show an increased prevalence with type 2 diabetes and vice versa [5, 9, 10]. These differences might be a reflection of the higher prevalence of the diabetes type in the respective study populations. Interestingly, the age of onset of CN is similar in both type 1 and type 2 diabetes though the duration of diabetes before symptom onset is longer for type 1 diabetes.

Diabetic CN III Cranial Neuropathy

Most of the literature in diabetic cranial neuropathies discusses CN III cranial neuropathy. These patients generally are in their 60s, with a slight male preponderance, but without a relationship to diabetes duration or control [7, 9, 21, 23, 24]. Pain is a common feature of diabetic ophthalmoplegia and is associated more with CN III cranial neuropathy. The pain is homolateral to the side of the palsy, located above or behind the eye, and resolves when diplopia sets in [17]. The pain could be due to concomitant involvement of the ophthalmic division of the trigeminal nerve or due to ischemia of CN III.

The classical teaching is that the pupil is spared in diabetic CN III cranial neuropathy, perhaps due to ischemia, whereas a dilated pupil is an ominous sign of a compressive etiology. However, mild anisocoria is described in many patients. With careful pupillary size measurements, some degree of anisocoria was seen in 25–50% of patients with isolated diabetic CN III cranial neuropathy [23, 24]. With less stringent measurement, anisocoria was still evident in 14–32%, but a fully dilated unreactive pupil does not support a diagnosis of diabetic CN III cranial neuropathy and should prompt investigation for alternate causes [23–25]. The anisocoria ranges from 0.5 mm to 2.5 mm, with most having about a 1-mm difference in size. Maximum anisocoria is found within 14 days of the development of diplopia and improves but lags behind the improvement of ophthalmoplegia [23]. Although diabetic CN III cranial neuropathy can be diagnosed clinically, an MRI of the brain excludes other more concerning causes of painful ophthalmoplegia.

Pathological studies from the 1950s and 1970s in patients with diabetic ocular cranial neuropathies showed striking myelin pallor in the proximal intracavernous section of CN III, suggestive of focal demyelination. Nerve enlargement and inflammation were not observed, but microfasciculation at the edge of nerve fibers was present [26, 27]. The intraneural vessels showed diffuse thickening and hyalinization without occlusion, pointing to ischemia as the primary cause for the observed demyelination [28]. The peripheral location of pupillomotor fibers in CN III, with concomitant peripheral sparing, in ischemia of the centrally located vessels explains the characteristic pupillary sparing found in diabetic CN III cranial neuropathy.

Diabetic CN VI Cranial Neuropathy

Abducens nerve palsy is the most common of the diabetic cranial neuropathies in many series. A sixfold increase of diabetes and an eightfold increase of combined diabetes and hypertension was seen in cases compared to controls, while there was no association with hypertension alone [29]. Pain is not a distinctive feature of diabetic CN VI cranial neuropathy and can be seen in both diabetics and nondiabetics [30]. Postmortem series from the lateral rectus muscle in diabetic CN VI cranial neuropathy showed both axonal and demyelinating changes, which did not correlate with duration, severity, treatment of diabetes, or presence of diabetic retinopathy [31]. Concomitant vascular changes suggestive of ischemia were found in about 80% of cases. Notable is the absence of inflammatory changes in the nerves and vessels [17, 28, 31]. It may be hypothesized from these findings that mild, noninflammatory ischemia leads to focal demyelination, which has a favorable prognosis for recovery [26]. Diabetic ophthalmoplegia has a good prognosis, with 80% recovering by 9–10 weeks, although data specific for diabetic CN VI cranial neuropathy is lacking [32].

Botulinum toxin A injections of the antagonistic medial rectus within 2–3 weeks of onset can hasten recovery from CN VI nerve palsy, especially in significantly disabled patients [33].

Diabetic CN IV Cranial Neuropathy

Isolated CN IV cranial neuropathies are the least common cause of diabetic ophthalmoplegia, despite CN IV having the longest intracranial course. CN IV neuropathies are more common than simultaneous multiple cranial neuropathies [8, 22]. Conversely, in a series of isolated CN IV neuropathies, diabetes in isolation was infrequent, but diabetes in combination with hypertension and other vascular risk factors was much more common [34, 35]. In keeping with other diabetic cranial neuropathies, the prognosis is favorable, with near complete recovery in 6 months [34].

Diabetic CN VII Cranial Neuropathy

The incidence of idiopathic CN VII cranial neuropathies (Bell's palsy) in the general population is 11–40 per 100,000 per year, while the global prevalence of type 2 diabetes is 6059 cases per 100,000 [36–38]. Thus, given the high frequency of these two conditions, a causal relationship between CN VII cranial neuropathy and diabetes might be suspected. Initial case series showed an increase in prevalence of diabetes in patients with Bell's palsy, but the frequency ranged from 11.4 to 66% because of differences in interpretation of the glucose tolerance tests [39–41]. The prevalence was higher with increasing age, mainly above 40 years, and also in recurrent Bell's palsy. More recent studies on larger patient cohorts have confirmed the association, with diabetes being the most common comorbidity seen in 30–40% of patients with CN VII cranial neuropathy [42, 43]. Thus, testing for diabetes is advisable in patients presenting with Bell's palsy, especially in those older than 40 [44].

There are some subtle clinical and possibly pathological distinctions between the idiopathic (Bell's palsy) and diabetes-related CN VII nerve palsies. Histological examination of facial nerve in Bell's palsy showed diffuse inflammatory infiltrate of chorda tympani and the main trunk, with normal perineurial vessels [45]. While autopsy studies are not available, the pathomechanism in diabetes-related CN VII cranial neuropathy is likely primary ischemia due to vasculopathy and ensuing nerve edema which results in nerve compression in the narrow fallopian canal, a mechanism of nerve injury confirmed in animal models [46, 47].

A distinct clinical feature in diabetes-related CN VII cranial neuropathies is the preservation of taste in most cases. Impaired taste sensation was found in 14% of those with diabetes compared to 60% in nondiabetes Bell's palsy, signifying in diabetes a lesion distal to the chorda tympani which joins the facial nerve about 5–6 mm proximal to the stylomastoid foramen [42]. The ischemia can produce focal demyelination with a good prognosis, but in severe cases of ischemia producing axonopathy and Wallerian degeneration, there are only minimal chances of recovery. As with other cranial neuropathies, the duration and severity of diabetes was not marked, and the Bell's palsy is independent of the presence of DSP [42]. Although the severity of CN VII cranial neuropathy has correlated with HbA1c levels in some studies, the presence of diabetes or glycemic control does not appear to correlate with prognosis, and at 6 months patients recovered to the same extent with and without diabetes, although some debate still exists in this matter [48–50]. Patients with Bell's palsy may have fewer diabetic complications and cardiovascular risk factors compared to those with CN III or VI cranial neuropathies, although the explanation of these differences remains obscure [9].

Simultaneous Multiple Cranial Neuropathies

A polyneuritis cranialis presentation is rare but well recognized in diabetes, but this presentation necessitates detailed investigations to exclude alternate causes. In most case series of diabetic cranial neuropathies, simultaneous multiple cranial neuropathies comprise 2.6–15% of cases [7, 9, 10, 51]. The combination of CN III and VI cranial neuropathies were the most common combination. In multiple diabetic cranial neuropathies, there is no correlation with severity of hyperglycemia, or the presence of retinopathy or other complications of diabetes. The mean time for recovery was about 13 weeks, marginally longer than with isolated cranial neuropathies [51].

Other Cranial Neuropathies Less Frequently Associated with Diabetes

Associations with diabetes have been noted in other cranial neuropathies, albeit with limited evidence [52]. Olfactory impairment has a significant association with diabetes, with the odds of having impairment 1.58 times more in diabetes compared to controls irrespective of subtype of diabetes [53]. While there could be multiple factors ranging from central to peripheral mechanisms, an association with diabetic neuropathy has not been clearly proven.

A variety of visual impairments is associated with diabetes and is beyond the scope of this chapter. Diabetic retinopathy is by far the most prevalent and is the prototype example for the microvascular complications. While it does not constitute optic neuropathy in the true sense, long-standing and severe diabetic retinopathy can lead to progressive loss of retinal ganglion cells and multiple retinal nerve fiber layer infarcts leading to optic atrophy [54]. The Wolfram syndrome of type 1 diabetes mellitus, diabetes insipidus, optic atrophy, and deafness is encountered in the pediatric population and can be missed unless the physician is aware of this association [55].

Diabetic papillopathy is a usually self-limiting, unilateral or bilateral, acute optic disc edema in younger patients with either type 1 or type 2 diabetes. The visual symptoms when present are mild and resolve over 2–10 months, with minimal visual sequelae unless coexisting with maculopathy. Normal intracranial pressure, absence of inflammation, and a lack of substantial optic nerve dysfunction are necessary for diagnosis [56]. Intravitreal VEGF injections have been used in its treatment. Some authors consider diabetic papillopathy to be a milder variant of ischemic optic neuropathy [57]. Non-arteritic anterior ischemic optic neuropathy (NA-AION),

on the other hand, is at the severe end of the spectrum and causes profound and mostly irreversible visual loss. Meta-analysis has shown an increase of NA-AION in patients with diabetes, with an odds ratio of 1.68 [58]. Certain demographic and clinical differences, such as increased vascular disease, increased risk of contralateral eye involvement, and characteristic telangiectatic vessels, in NA-AION are associated with diabetes. Visual acuity at the end of 6 months did not significantly differ in those with and without diabetes [59].

An association exists between diabetes and trigeminal neuralgia, as shown in a recent large series of classical trigeminal neuralgia, where the prevalence of diabetes was nearly double that of the control population [60]. Rare reports of bilateral painful trigeminal neuralgia affecting ophthalmic and maxillary divisions and improving with glycemic control have been described [61]. Interestingly, diabetes and glycemic control were major determinants of resistance to carbamazepine in trigeminal neuralgia and may be related to the alteration of sodium channel kinetics by diabetes [62].

Data show that sensorineural hearing loss also has an association with diabetes, with an odds ratio of nearly 2, and the association was irrespective of age and type of diabetes, though the association was stronger in the younger population [63]. Glossopharyngeal neuralgia with bilateral orofacial pain has been rarely reported with diabetes, and in such cases a younger age of presentation compared to other causes for glossopharyngeal neuralgia was noted [64].

CN X, which accounts for 75% of all parasympathetic activity, is the longest CN and additionally is the longest autonomic nerve. It is involved early in diabetes, as reflected in the early parasympathetic attenuation and resulting sympathetic overtone, although clinical symptoms are not evident in most patients [65]. Although the prevalence of CN X cranial neuropathies in diabetes has not been examined directly, if autonomic neuropathy is considered to be due to vagal involvement, then the tenth CN may be the most common, as autonomic neuropathy ranges from 16 to 22% in diabetes. Clinical features of resting tachycardia and decreased heart rate variability, corresponding to the imbalance between sympathetic and parasympathetic activity, may be ascertained on examination, even at diagnosis of diabetes [2]. Poor glycemic control has a negative correlation with vagal dysfunction and also with sympathetic activity [66]. Rare instances of vagal neuropathy presenting with subacute onset dysphagia have been reported in newly detected diabetes, but the association is presumptive [67, 68]. Diabetes-related unilateral and bilateral vocal cord palsies have been reported and usually tend to have a good prognosis with complete recovery [69, 70]. A single case report of unilateral hypoglossal nerve palsy presumed to be of diabetic etiology has also been reported [71].

Cranial Autonomic Dysfunction

Though diabetic autonomic neuropathy encompasses a distinct spectrum of diabetic neuropathy, since the parasympathetic outputs are mediated through the various cranial nerves, a brief overview of autonomic dysfunction involving cranial segments is warranted. The parasympathetic cranial outflow mediates pupillary constriction through CN III to the ciliary ganglion, lacrimation and salivation through CNs VII and IX via sphenopalatine and otic ganglia, and cardiac, pulmonary, and enteric nervous plexuses through CN X [72]. Sweating of the face is mediated through the sympathetic nervous system, where the spinal innervation for the face arises from T1 to T4 and is supplied via the superior cervical ganglion, which also supplies the pupillary constrictor [73].

Though most patients may be asymptomatic, smaller pupillary size with sluggish mydriasis is a well-documented feature of early autonomic neuropathy and is more common in complicated diabetes. Topical pharmacological tests localize the lesion to a mixed pre- and postganglionic dysfunction of the sympathetic plexus [74].

Consistent with clinical experiences, a recent systematic review confirmed xerostomia, hyposalivation, and decreased salivary flow rate to be more common in diabetes than nondiabetes

[75]. Diabetic neuropathy is a definite causative factor, but there might be other contributory factors as well [76].

Gustatory sweating, which often can be profuse and socially embarrassing, is occasionally encountered in patients with diabetic autonomic neuropathy. It usually begins a few seconds after chewing food, starts in the forehead, and quickly spreads to most of the face, with the tips of the nose and chin often spared. The sweating can spread to the neck and sometimes extend to the shoulders and chest. There is a predilection with certain stimuli, such as cheese, which evokes a maximal response, while chewing inert substances can be asymptomatic [77]. The majority of patients have severe diabetic autonomic neuropathy, which is the most significant predictor [78]. Various theories include regenerating fibers from CN X that follow the sympathetic fibers to facial sweat glands, impaired tonic suppression of facial sweating, antisympathetic ganglia antibodies, and altered central autonomic responses [78]. A close link with diabetic nephropathy has also been noted, with patients reporting significant improvement after renal transplant.

Recommendation

Diabetic cranial neuropathy disorders are far less prevalent than other forms of diabetic neuropathy but can be no less symptomatic. With a generally favorable prognosis, patients can be reassured regarding a good chance of recovery for CN III, IV, VI, and VII palsies. The clinical features and limited pathological evidence raise questions concerning the presumptive microvascular pathogenesis. Since pathologic evaluation of the affected nerves is not possible, further research in animal models may be needed to fully elucidate the perpetrating mechanisms.

References

1. Tesfaye S, Selvarajah D. Advances in the epidemiology, pathogenesis and management of diabetic peripheral neuropathy. Diabetes Metab Res Rev [Internet].

2012 [cited 2021 Feb 18];28(S1):8–14. https://onlinelibrary.wiley.com/doi/abs/10.1002/dmrr.2239.

2. Boulton AJM, Vinik AI, Arezzo JC, Bril V, Feldman EL, Freeman R, et al. Diabetic neuropathies: a statement by the American Diabetes Association. Diabetes Care [Internet]. 2005 [cited 2021 Feb 17];28(4):956–62. https://care.diabetesjournals.org/content/28/4/956.

3. Vinik AI, Maser RE, Mitchell BD, Freeman R. Diabetic autonomic neuropathy. Diabetes Care [Internet]. 2003 [cited 2021 Apr 24];26(5):1553–79. https://care.diabetesjournals.org/content/26/5/1553.

4. Dyck PJ, Kratz KM, Karnes JL, Litchy WJ, Klein R, Pach JM, et al. The prevalence by staged severity of various types of diabetic neuropathy, retinopathy, and nephropathy in a population-based cohort: the Rochester diabetic neuropathy study. Neurology. 1993;43(4):817–24.

5. O'Hare JA, Abuaisha F, Geoghegan M. Prevalence and forms of neuropathic morbidity in 800 diabetics. Ir J Med Sci [Internet]. 1994 [cited 2021 Feb 17];163(3):132–5. https://doi.org/10.1007/BF02965972.

6. Waite JH, Beetham WP. The visual mechanism in diabetes mellitus. N Engl J Med [Internet]. 1935 [cited 2021 Feb 18];212(9):367–79. https://doi.org/10.1056/NEJM193502282120901.

7. Watanabe K, Hagura R, Akanuma Y, Takasu T, Kajinuma H, Kuzuya N, et al. Characteristics of cranial nerve palsies in diabetic patients. Diabetes Res Clin Pract. 1990;10(1):19–27.

8. Al Kahtani ES, Khandekar R, Al-Rubeaan K, Youssef AM, Ibrahim HM, Al-Sharqawi AH. Assessment of the prevalence and risk factors of ophthalmoplegia among diabetic patients in a large national diabetes registry cohort. BMC Ophthalmol [Internet]. 2016 [cited 2021 Apr 2];16. https://www.ncbi.nlm.nih.gov/pmc/articles/PMC4957375/.

9. Greco D, Gambina F, Pisciotta M, Abrignani M, Maggio F. Clinical characteristics and associated comorbidities in diabetic patients with cranial nerve palsies. J Endocrinol Invest [Internet]. 2012 [cited 2021 Feb 18];35(2):146–9. https://doi.org/10.3275/7574.

10. Trigler L, Siatkowski RM, Oster AS, Feuer WJ, Betts CL, Glaser JS, et al. Retinopathy in patients with diabetic ophthalmoplegia. Ophthalmology. 2003;110(8):1545–50.

11. Rush JA, Younge BR. Paralysis of cranial nerves III, IV, and VI. Cause and prognosis in 1000 cases. Arch Ophthalmol. 1981;99(1):76–9.

12. Richards BW, Jones FR, Younge BR. Causes and prognosis in 4,278 cases of paralysis of the oculomotor, trochlear, and Abducens cranial nerves. Am J Ophthalmol [Internet]. 1992 [cited 2021 Feb 18];113(5):489–96. https://www.sciencedirect.com/science/article/pii/S000293941474718X.

13. Keane JR. Multiple cranial nerve palsies: analysis of 979 cases. Arch Neurol [Internet]. 2005 [cited 2021 Feb 17];62(11):1714–7. https://doi.org/10.1001/archneur.62.11.1714.

14. Said G. Diabetic neuropathy—a review. Nat Clin Pract Neurol. 2007;3(6):331–40.

15. Lajmi H, Hmaied W, Ben Jalel W, Chelly Z, Ben Yakhlef A, Ben Zineb F, et al. Oculomotor palsy in diabetics. J Fr Ophtalmol. 2018;41(1):45–9.

16. Liu X, Xu Y, An M, Zeng Q. The risk factors for diabetic peripheral neuropathy: a meta-analysis. PLoS One [Internet]. 2019 [cited 2021 Feb 19];14(2). https://www.ncbi.nlm.nih.gov/pmc/articles/PMC6382168/.

17. Said G. Focal and multifocal diabetic neuropathies. Arq Neuropsiquiatr [Internet]. 2007 [cited 2021 Feb 18];65(4B):1272–8. http://www.scielo.br/scielo.php?script=sci_abstract&pid=S0004-282X2007000700037&lng=en&nrm=iso&tlng=en.

18. Feldman EL, Callaghan BC, Pop-Busui R, Zochodne DW, Wright DE, Bennett DL, et al. Diabetic neuropathy. Nat Rev Dis Primer [Internet]. 2019 [cited 2021 Feb 19];5(1):42. https://www.ncbi.nlm.nih.gov/pmc/articles/PMC7096070/.

19. Acaroglu G, Akinci A, Zilelioglu O. Retinopathy in patients with diabetic ophthalmoplegia. Ophthalmology. 2008;222(4):225–8.

20. Lazzaroni F, Laffi GL, Galuppi V, Scorolli L. [Paralysis of oculomotor nerves in diabetes mellitus. A retrospective study of 44 cases]. Rev Neurol (Paris). 1993;149(10):571–573.

21. Goldstein JE, Cogan DG. Diabetic ophthalmoplegia with special reference to the pupil. Arch Ophthalmol. 1960;64:592–600.

22. Greco D, Gambina F, Maggio F. Ophthalmoplegia in diabetes mellitus: a retrospective study. Acta Diabetol [Internet]. 2008 [cited 2021 Feb 18];46(1):23. https://doi.org/10.1007/s00592-008-0053-8.

23. Dhume KU, Paul KE. Incidence of pupillary involvement, course of anisocoria and ophthalmoplegia in diabetic oculomotor nerve palsy. Indian J Ophthalmol [Internet]. 2013 [cited 2021 Feb 21];61(1):13–7. https://www.ncbi.nlm.nih.gov/pmc/articles/PMC3554988/.

24. Jacobson DM. Pupil involvement in patients with diabetes-associated oculomotor nerve palsy. Arch Ophthalmol. 1998;116(6):723–7.

25. Shih MH, Huang FC, Tsai RK. Ischemic ophthalmoplegia in diabetic mellitus. Neuroophthalmology [Internet]. 2002 [cited 2021 Feb 20];26(3):181–91. https://doi.org/10.1076/noph.26.3.181.13974.

26. Dreyfus PM, Hakim S, Adams RD. Diabetic ophthalmoplegia; report of case, with postmortem study and comments on vascular supply of human oculomotor nerve. AMA Arch Neurol Psychiatry. 1957;77(4):337–49.

27. Smith BE, Dyck PJ. Subclinical histopathological changes in the oculomotor nerve in diabetes mellitus. Ann Neurol. 1992;32(3):376–85.

28. Asbury AK, Aldredge H, Hershberg R, Fisher CM. Oculomotor palsy in diabetes mellitus: a clinico-pathological study. Brain J Neurol. 1970;93(3):555–66.

29. Patel SV, Holmes JM, Hodge DO, Burke JP. Diabetes and hypertension in isolated sixth nerve palsy: a population-based study. Ophthalmology. 2005;112(5):760–3.

30. Wilker SC, Rucker JC, Newman NJ, Biousse V, Tomsak RL. Pain in ischemic ocular motor cranial nerve palsies. Br J Ophthalmol [Internet]. 2009 [cited 2021 Apr 2];93(12):1657–9. https://www.ncbi.nlm.nih.gov/pmc/articles/PMC2998753/.

31. Zrůstová M, Vrabec F, Rostlapil J. Diabetic changes of the extra-ocular muscles in man. Acta Diabetol Lat. 1979;16(1):55–62.

32. King AJ, Stacey E, Stephenson G, Trimble RB. Spontaneous recovery rates for unilateral sixth nerve palsies. Eye [Internet]. 1995 [cited 2021 Apr 2];9(4):476–8. https://www.nature.com/articles/eye1995110.

33. Ganesh S, Anilkumar SE, Narendran K. Botulinum toxin A in the early treatment of sixth nerve palsy in type 2 diabetes. Indian J Ophthalmol. 2019;67(7):1133–6.

34. Mollan SP, Edwards JH, Price A, Abbott J, Burdon MA. Aetiology and outcomes of adult superior oblique palsies: a modern series. Eye (Lond). 2009;23(3):640–4.

35. Dosunmu EO, Hatt SR, Leske DA, Hodge DO, Holmes JM. Incidence and etiology of presumed fourth cranial nerve palsy: a population-based study. Am J Ophthalmol [Internet]. 2018 [cited 2021 Apr 3];185:110–4. https://www.ncbi.nlm.nih.gov/pmc/articles/PMC5784757/.

36. McCaul JA, Cascarini L, Godden D, Coombes D, Brennan PA, Kerawala CJ. Evidence based management of Bell's palsy. Br J Oral Maxillofac Surg. 2014;52(5):387–91.

37. Khan MAB, Hashim MJ, King JK, Govender RD, Mustafa H, Al Kaabi J. Epidemiology of type 2 diabetes—global burden of disease and forecasted trends. J Epidemiol Glob Health [Internet]. 2020 [cited 2021 Mar 31];10(1):107–11. https://www.ncbi.nlm.nih.gov/pmc/articles/PMC7310804/.

38. Fazeli Farsani S, van der Aa MP, van der Vorst MMJ, Knibbe CAJ, de Boer A. Global trends in the incidence and prevalence of type 2 diabetes in children and adolescents: a systematic review and evaluation of methodological approaches. Diabetologia [Internet]. 2013 [cited 2021 Mar 31];56(7):1471–1488. https://doi.org/10.1007/s00125-013-2915-z.

39. Korczyn AD. Bell's palsy and diabetes mellitus. Lancet. 1971;1(7690):108–9.

40. Adour K, Wingerd J, Doty HE. Prevalence of concurrent diabetes mellitus and idiopathic facial paralysis (Bell's palsy). Diabetes. 1975;24(5):449–51.

41. Korczyn AD. Prevalence of diabetes mellitus in Bell's palsy. Lancet. 1971;2(7722):489.

42. Pecket P, Schattner A. Concurrent Bell's palsy and diabetes mellitus: a diabetic mononeuropathy? J Neurol Neurosurg Psychiatry [Internet]. 1982 [cited 2021 Mar 31];45(7):652–5. https://www.ncbi.nlm.nih.gov/pmc/articles/PMC491483/.

43. Zhao H, Zhang X, da Tang Y, Zhu J, Wang XH, Li ST. Bell's palsy: clinical analysis of 372 cases and review of related literature. Eur Neurol [Internet]. 2017 [cited 2021 Mar 31];77(3–4):168–72. https://www.karger.com/Article/FullText/455073.

44. Tiemstra JD, Khatkhate N. Bell's palsy: diagnosis and management. Am Fam Physician [Internet]. 2007 [cited 2021 Apr 1];76(7):997–1002. https://www.aafp.org/afp/2007/1001/p997.html.

45. Liston SL, Kleid MS. Histopathology of Bell's palsy. Laryngoscope. 1989;99(1):23–6.

46. Pecket P, Schattner A. Concurrent Bell's palsy and diabetes mellitus: a diabetic mononeuropathy? J Neurol Neurosurg Psychiatry. 1982;45(7):652–5.

47. Zhang W, Xu L, Luo T, Wu F, Zhao B, Li X. The etiology of Bell's palsy: a review. J Neurol. 2020;267(7):1896–905.

48. Riga M, Kefalidis G, Danielides V. The role of diabetes mellitus in the clinical presentation and prognosis of Bell palsy. J Am Board Fam Med [Internet]. 2012 [cited 2021 Apr 1];25(6):819–26. https://www.jabfm.org/content/25/6/819.

49. Hohman MH, Hadlock TA. Etiology, diagnosis, and management of facial palsy: 2000 patients at a facial nerve center. Laryngoscope. 2014;124(7):E283–93.

50. Şevik Eliçora S, Erdem D. Does type 2 diabetes mellitus affect the healing of Bell's palsy in adults? Can J Diabetes. 2018;42(4):433–6.

51. Eshbaugh CG, Siatkowski RM, Smith JL, Kline LB. Simultaneous, multiple cranial neuropathies in diabetes mellitus. J Neuroophthalmol. 1995;15(4):219–24.

52. Boulton AJM, Malik RA, Arezzo JC, Sosenko JM. Diabetic somatic neuropathies. Diabetes Care [Internet]. 2004 [cited 2021 Apr 8];27(6):1458–86. https://care.diabetesjournals.org/content/27/6/1458.

53. Kim SJ, Windon MJ, Lin SY. The association between diabetes and olfactory impairment in adults: a systematic review and meta-analysis. Laryngoscope Investig Otolaryngol [Internet]. 2019 [cited 2021 Apr 8];4(5):465–75. https://www.ncbi.nlm.nih.gov/pmc/articles/PMC6793600/.

54. Sadun AA. Neuro-ophthalmic manifestations of diabetes. Ophthalmology [Internet]. 1999 [cited 2021 Apr 23];106(6):1047–1048. https://www.aaojournal.org/article/S0161-6420(99)90242-7/abstract.

55. Medlej R, Wasson J, Baz P, Azar S, Salti I, Loiselet J, et al. Diabetes mellitus and optic atrophy: a study of Wolfram syndrome in the Lebanese population. J Clin Endocrinol Metab. 2004;89(4):1656–61.

56. Gian PG, Ama S, Peter YC, Rafael TC. Diabetic papillopathy: current and new treatment options. Curr Diabetes Rev [Internet]. 2011 [cited 2021 Apr 22];7(3):171–5. https://www.eurekaselect.com/74265/article.

57. Hayreh SS. Diabetic papillopathy and nonarteritic anterior ischemic optic neuropathy. Surv Ophthalmol. 2002;47(6):600–2; author reply 602.

58. Chen T, Song D, Shan G, Wang K, Wang Y, Ma J, et al. The association between diabetes mellitus and

nonarteritic anterior ischemic optic neuropathy: a systematic review and meta-analysis. PLoS One [Internet]. 2013 [cited 2021 Apr 23];8(9):e76653. https://journals.plos.org/plosone/article?id=10.1371/journal.pone.0076653.

59. Hayreh SS, Zimmerman MB. Nonarteritic anterior ischemic optic neuropathy: clinical characteristics in diabetic patients versus nondiabetic patients. Ophthalmology [Internet]. 2008 [cited 2021 Apr 23];115(10):1818–25. https://www.sciencedirect.com/science/article/pii/S0161642008003047.

60. Xu Z, Zhang P, Long L, He H, Zhang J, Sun S. Diabetes mellitus in classical trigeminal neuralgia: a predisposing factor for its development. Clin Neurol Neurosurg. 2016;151:70–2.

61. Takayama S, Osawa M, Takahashi Y, Iwamoto Y. Painful neuropathy with trigeminal nerve involvement in type 2 diabetes. J Int Med Res. 2006;34(1):115–8.

62. Zhang A, Zhang W, Xu H, Guo C, Yuan L, Xu Y, et al. Diabetes mellitus contributes to carbamazepine resistance in patient with trigeminal neuralgia. Neurosurg Rev [Internet]. 2020 [cited 2021 Apr 8]. https://doi.org/10.1007/s10143-020-01304-4.

63. Baiduc RR, Helzner EP. Epidemiology of diabetes and hearing loss. Semin Hear. 2019;40(4):281–91.

64. Matsumoto F, Momota Y, Takano H, Matsuka Y. Glossopharyngeal neuralgia caused by diabetes mellitus: a case report. Jpn J Orofac Pain. 2016;9(1):81–5.

65. Pop-Busui R. Cardiac autonomic neuropathy in diabetes. Diabetes Care [Internet]. 2010 [cited 2021 Apr 8];33(2):434–41. https://www.ncbi.nlm.nih.gov/pmc/articles/PMC2809298/.

66. Yu Y, Hu L, Xu Y, Wu S, Chen Y, Zou W, et al. Impact of blood glucose control on sympathetic and vagus nerve functional status in patients with type 2 diabetes mellitus. Acta Diabetol. 2020;57(2):141–50.

67. Berry H, Blair RL. Isolated vagus nerve palsy and vagal mononeuritis. Arch Otolaryngol [Internet]. 1980 [cited 2021 Apr 8];106(6):333–8. https://europepmc.org/article/med/7378018.

68. Mathew J, Mohan M, Menon A. Multiple cranial neuropathies in a patient with diabetes mellitus. Ann Indian Acad Neurol [Internet]. 2019 [cited 2021 Apr 8];22(3):353–5. https://www.ncbi.nlm.nih.gov/pmc/articles/PMC6613403/.

69. Sommer DD, Freeman JL. Bilateral vocal cord paralysis associated with diabetes mellitus: case reports. J Otolaryngol. 1994;23(3):169–71.

70. Ravi R, Gunjawate DR. Effect of diabetes mellitus on voice: a systematic review. Pract Diabetes. 2019;36(5):177–80.

71. Kenmegne C, Kamdem F, Jingi AM, Choukem SP. Hypoglossal nerve paralysis revealing type 2 diabetes mellitus: a case report. Rev Méd Pharm. 2016;6(2):617–21.

72. Benarroch EE. Physiology and pathophysiology of the autonomic nervous system. Continuum (Minneap Minn). 2020;26(1):12–24.

73. Coon EA, Cheshire WP. Sweating disorders. Continuum (Minneap Minn). 2020;26(1):116–37.

74. Pittasch D, Lobmann R, Behrens-Baumann W, Lehnert H. Pupil signs of sympathetic autonomic neuropathy in patients with type 1 diabetes. Diabetes Care [Internet]. 2002 [cited 2021 Apr 4];25(9):1545–50. https://care.diabetesjournals.org/content/25/9/1545.

75. López-Pintor RM, Casañas E, González-Serrano J, Serrano J, Ramírez L, de Arriba L, et al. Xerostomia, hyposalivation, and salivary flow in diabetes patients. J Diabetes Res [Internet]. 2016 [cited 2021 Apr 3];2016. https://www.ncbi.nlm.nih.gov/pmc/articles/PMC4958434/.

76. Moore PA, Guggenheimer J, Etzel KR, Weyant RJ, Orchard T. Type 1 diabetes mellitus, xerostomia, and salivary flow rates. Oral Surg Oral Med Oral Pathol Oral Radiol Endod. 2001;92(3):281–91.

77. Watkins PJ. Facial sweating after food: a new sign of diabetic autonomic neuropathy. Br Med J [Internet]. 1973 [cited 2021 Apr 3];1(5853):583–7. https://www.bmj.com/content/1/5853/583.

78. Shaw JE, Parker R, Hollis S, Gokal R, Boulton AJ. Gustatory sweating in diabetes mellitus. Diabet Med. 1996;13(12):1033–7.

Bullet Points

- Patients with malignancy can develop cranial nerve (CN) involvement directly due to infiltration or local compression of the nerve trunk by the tumor mass or indirectly via treatment-related neurotoxicity, metabolic and endocrine complications, virus infections, and paraneoplastic involvement.
- Paraneoplastic optic neuropathy (PON) is the most frequent cranial neuropathy and has been associated with small cell lung cancer (SCLC).
- Brainstem encephalitis may present as isolated syndrome or be associated with a more widespread encephalomyelitis, and any part of the brainstem can be affected, with features usually depending on the type of antibody involved.
- Cancer immunotherapy with immune checkpoint inhibitors may trigger cranial neuropathies.

Introduction

Patients with malignancy can develop cranial nerve (CN) involvement due to different mechanisms. The most frequent is the direct infiltration or local compression of the nerve trunk by tumor mass. Other indirect mechanisms include treatment-related neurotoxicity, metabolic and endocrine complications, virus infections, and paraneoplastic involvement [1]. In this chapter we investigated the paraneoplastic involvement and the immunological complication of the cancer treatments with immune checkpoint inhibitors.

Paraneoplastic Neurological Syndrome with Cranial Nerve Involvement

Paraneoplastic neurological syndromes are a group of uncommon disorders strongly associated with systemic cancers. They are not caused by direct involvement of nervous system, endocrine, metabolic, iatrogenic, or infectious complications, but are determined by an aberrant immune-mediated response triggered by the cancer itself [2]. Tumors may in fact express individual neuronal proteins or contain mature/immature neuronal tissue, and this ectopic expression triggers an immune response misdirected against the nervous system through cross-

Authors of this chapter: Silvia Casagrande and Bruno Giometto.

reactivity phenomena [3]. In addition, the malignancy may originate from an organ directly involved in immune system regulation (such as thymomas), leading to the loss of self-tolerance mechanisms [4].

Paraneoplastic neurological syndromes usually present with serum and/or cerebrospinal fluid (CSF) autoantibodies (Abs) to neuronal antigens, mostly located inside the neurons. Considering the co-expression of these antigens, both by the nervous system and by the neoplasms, these Abs are often defined as "onco-neuronal Abs" [5]. Due to their intracellular localization, antigens are not directly exposed to Abs that represent a non-pathogenetic epiphenomenon of a cell-mediated response. Several findings indeed suggest a predominant cytotoxic T-cell pathogenesis, with activated CD8+ T cells responsible for neuronal damage [6]. Despite the negative effect on the nervous system, this aberrant immune response also inhibits the growth of the malignancy, which may be so small it remains unknown until the diagnosis of the paraneoplastic neurological syndrome leads to oncological screening. Neurological symptoms usually appear before the cancer has been identified, and in 90% of patients the underlying malignancy is discovered during the first years after the appearance of the neurological picture [2]. Timely recognition of these disorders facilitates the early detection of an unsuspected cancer, improving patients' survival.

Treatment is mainly based on removal of the trigger of the aberrant immune response. For most of the paraneoplastic neurological syndromes, the most effective approach is cancer treatment, where possible. A stabilization or a slight improvement of the clinical picture may be obtained with immunotherapy, but usually with only partial response [2]. Paraneoplastic neurological syndromes may affect each part of the peripheral and central nervous system with different clinical picture, and tumor association depends on antigen localization/Ab specificity. Each Ab may in fact be associated with a limited number of clinical manifestations and appear within some defined oncological forms [5].

Paraneoplastic CN disorders may present as individual or multiple cranial neuropathies, or in the context of a more widespread encephalitis mostly with brainstem involvement.

Paraneoplastic Cranial Neuropathies

Paraneoplastic cranial neuropathies are rare, and except for paraneoplastic optic neuropathy (PON), they have been mostly described in individual case reports. Considering their low frequency, only PON has been mentioned in the previous and updated diagnostic criteria for paraneoplastic neurological syndromes but is considered as a nonclassical syndrome [7, 8]. Symptoms depend on the CNs affected. Possible imaging findings include enhancement and/or enlargement of the involved CNs but magnetic resonance imaging (MRi) can also be unremarkable [9]. Although uncommon, a paraneoplastic etiology should be considered in all patients with malignancy and exclusion of alternative causes, especially in the setting of small cell lung cancer.

Paraneoplastic optic neuropathy (PON): Paraneoplastic syndromes affecting the visual system include cancer-associated retinopathy, melanoma-associated retinopathy, bilateral diffuse uveal melanocytic proliferation, and PON [10]. Compared to other paraneoplastic neurological syndromes, they are rare, affecting about 0.01% of oncological patients [10]. The first description of paraneoplastic nerve involvement dates to 1989 by Hoogenraadet et al., but a possible immunologic pathogenesis was first suggested in 1992 by Malik et al. with the identification of a serum IgG which reacted both with neuronal and glial cytoplasm and with patient's tumor [11, 12]. Since then, several cases of PON have been reported, mostly associated with small cell lung cancer (SCLC) [10, 13].

Clinical presentation is characterized by subacute onset and rapid progression of bilateral, painless visual deficits. Visual field evaluation may reveal enlarged blind spots and variable visual field defects, such as arcuate or paracentral scotomas, altitudinal defects, or peripheral constriction [13]. Ophthalmoscopy usually displays subacute or chronic optic disc swelling in the first phases, often along with nerve fiber layer hemorrhages, with possible atrophy development in later stages [13]. Fluorescein angiography shows optic disc hyperfluorescence consistent with leakage and in some cases subretinal accumulation of fluid [13]. Reactive inflammatory lymphocytic infiltrates at vitreous biopsy have been reported [13]. The triad of optic neuritis, retinal vascular leakage, and vitreous cell is thus considered the hallmark of PON [10]. MRI may be unremarkable or show enhancement of the optic nerve, similarly to other optic neuritis, sometimes along with matter lesions [13].

In most of patients, PON occurs in the context of a SCLC, but other less common associations have been reported, including B-cell lymphoma, thymomas, pancreatic neuroendocrine and thyroid tumors, breast neoplasms, and non-SCLCs [13–20]. CSF analysis usually shows lymphocytic pleocytosis and hyperproteinorrachia, and oligoclonal bands have also been described [13]. In most patients, Abs against a neuronal antigen called collapsing response-mediating protein-5 (CRMP5) or CV2 are detectable in serum and or/ CSF, sometimes along with other onconeuronal Abs (anti-Hu, anti-amphiphysin, or anti-glutamic acid decarboxylase), but seronegative cases have also been reported [13, 21, 22]. PON may be the only manifestation, but usually occurs in the setting of a more complex paraneoplastic neurological syndrome. CRMP5 is in fact expressed not only by the retina and optic nerve, but also widespread throughout the central and peripheral nervous systems [13, 23]. Most of patients with this Ab present a multifocal neurological dysfunction with signs of cerebellar degeneration, brainstem encephalitis, and/or peripheral neuropathy, and PON is encountered in 9% of cases [23]. For example, in the cohort of PON published by Cross et al., despite prominent involvement of the optic nerve, other slight neurological symptoms were reported, mostly consistent with coexistent peripheral nervous system involvement, such as peripheral neuropathy (33%) or polyradiculoneuropathy (13%). In addition, some patients with PON present a concomitant myelopathy with a clinical picture resembling

those of neuromyelitis optica spectrum disorders [13, 24, 25].

Tumor treatment/removal, where possible, lead to stabilization or improvement of visual deficit in some patients, but severe visual loss despite cancer treatment has also been reported [13, 14, 26–29]. Immunotherapy alone is usually not enough to achieve a good outcome, but efficacy of steroid therapy along with cancer treatment has been reported in several cases [13, 30, 31].

Other cranial mono- and multi-neuropathies: Compared to the optic nerve, other CNs are less commonly affected by paraneoplastic mechanisms.

Involvement of the trigeminal nerve, in the form of an isolated paraneoplastic sensory neuropathy, has been reported in several cases of cancer patients, mostly with anti-Hu Abs [32–36]. Trigeminal neuropathy may be the first manifestation, but patients later develop signs and symptoms of a more widespread anti-Hu syndrome, with subsequent occurrence of encephalomyelitis/sensory neuropathy. Patients usually complain of unilateral facial pain or numbness, and "numb cheek syndrome" has also been reported [32–35]. MRI may be unremarkable or show contrast enhancement of one or both trigeminal nerves [32–35]. CSF analysis usually displays elevated protein, with or without lymphocytic pleocytosis and oligoclonal bands [32–34]. Facial pain or numbness has been also reported as a symptom of paraneoplastic brainstem encephalitis and in most patients is therefore not easy to discriminate between nerve trunk/ganglion and central involvement, particularly if MRI is unremarkable [36]. Only anecdotal case reports exist on paraneoplastic trigeminal neuropathy without anti-Hu Abs, but a paraneoplastic origin has been hypothesized for "numb chin syndrome" in seronegative oncological patients without evidence of local tumor infiltration/compression [37, 38].

Subacute sensorineural bilateral hearing loss is the most common cranial neuropathy in anti-Hu-related paraneoplastic neurologic syndrome [39, 40]. As for the trigeminal nerve, the exact localization of the pathological process is often not reported, and most patients present other neurological symptoms consistent with encephalomyelitis/sensory neuropathy. In a large case series of patients with anti-Hu Abs, involvement of CN VIII accounted for half of the cranial neuropathies [40].

Oculomotor nerve and facial nerve involvement has been rarely reported without coexistent signs and symptoms of brainstem encephalitis. One case of anti-Hu paraneoplastic syndrome presenting as isolated bilateral CN VI palsies has been described [41]. Another case of bilateral peripheral facial nerve palsy has been reported in a patient with anti-amphiphysin Abs and breast cancer [42].

Several cases of paraneoplastic multiple cranial neuropathies have been described in association with different onconeuronal Abs and cancer subtypes [43–45]. All CNs may be affected, except for the optic nerve, which more frequently associates with symptoms of central nervous system involvement [10]. Patients with anti-Hu Abs usually present multiple cranial neuropathies along with systemic sensory neuronopathy in the context of SCLCs, whereas the only reported case with anti-Ri Abs presented isolated CN involvement with breast cancer [43–45]. In addition, in some patients with cranial neuropathies and other neurological symptoms, Abs targeting neurofilament light chain (NfL) may be found [46]. Eventually, anecdotal cases without known Abs were also reported [47, 48].

Paraneoplastic Brainstem Encephalitis

Paraneoplastic CN involvement more frequently occurs in the context of a paraneoplastic brainstem encephalitis, probably due to damage of CN nuclei. Brainstem encephalitis may present as an isolated syndrome or may be associated with a more widespread encephalomyelitis. Each part of the brainstem can be affected by the inflammatory process, but usually, depending on onconeuronal Abs specificity, different clinical features can be observed [49].

Brainstem encephalitis with anti-Hu Abs: In cases with anti-Hu Abs, brainstem involvement may appear as isolated paraneoplastic neurological syndromes or in the context of a more widespread multifocal encephalomyelitis, sometimes with peripheral nervous system involvement [36, 50]. Most of patients with brainstem encephalitis and anti-Hu Abs show a predominant involvement of the medulla, characterized by subacute onset of dysfunction of the caudal CNs with dysarthria, dysphagia, and development of central hypoventilation [50]. Less frequently, patients present with a ponto-mesencephalic syndrome, but a rapid downward progression to a bulbar syndrome can be observed in all patients [36]. As in other anti-Hu-associated paraneoplastic neurological syndromes, affected patients are usually males over the age of 40 years with SCLC or, more rarely, neuroendocrine tumors [36, 50]. MRI is usually unremarkable, and in most patients CSF analysis only displays a mild hyperproteinorrachia without pleocytosis [50]. Overall, the prognosis is poor. Tumor treatment seems to have more effect on the neurological outcome than the use of immunotherapies, but only rarely is a stabilization observed, mostly in patients with isolated medullary involvement without central hypoventilation [50].

Brainstem encephalitis with anti-Ma2 Abs: Anti-Ma2 Abs are usually detectable in patients with a specific brainstem encephalitis with prominent upper brainstem involvement. Typical symptoms are vertical gaze palsy, extrapyramidal signs, and involvement of CNs with ponto-mesencephalic origin (eyelid ptosis, ataxia, sensorineural hearing loss, facial palsy, and later bulbar signs). In most patients, signs and symptoms of diencephalic involvement are present, such as extensive daytime sleepiness, hyperphagia, hyperthermia, and hypothalamic–pituitary hormonal dysfunctions [51]. In addition, some patients show a coexistent limbic encephalitis, with psychiatric symptoms, memory deficits, and focal temporal seizures [51, 52]. Onset is usually subacute and slower than that of other paraneoplastic limbic encephalitis [51]. Patients younger than 50 years are typically males with testicular germ cell tumors, whereas no gender predominance exists in older cases who usually present with SCLC or breast cancer [51, 52]. In most cases, MRI reveals abnormalities in the affected site, and inflammatory signs are detectable on CSF analysis. Overall, in half of subjects there is a clear response to immunotherapy and/or tumor treatment, with stabilization or improvement of the neurological picture. Prognosis is thus better than in the anti-Hu form [51].

Brainstem encephalitis with anti-CRMP5 Abs: Anti-CRMP5 Abs can be found in the context of almost all paraneoplastic neurological syndromes that may occur alone or in variable associations. In patients with anti-CRMP5 Abs, isolated brainstem encephalitis is uncommon [13, 23]. More frequently, patients present a more widespread encephalomyelitis, with basal ganglia, optic nerve, and spinal cord involvement [13, 23]. CNs are often affected in the form of pure CN neuropathy or due to brainstem involvement. In a large series of 116 patients published in 2001 by Yu et al., 17% of patients presented with signs and symptoms of CN involvement, mostly with PON. Other manifestations of CN involvement were olfactory/taste loss, bilateral hearing loss, facial palsy, and oculomotor nerve dysfunction [23]. Most subjects develop SCLC or thymomas. Prognosis is similar to that described for anti-Hu Abs [13, 23].

Brainstem encephalitis with anti-Ri Abs: Anti-Ri Abs were initially described in patients with paraneoplastic opsoclonus–myoclonus and breast cancer [53]. However, these Abs are also associated with brainstem dysfunction that may appear alone or in association with opsoclonus–myoclonus syndrome [54, 55]. Paraneoplastic brainstem encephalitis with anti-Ri Abs is usually characterized by frequent ocular motor dysfunction, even in the absence of opsoclonus, that may occur due to conjugate gaze paresis, ocular flutter, reduced saccadic velocities, internuclear ophthalmoplegia, or CN palsy. Involvement of one of the oculomotor nerves is reported in 18% of patients, along with other manifestations [54, 55]. Other typical symptoms are trunk ataxia and postural instability [54, 55]. Less frequently, patients complain of muscle rigidity, with superimposed painful spasms similar to those reported in stiff-person syndrome [55]. Some patients show laryngospasms and/or jaw dystonia, with consequent nutritional and respiratory deficits due to the impossibility in opening the mouth [56]. Most subjects are females with breast cancer, whereas lung cancer is the most frequent association in males [55]. CSF analysis reveals mild pleocytosis in 40% and elevated protein in 70% of patients. More than 80% of subjects have no abnormalities on MRI. Immunotherapy and tumor treatment may improve opsoclonus–myoclonus, but trunk ataxia and other brainstem symptoms rarely disappear, and good prognosis is rare [53–55].

Brainstem encephalitis with anti-KLHL11: Abs against Kelch-like protein 11 (KLHL11) were discovered in 2019 and are mainly associated with a paraneoplastic brainstem–cerebellar encephalitis [57]. Patients usually present with gait instability, limb ataxia, nystagmus, and ocular motor symptoms. Diplopia due to involvement of CNs occurs in more than 50% of patients. Another hallmark of this syndrome is vestibulocochlear symptoms, like vertigo, sensorineural hearing loss, and tinnitus [57, 58]. Hearing deficits and tinnitus often precede other neurological manifestations and are the most frequent onset symptom. Less frequently, these Abs are detectable in isolated limbic encephalitis [58]. Anti-KLHL11 Abs were initially described in male patients with paraneoplastic brainstem encephalitis and testicular seminoma [57]. However, subsequent case series have expanded the clinical spectrum associated with anti-KLHL11 Abs, showing different oncological associations [58, 59]. They are also detectable in female patients, which usually present with ovarian teratomas, and in 28% of cases no cancer can be found at neurological presentation [59]. In most cases, MRI reveals T2/FLAIR hyperintensity in the temporal lobes, cerebellum, and/or brainstem, consistent with clinical symptoms [58]. CSF analysis displays inflammatory signs in more than 80% of cases, with pleocytosis and oligoclonal bands [58]. Response to immunotherapy and tumor treatment is suboptimal, but overall, half of subjects show a clear improvement of the neurological picture [57, 58].

Cranial Nerve Disorders Associated with Immune Checkpoint Inhibitors

Paraneoplastic neurological syndromes may be also triggered by cancer immunotherapy, particularly immune checkpoint inhibitors (ICIs) [60]. Immune checkpoints are key regulators of the immune system and are crucial for self-tolerance mechanisms. They are usually expressed on activated immune cells and when stimulated prevent the indiscriminate activation of the immune system against self-antigens. Tumor cells can overexpress immune checkpoint ligands, downregulating the immune response and thus escaping the tumor immune surveillance. ICIs, blocking either checkpoint molecules or their ligands, restore immune system function and result in an effective and prolonged immune response to the cancer [61]. Given that ICIs result in generalized immune activation, they carry a high risk of immune-related adverse events (irAEs), some of which may involve the nervous system [60]. The pathophysiology of these forms is still to be elucidated. One hypothesis is a facilitation of the immune response against antigens shared between cancer and neural tissue, as in classical paraneoplastic syndromes. An alternative hypothesis is the presence of a preexisting autoimmune predisposition or a silent autoimmune condition independent of the neoplastic pathology, which may result in a clinically manifested disease only after ICI-mediated immune activation [60]. Neurological irAEs are not common and have an estimated incidence of 1–3% [62, 63]. Some neurological irAEs present with the clinical phenotype of classical paraneoplastic neurological syndromes, often along with onconeuronal Abs, and should be considered of paraneoplastic etiology. Some other neurological irAEs present with the clinical phenotype of other autoimmune disorders and should therefore not be considered as properly paraneoplastic.

Compared to other neurological irAEs, ICI-related CN involvement has emerged as a common phenotype [64, 65]. Cranial neuropathies may be isolated or associated with other neurological manifestations. Usually, one single CN is affected, but rare cases with involvement of two different CNs have been also reported [64, 65]. The most common cranial neuropathy is facial palsy, representing 33% of the described ICI-related cranial neuropathies. Other frequently involved nerves were the vestibulocochlear and optic nerves. Oculomotor nerves are less commonly involved and usually present with abducens nerve palsy. Cases of trigeminal and glossopharyngeal nerves have been also described [65]. As for other neurological irAEs, some cranial neuropathies present with onconeuronal Abs and may be properly considered as paraneoplastic. Other CN disorders instead represent a non-paraneoplastic autoimmune disorder, triggered by ICI administration in the context of a Guillain–Barré or Miller Fisher syndrome [64, 65]. Some features of ICI-related cranial neuropathies are different from their classical inflammatory counterparts not triggered by ICIs. Optic nerve involvement, for example, mainly occurs without detectable onconeuronal Abs, but does not show the clinical picture of a demyelinating optic neuritis, presenting with painless visual loss and poor outcome, more resembling classical PON [65]. Treatment of ICI-related cranial neuropathies is based on ICI withdrawal/discontinuation and/or immunotherapies, mainly corticosteroids and intravenous immunoglobulins, but also plasma exchange and other immunosuppressive agents [65]. Outcome depends on the CN involved. Facial palsy usually presents a good outcome, but approximately one-third of patients with ICI-related cranial neuropathy show persisting deficits, most frequently involving hearing and vision loss [65].

References

1. Antoine JC, Camdessanché JP. Peripheral nervous system involvement in patients with cancer. Lancet Neurol. 2007;6(1):75–86. https://doi.org/10.1016/S1474-4422(06)70679-2.

2. Darnell RB, Posner JB. Paraneoplastic syndromes involving the nervous system. N Engl J Med. 2009;349:1543–54. https://doi.org/10.1056/NEJMRA023009.

3. DeLuca I, Blachére NE, Santomasso B, Darnell RB. Tolerance to the neuron-specific paraneoplastic

HuD antigen. PLoS One. 2009;4:e5739. https://doi.org/10.1371/JOURNAL.PONE.0005739.

4. Shelly S, Agmon-Levin N, Altman A, Shoenfeld Y. Thymoma and autoimmunity. Cell Mol Immunol. 2011;8:199–202. https://doi.org/10.1038/CMI.2010.74.

5. Melzer N, Meuth SG, Wiendl H. Paraneoplastic and non-paraneoplastic autoimmunity to neurons in the central nervous system. J Neurol. 2013;260(5):1215–33. https://doi.org/10.1007/s00415-012-6657-5.

6. Melzer N, Meuth SG, Wiendl H. CD8+ T cells and neuronal damage: direct and collateral mechanisms of cytotoxicity and impaired electrical excitability. FASEB J. 2009;23:3659–73. https://doi.org/10.1096/FJ.09-136200.

7. Graus F, Delattre JY, Antoine JC, et al. Recommended diagnostic criteria for paraneoplastic neurological syndromes. J Neurol Neurosurg Psychiatry. 2004;75:1135. https://doi.org/10.1136/JNNP.2003.034447.

8. Graus F, Vogrig A, Muñiz-Castrillo S, et al. Updated diagnostic criteria for paraneoplastic neurologic syndromes. Neurology - Neuroimmunology Neuroinflammation. 2021;8:e1014. https://doi.org/10.1212/NXI.0000000000001014.

9. Madhavan AA, Carr CM, Morris PP, et al. Imaging review of paraneoplastic neurologic syndromes. AJNR Am J Neuroradiol Dec. 2020;41(12):2176–87. https://doi.org/10.3174/ajnr.A6815.

10. Rahimy E, Sarraf D. Paraneoplastic and non-paraneoplastic retinopathy and optic neuropathy: evaluation and management. Surv Ophthalmol. 2013;58(5):430–58. https://doi.org/10.1016/j.survophthal.2012.09.001.

11. Hoogenraad TU, Sanders EACM, Tan KEWP. Paraneoplastic optic neuropathy with histopathological verification of absence of meningeal metastases. Neuroophthalmology. 1989;9:247–50.

12. Malik S, Furlan AJ, Sweeney PJ, et al. Optic neuropathy: a rare paraneoplastic syndrome. J Clin Neuroophthalmol. 1992;12:137–41.

13. Cross SA, Salomao DR, Parisi JE, et al. Paraneoplastic autoimmune optic neuritis with retinitis defined by CRMP-5- IgG. Ann Neurol. 2003;54:38–50.

14. Luiz JE, Lee AG, Keltner JL, et al. Paraneoplastic optic neuropathy and autoantibody production in small-cell carcinoma of the lung. J Neuroophthalmol. 1998;18:178–81.

15. Richter RB, Moore RY. Non-invasive central nervous system disease associated with lymphoid tumors. Johns Hopkins Med J. 1968;122:271–83. Leuk Res 2011;35:e111–3.

16. Lambrecht ER, van der Loos TL, van der Eerden AH. Retrobulbar neuritis as the first sign of the glucagonoma syndrome. Int Ophthalmol. 1987;11:13–5.

17. Pulido J, Cross SA, Lennon VA, et al. Bilateral autoimmune optic neuritis and vitreitis related to CRMP-5-IgG: intravitreal triamcinolone acetonide therapy of four eyes. Eye (Lond). 2008;22:1191–3.

18. Antoine JC, Honnorat J, Vocanson C, et al. Posterior uveitis, paraneoplastic encephalomyelitis and auto-antibodies reacting with developmental protein of brain and retina. J Neurol Sci. 1993;117:215–23.

19. Asproudis IC, Nikas AN, Psilas KG. Paraneoplastic optic neuropathy in a patient with a non-small cell lung carcinoma: a case report. Eur J Ophthalmol. 2005;15:420–3.

20. Murakami Y, Yoshida S, Yoshikawa H, et al. CRMP-5-IgG in patient with paraneoplastic optic neuritis with lung adenocarcinoma. Eye (Lond). 2007;21:860.

21. Honnorat J, Antoine JC, Derrington E, et al. Antibodies to a subpopulation of glial cells and a 66 kDa developmental protein in patients with paraneoplastic neurological syndromes. J Neurol Neurosurg Psychiatry. 1996;61:270–8.

22. Cheung SSL, Lau GKK, Chan KH, et al. Optic neuritis as the initial clinical presentation of limbic encephalitis: a case report. J Med Case Rep. 2018;12:357. https://doi.org/10.1186/s13256-018-1893-7.

23. Yu Z, Kryzer TJ, Griesmann GE, et al. CRMP-5 neuronal autoantibody: marker of lung cancer and thymoma-related autoimmunity. Ann Neurol. 2001;49:146–54.

24. De Santis G, Caniatti L, De Vito A, et al. A possible paraneoplastic neuromyelitis optica associated with lung cancer. Neurol Sci. 2009;30:397–400.

25. Nakayama-Ichiyama S, Yokote T, Hiraoka N, et al. A paraneoplastic neuromyelitis optica spectrum disorder associated with a mature B-cell neoplasm. Leuk Res. 2011;35:e111–3.

26. Rosencher L, Maisonobe T, Lavole A, et al. Neurologic paraneoplastic syndrome with anti-CV2/CRMP5 antibodies revealing a small cell lung cancer. Effectiveness of the lung cancer treatment. Rev Neurol (Paris). 2012;168:371–4.

27. Chan JW. Paraneoplastic retinopathies and optic neuropathies. Surv Ophthalmol. 2003;48:12–38.

28. Sheorajpanday R, Slabbynck H, Van De Sompel W, et al. Small cell lung carcinoma presenting as collapsin response mediating protein (CRMP) -5 paraneoplastic optic neuropathy. J Neuroophthalmol. 2006;26:168–72.

29. Pau D, Yalamanchili S, Lee AG. Long-term survivor of paraneoplastic optic neuropathy. J Neuroophthalmol. 2010;30:387.

30. Moss HE, Liu GT, Dalmau J. Glazed (vision) and confused. Surv Ophthalmol. 2010;55:169–73.

31. Hoh ST, Teh M, Chew SJ. Paraneoplastic optic neuropathy in nasopharyngeal carcinoma. Report of a case. Singap Med J. 1991;32:170–3.

32. Raaphorst J, Vanneste J. Numb cheek syndrome as the first manifestation of anti-Hu paraneoplastic neuronopathy. J Neurol. 2006;253:664–5.

33. De Schamphelaere E, Sieben A, Heyndrickx S, et al. Long lasting trigeminal neuropathy, limbic encephalitis and abdominal ganglionitis without primary cancer: an atypical case of Hu-antibody syndrome. Clin Neurol Neurosurg. 2020;194:105849.

34. Kalanie H, Harandi AA, Mardani M, Shahverdi Z, Morakabati A, Alidaei S, et al. Trigeminal neuralgia as the first clinical manifestation of anti-Hu para-

neoplastic syndrome induced by a borderline ovarian mucinous tumor. Case Rep Neurol. 2014;6:7.

35. Demarquay G, Didelot A, Rogemond V. Facial pain as first manifestation of anti-Hu paraneoplastic syndrome. J Headache Pain. 2010;11(4):355–7. https://doi.org/10.1007/s10194-010-0212-5. Epub 2010 Apr 13.

36. Graus F, Keime-Guibert F, Reñe R, et al. Anti-Hu-associated paraneoplastic encephalomyelitis: analysis of 200 patients. Brain. 2001;124:1138–48. https://doi.org/10.1093/BRAIN/124.6.1138.

37. Gaughran J, Lyne T, Sayasneh A. Trigeminal neuralgia leading to a diagnosis of ovarian cancer: a timely coincidence or a case of paraneoplastic syndrome? BMJ Case Rep. 2021;14(7):e243480. https://doi.org/10.1136/bcr-2021-243480.

38. Lossos A, Siegal T. Numb chin syndrome in cancer patients: etiology, response to treatment, and prognostic significance. Neurology. 1992;42:1181. https://doi.org/10.1212/WNL.42.6.1181.

39. Renna R, Plantone D, Batocchi AP. Teaching neuroimages: a case of hearing loss in a paraneoplastic syndrome associated with anti-Hu antibody. Neurology. 2012;79:e134.

40. Lucchinetti C, Kimmel DW, Lennon VA. Paraneoplastic and oncologic profiles of patients seropositive for type 1 antineuronal nuclear autoantibodies. Neurology. 1998;50:652–7.

41. Hammam T, McFadzean RM, Ironside JW. Anti-hu paraneoplastic syndrome presenting as bilateral sixth cranial nerve palsies. J Neuroophthalmol. 2005;25(2):101–4.

42. Kwatra V, Charakidis M, Karanth NV. Bilateral facial nerve palsy associated with amphiphysin antibody in metastatic breast cancer: a case report. J Med Case Rep. 2021;15(1):158. https://doi.org/10.1186/s13256-021-02727-3.

43. Fujimoto S, Kumamoto T, Ito T, et al. Clinicopathological study of a patient with anti-Hu-associated paraneoplastic sensory neuronopathy with multiple cranial nerve palsies. Clin Neurol Neurosurg. 2002;104(2):98–102. https://doi.org/10.1016/s0303-8467(01)00190-1.

44. Yamada M, Inaba A, Yamawaki M, et al. Paraneoplastic encephalo-myelo-ganglionitis: cellular binding sites of the antineuronal antibody. Acta Neuropathol. 1994;88(1):85–92. https://doi.org/10.1007/BF00294364.

45. Tazi R, Salimi Z, Fadili H, et al. Anti-Ri-associated paraneoplastic neurological syndrome revealing breast cancer: a case report. Cureus. 2022;14(1):e21106. https://doi.org/10.7759/cureus.21106. eCollection 2022 Jan.

46. Basal E, Zalewski N, Kryzer TJ, et al. Paraneoplastic neuronal intermediate filament autoimmunity. Neurology. 2018;91:e1677–89. https://doi.org/10.1212/WNL.0000000000006435.

47. Kaido M, Yuasa Y, Yamamoto T, et al. A case of possible paraneoplastic neurological syndrome presenting as multiple cranial nerve palsies associated with gallbladder cancer. Rinsho Shinkeigaku. 2016;56:617–21.

48. Nomiyama K, Uchino A, Yakushiji Y, Kosugi M, Takase Y, Kudo S. Diffuse cranial nerve and cauda equina lesions associated with breast cancer. Clin Imaging. 2007;31:202–5. https://doi.org/10.1016/j.clinimag.2007.01.006.

49. Blaes F. Paraneoplastic brain stem encephalitis. Curr Treat Options Neurol. 2013;15(2):201–9. https://doi.org/10.1007/s11940-013-0221-1.

50. Saiz A, Bruna J, Stourac P, et al. Anti-Hu-associated brainstem encephalitis. J Neurol Neurosurg Psychiatry. 2009;80(4):404–7.

51. Dalmau J, Graus F, Villarejo A, et al. Clinical analysis of anti-Ma2-associated encephalitis. Brain. 2004;127:1831–44. https://doi.org/10.1093/BRAIN/AWH203.

52. Rosenfeld MR, Eichen JG, Wade DF, et al. Molecular and clinical diversity in paraneoplastic immunity to Ma proteins. Ann Neurol. 2001;50:339–48. https://doi.org/10.1002/ANA.1288.

53. Luque FA, Furneaux HM, Ferziger R, et al. Anti-Ri: an antibody associated with paraneoplastic opsoclonus and breast cancer. Ann Neurol. 1991;29:241–51. https://doi.org/10.1002/ANA.410290303.

54. Sutton IJ, Barnett MH, Watson JD, Ell JJ, Dalmau J. Paraneoplastic brain stem encephalitis and anti-Ri antibodies. J Neurol. 2002;249(11):1597–8.

55. Simard C, Vogrig A, Joubert B, Muñiz-Castrillo S, Picard G, Rogemond V, et al. Clinical spectrum and diagnostic pitfalls of neurologic syndromes with Ri antibodies. Neurol Neuroimmunol Neuroinflamm. 2020;7(3):e699. https://doi.org/10.1212/NXI.0000000000000699.

56. Pittock SJ, Parisi JE, McKeon A, et al. Paraneoplastic jaw dystonia and laryngospasm with antineuronal nuclear autoantibody type 2 (anti-Ri). Arch Neurol. 2010;67(9):1109–15.

57. Mandel-Brehm C, Dubey D, Kryzer TJ, et al. Kelch-like protein 11 antibodies in seminoma-associated paraneoplastic encephalitis. N Engl J Med. 2019;381:47–54.

58. Dubey D, Wilson MR, Clarkson B, et al. Expanded clinical phenotype, oncological associations, and immunopathologic insights of paraneoplastic Kelch-like Protein-11 encephalitis. JAMA Neurol. 2020;77(11):1420–9. https://doi.org/10.1001/jamaneurol.2020.2231.

59. Maudes E, Landa J, Muñoz-Lopetegi A, et al. Clinical significance of Kelch-like protein 11 antibodies. Neurol Neuroimmunol Neuroinflamm. 2020;7(3):e666. https://doi.org/10.1212/NXI.0000000000000666. Print 2020 May.

60. Vogrig A, Muñiz-Castrillo S, Desestret V, et al. Pathophysiology of paraneoplastic and auto-

immune encephalitis: genes, infections, and checkpoint inhibitors. Ther Adv Neurol Disord. 2020;13:1756286420932797. https://doi.org/10.1177/1756286420932797.

61. Ribas A, Wolchok JD. Cancer immunotherapy using checkpoint blockade. Science. 2018;359:1350–5. https://doi.org/10.1126/SCIENCE.AAR4060.

62. Marini A, Bernardini A, Gigli GL, et al. Neurologic adverse events of immune checkpoint inhibitors: a systematic review. Neurology. 2021;96:754–66. https://doi.org/10.1212/WNL.0000000000011795.

63. Dubey D, David WS, Reynolds KL, Chute DF, Clement NF, Cohen JV, et al. Severe neurological toxicity of immune checkpoint inhibitors: growing spectrum. Ann Neurol. 2020;87:659–69. https://doi.org/10.1002/ana.25708.

64. Dubey D, David WS, Amato AA, Reynolds KL, Clement NF, Chute DF, et al. Varied phenotypes and management of immune checkpoint inhibitor-associated neuropathies. Neurology. 2019;93:e1093–103. https://doi.org/10.1212/WNL.0000000000008091.

65. Vogrig A, Muñiz-Castrillo S, Joubert B, Picard G, Rogemond V, Skowron F, et al. Cranial nerve disorders associated with immune checkpoint inhibitors. Neurology. 2021;96:e866–75. https://doi.org/10.1212/WNL.0000000000011340.

Introduction

Toxicity is usually considered to occur as a cumulative and often dose-dependent effect. The potential toxin is identified using the Bradford criteria [1] or further developments thereof. Toxins, substances, and often drugs, including some recreational and occupational substances, have toxic effects on the CNs. These effects not only act on myelin and axons according to the toxin's biochemical properties, but can also involve ion channels and neuromuscular transmission.

Toxins can be identified in the environment (e.g., arsenic, lead, mercury, and organophosphorus), be industrial agents (e.g., hexane, carbon disulfide, and newer chlorofluorocarbon replacing agents like 1-bromopropane), or be intentionally given poisons (e.g., As, thallium) or drugs. There is a long list of potential neurotoxic side effects of drugs, and the frequent issue of toxicity associated with cancer chemotherapy will be discussed in Chap. 23.

Exposures to biological toxins (animals, bacteria, and plants) are to be considered as neurotoxicity. Animal toxins can originate from snakes, arthropods, and marine creatures including poisonous shellfish and fish. There are several plant toxins, such as curare, and also bacterial toxins, such as botulinum toxin. In bioterrorism, biological toxins can be used as biological warfare agents and are classified into categories A–C [2].

In addition to direct toxic effects, indirect mechanisms of toxicity can also occur, such as vasculitis induced by substances in drug abuse [3, 4] and in the historic Spanish toxic oil syndrome [5]. Also, the frequently used sulfonamides may be involved in causing vasculitis.

Drug toxicity of CNs seems to most frequently affect the olfactory nerve, optic nerve, and acoustic and vestibular nerves and can be a dose-limiting factor in chronic drug treatment. Well-known examples are dose-limiting toxic

Authors of this chapter: Anna Grisold, Stacey A. Sakowski, and Wolfgang Grisold.

Table 22.1 Toxicity in relation to time course

	Acute toxicity	Cumulative	Delayed	Not directly related	Late
Examples	Oxaliplatin Venoms	Most toxins, drugs Chronic exposure	Immune checkpoint inhibitors	Vasculitis induced by substances	Chemotherapy-induced neuropathy

CN effects on the auditory nerve in platinum therapies or ototoxicity with antibiotics such as aminoglycosides.

Toxic substances can be ingested, received parenterally, inhaled, or absorbed via the skin (dermal and ocular) [6]. Local toxic effects are also seen following various types of contact, injection, local anesthesia, and others.

The important question for the clinician is the clinical context in the appearance of a CN lesion. Usually, other causes must be ruled out. Toxic CN lesions occur either isolated or in the context of a generalized neuropathy, such as in cis-platinum neuropathy with hearing loss or in organophosphate intoxications.

Exposure to physical agents, such as heat or cold, or exposure to radiation and radiotherapy is also considered a neurotoxic effect [7, 8]. The radiation therapy-induced effects are usually distinguished into acute, subacute, and long-term effects and are characteristically delayed effects.

Time Course

A time course of various toxins is illustrated in Table 22.1.

The time course follows the type of intoxication and the mechanisms and is substance dependent. Most frequently, a cumulative toxicity with various time courses is observed.

The toxicity of highly diluted substances in well and drinking water, as well as exposure of healthcare professionals to diluted substances, is debated but may be important for vulnerable individuals.

CNs Affected

The most frequently reported CNs in regard to drug toxicity are CN I, II, and VIII. This is a dif-

Table 22.2 Mechanisms of focal toxicity

Mechanisms	Interventions
Local aesthetics	Interventions in the head
Perfusion	Tumor therapy
Embolism (therapeutic in tumor therapy)	Tumor therapy
Skin, eye, and mucous membranes	Exposition
Direct: venoms	Bites and exposure to biological toxins
Direct: grouting	Industrial procedures
Radiotherapy	Following the pattern of acute, delayed, and late effects, e.g., Optic nerve

ferent spectrum than in diabetes mellitus (see Chap. 20).

Isolated Cn Lesions or as Part of a Generalized Neuropathy

Toxic CN lesions can appear in isolation, requiring thorough differential diagnostic considerations, or can be part of a generalized neuropathy.

Focal Toxicity

Focal toxicity is often neglected and can be due to local interventions (injections, infiltrations, perfusion), animal venoms, or physical influences such as heat, cold, or radiotherapy.

There are numerous reports on CN toxicity by various mechanisms. Table 22.2 focuses on drugs, other substances, and other possible mechanisms. This mirrors the most frequently affected CN and excludes chemotherapy-induced lesions; these are mentioned separately in Chap. 23.

Table 22.3 Toxic effects on CNs

CN	Drugs	CIPN	Toxic substances	Other
1[a]	++	++	+	+
2	++	+	++	+
3	+			?
4				
5	?	?	+	
6	+			+
7				?
8	++	++	+	+
9				+
10				+
11				+
12				+

[a] Taste misperception is often associated with lesions of the olfactory nerve but is more complex; see Chap. 18—tongue

Individual CNs

The individual CNs can be affected by drugs, chemicals, and other influences and will be systematically discussed.

Table 22.3 includes a systematic list of CNs classified according to drugs, toxic substances, and others. The distribution is estimated and concurs with most assumptions.

Olfactory Nerve

The olfactory nerve can be impacted by several drugs, and in addition to smell, taste is also generally impaired [9, 10]. The effects of chemotherapy will be discussed in Chap. 23. In addition, several chemicals can cause smell disorders, and radiation therapy can cause immediate and late effects [11].

Drugs: Allopurinol, analgesics, antibiotics (amphotericin B, ampicillin, crizotinib [12], ethambutol, lincomycin, tetracycline), antihelminthics, local anesthetics, anticancer chemotherapy (see Chap. 23), colchicine, diuretics, immunosuppressants (azathioprine), muscle relaxants, opiates, and statins.

Substances: Chemicals (e.g., benzene, carbon disulfide, heavy metals, menthol, pesticides), solvents [13], sulfur dioxide, zinc.

Different mechanisms: Examples of physical influences include local radiotherapy at the frontal base of the skull or radiation therapy of nasopharyngeal carcinoma.

Optic Nerve

Toxic optic neuropathies can be caused by several recreational substances, drugs, chemicals, and physical impacts, such as radiation therapy which causes damage to the optic nerve focally.

The topic of visual dysfunction and the respective differential diagnosis is of eminent clinical importance. Usually loss of vision is the symptom, and effects on color vision can appear with some substances [14–17].

Drugs: Antibiotics (chloramphenicol, ethambutol influences color perception [18], isoniazid, linezolid, streptomycin sulfonamide, vancomycin [19]).

Anticancer drugs: See Chap. 23; gemcitabine, platinum [20].
Antimalaria drugs: Chloroquine, hydroxychloroquine, quinine.
Antiarrhythmics: Amiodarone, digitalis.
Immune suppressants: Tacrolimos [21].
Phosphodiesterase inhibitors: Sildenafil.

Substances: Alcohol (methylalcohol [22]), heavy metals (arsenic, lead, mercury, thallium), other substances (aniline dye, carbon monoxide, carbon tetrachloride, tobacco), nitrous oxide [14], nicotine [23].

Nutritive: Alcohol ingestion, B1 deficiency, B12 anemia, "Cuban" neuropathy, folic acid deficiency, Strachan's syndrome (malnourishment).
Radiation: Radiation therapy of brain tumors, pituitary tumors, metastases, or ENT tumors can cause unilateral or bilateral loss of vision appearing after long latencies.

Oculomotor Nerve

Clinically, CN III paresis presents with diplopia and ptosis and is rarely caused by toxicity, although a few substances have been mentioned.

Drugs: Vincristine, [24] retinoids.

Toxic: Alcohol, arsenic, carbon monoxide, and lead; carbon disulfide or dinitrophenol poisoning.

Local toxins: Botulinum toxin.

Trochlear Nerve

The same as for CN III is true for the trochlear nerve, and isolated intoxications are not likely.

Trigeminal Nerve

The trigeminal nerve is rarely affected by toxicity, and usually the sensory part is affected.

Drugs: Pyridoxine toxicity.

Substances: Solvents, trichloroethylene, trilene, thallium, arsenic.Local effects: Local infiltrations, interventions, skin and contact poisons. Radiation therapy. Therapeutic interventions such as alcohol instillation in the ganglion Gasseri in trigeminal neuralgia.

Abducens Nerve

Toxic causes of abducens nerve lesions are rare.

Drugs: Capecitabine, etanercept [25], pembrolizumab [26, 27], retinoids [28], vincristine therapy [29–31].

Toxic: Glufosinate herbicide [32].

Local toxicity: Local anesthetics to treat the maxillary nerve cause transient diplopia with ipsilateral abducent nerve palsy [33].

Facial Nerve

Facial nerve damage by toxicity is infrequently described.

Drugs: Bilateral CN VII palsy after paclitaxel therapy [34] has been described.

Substances: Dichloromethane [35, 36].

Others: Local anesthetics (neurotoxic effects of selectively applied local anesthetics), botulinum toxins, radiation therapy, gamma knife therapy.

Auditory Nerve

The auditory nerve is one of the most frequently affected CNs by toxicity, usually by systemic effects of drugs or substances. Focal effects such as radiation therapy and other intervention also cause vestibulocochlear damage [31]. The combination of several ototoxicants increases the risk of hearing loss.

Drugs: Antibiotics (aminoglycosides, chloramphenicol, colistin, erythromycin, ethambutol, isoniazid, streptomycin, sulfonamides, tetracyclines, vancomycin, and other antibacterial agents [37]), anticancer drugs (carboplatin, platinum, vinca alkaloids, thalidomide; see Chap. 23 [38]), chinin [39], diuretics, immune checkpoint inhibitors [31], quinine, salicylates [40].

Substances: Carbon monoxide, heavy metals such as mercury and lead, pesticides, glue sniffing [41].

Other: Local radiation therapy of the head and neck [42].

Vestibular Nerve

Toxicity effects on the vestibular nerve is rarer than on the acoustic nerve [43].

Drugs: Aminoglycosides, chemotherapy (cisplatin), cyclophosphamide, hydroxyurea, platinum [44], vinblastine, heavy metals (lead, mercury), quinine, salicylate [45].

Substances: Alcohol.

Other: Radiation therapy.

Glossopharyngeal nerve:

Isolated lesions of the glossopharyngeal nerve are difficult to detect. Toxic lesions have been mentioned in the context of other caudal CN lesions.

Drugs: Nitrofurantoin, salvarsan intoxication. Neuromuscular transmission can be affected by tetanus toxin and local anesthetics [46].

Other: Iatrogenic, carotid operations, neck dissection (ENT and neurosurgical procedures), resection of aneurysms. Tonsillectomy is rarely a cause (0.1%), lesions of the lateral pharynx wall.

Vagus Nerve

The vagus nerve is difficult to examine in isolation from the other caudal CN functions. An exception is the recurrent vagal nerve, which has a typical clinical manifestation.

Drugs: Vincristine vocal cord [47], intrathecal drug toxicity [48]. Following vaccination [49, 50].

Toxic: Alcoholic polyneuropathy [51] and thallium aconitin.

Others: Local interventions, radiation therapy.

Accessory Nerve

This nerve is usually damaged by local interventions, such as surgery, or the influence of physical properties, such as radiation therapy.

Iatrogenic: Surgery in the neck (posterior cervical triangle), deep cervical lymph node removal, "neck dissection procedures," shunt implantation, fibrosis following radiotherapy, shoulder support in the Trendelenburg position.

Hypoglossal Nerve

Toxicity by drugs or chemicals is not to be expected, apart from local interventions (local anesthetics, embolization) and radiation therapy [52].

Multiple CN Lesions

In addition to individual CN lesions, multiple CN lesions have been described.

Multiple CN lesions have been reported in ethylene alcohol intoxications and in chemotherapy [53], organophosphate intoxications [54], [55], tricresyl phosphate [56], and delayed after radiation therapy [57].

Other Causes

Warfare agents: Warfare agents also act on the neuromuscular (neuromuscular transmission) system by producing a cholinergic toxidrome presenting with miosis and excessive lacrimation in addition to fasciculations, seizures, diarrhea, and respiratory arrest and coma [6, 58].

Venoms and snake bites: These instances are more heterogenous. Neuromuscular transmission is often affected [59] in snake bites [60], whereas shellfish [61, 62] seem to have other mechanisms [63]. Perioral dysesthesia is typical of ciguatera, among other symptoms [64].

Biological agents and venoms include brevetoxin, ciguatera, latratoxin, saxitoxin, snake and spider venoms, and tetrodotoxin and recently also the possible influence of drugs used in COVID-19 therapy.

Environment, drinking water, well water: Well and drinking water [65] are a concern in regard to contamination by several drugs, including cytostatic drugs, arsenic, and organophosphorus [66], among others [67–69].

Exposure of healthcare personnel is also a concern, and while the concentrations are low, even those doses may create a danger for vulnerable populations.

Antibacterial therapy: Toxicity of CNs is an important aspect in the differential diagnosis in drug treatment. Systemic effects usually need to be considered, as well as local interventions, such as local anesthetics and radiation therapy [70]. Also, toxicity affecting the CNs has been observed in COVID-19 therapy [71].

Conclusion

The olfactory nerve, the optic nerve, and the acoustic and vestibular nerves are most frequently affected by toxicity, albeit by various mechanisms. CN toxicity can be dose-limiting for various drugs, such as for the optic nerve in tuberculostatic therapy, the auditory nerve with platinum therapies, or ototoxicity with antibiotics such as aminoglycosides. Chemotherapy for cancer also involves potential neurotoxic side effects and will be discussed in Chap. 23. Also, exposures to biological toxins, animal toxins, and plant toxins need to be considered, as well as effects of biological warfare and the environment. Historically, several examples of indirect effects via induction of inflammatory changes on CN toxicity have been reported.

References

1. Fedak KM, Bernal A, Capshaw ZA, Gross S. Applying the Bradford Hill criteria in the 21st century: how data integration has changed causal inference in molecular epidemiology. Emerg Themes Epidemiol. 2015;12:14.
2. Bioterrorism agents/diseases. Centers for Disease Control and Prevention. https://emergency.cdc.gov/agent/agentlist-category.asp.
3. Neiman J, Haapaniemi HM, Hillbom M. Neurological complications of drug abuse: pathophysiological mechanisms. Eur J Neurol. 2000;7(6):595–606.
4. Stevens H, Restak R. Neurological complications of drug abuse. Ann Clin Lab Sci. 1976;6(6):514–20.
5. Gelpi E, de la Paz MP, Terracini B, Abaitua I, de la Camara AG, Kilbourne EM, et al. The Spanish toxic oil syndrome 20 years after its onset: a multidisciplinary review of scientific knowledge. Environ Health Perspect. 2002;110(5):457–64.
6. Chai PR, Boyer EW, Al-Nahhas H, Erickson TB. Toxic chemical weapons of assassination and warfare: nerve agents VX and sarin. Toxicol Commun. 2017;1(1):21–3.
7. Alice Thomas AL, Psimaras D, Bompaire F, Hoang-Xuan K, Ricard D. 1.2 Radiotherapy including hyperthermia and brain toxicity. In: Grisold W, Soffietti R, Oberndorfer S, Cavaletti G. Effects of cancer treatment on the nervous system, vol. 2. Cambridge Scholar Publishing. p. 31–70.
8. Dong Y, Ridge JA, Ebersole B, Li T, Lango MN, Churilla TM, et al. Incidence and outcomes of radiation-induced late cranial neuropathy in 10-year survivors of head and neck cancer. Oral Oncol. 2019;95:59–64.
9. Hummel T, Whitcroft KL, Andrews P, Altundag A, Cinghi C, Costanzo RM, et al. Position paper on olfactory dysfunction. Rhinol Suppl. 2017;54(26):1–30.
10. Aulisio MC, Glueck AC, Dobbs MR, Pasagic S, Han DY. Neurotoxicity and chemoreception: a systematic review of neurotoxicity effects on smell and taste. Neurol Clin. 2020;38(4):965–81.
11. Alvarez-Camacho M, Gonella S, Campbell S, Scrimger RA, Wismer WV. A systematic review of smell alterations after radiotherapy for head and neck cancer. Cancer Treat Rev. 2017;54:110–21.
12. Koizumi T, Fukushima T, Tatai T, Kobayashi T, Sekiguchi N, Sakamoto A, et al. Successful treatment of crizotinib-induced dysgeusia by switching to alectinib in ALK-positive non-small cell lung cancer. Lung Cancer. 2015;88(1):112–3.
13. Dick FD. Solvent neurotoxicity. Occup Environ Med. 2006;63(3):221–6, 179.
14. Grzybowski A, Zulsdorff M, Wilhelm H, Tonagel F. Toxic optic neuropathies: an updated review. Acta Ophthalmol. 2015;93(5):402–10.
15. Wasinska-Borowiec W, Aghdam KA, Saari JM, Grzybowski A. An updated review on the most common agents causing toxic optic neuropathies. Curr Pharm Des. 2017;23(4):586–95.
16. Baj J, Forma A, Kobak J, Tyczynska M, Dudek I, Maani A, et al. Toxic and nutritional optic neuropathies—an updated mini-review. Int J Environ Res Public Health. 2022;19(5):3092.
17. Dworak DP, Nichols J. A review of optic neuropathies. Dis Mon. 2014;60(6):276–81.
18. Nasemann J, Zrenner E, Riedel KG. Recovery after severe ethambutol intoxication—psychophysical and electrophysiological correlations. Doc Ophthalmol. 1989;71(3):279–92.
19. Todorich B, Faia LJ, Thanos A, Amin M, Folberg R, Wolfe JD, et al. Vancomycin-associated hemorrhagic occlusive retinal vasculitis: a clinical-pathophysiological analysis. Am J Ophthalmol. 2018;188:131–40.
20. Golombek T, Henker R, Rehak M, Quaschling U, Lordick F, Knodler M. A rare case of mixed adeno-neuroendocrine carcinoma (MANEC) of the gastro-esophageal junction with HER2/neu overexpression and distinct orbital and optic nerve toxicity after intravenous administration of cisplatin. Oncol Res Treat. 2019;42(3):123–7.
21. Venneti S, Moss HE, Levin MH, Vagefi MR, Brozena SC, Pruitt AA, et al. Asymmetric bilateral demyelinating optic neuropathy from tacrolimus toxicity. J Neurol Sci. 2011;301(1–2):112–5.
22. Bennett IL Jr, Cary FH, Mitchell GL Jr, Cooper MN. Acute methyl alcohol poisoning: a review based on experiences in an outbreak of 323 cases. Medicine (Baltimore). 1953;32(4):431–63.
23. Grzybowski A, Holder GE. Tobacco optic neuropathy (TON)—the historical and present concept of the disease. Acta Ophthalmol. 2011;89(5):495–9.
24. Chroni E, Monastirli A, Tsambaos D. Neuromuscular adverse effects associated with systemic retinoid der-

matotherapy: monitoring and treatment algorithm for clinicians. Drug Saf. 2010;33(1):25–34.

25. Lai CC, Hsiao KH, Chang YS, Tsai CY, Chou CT. Etanercept-associated right abducens nerve palsy in rheumatoid arthritis. Int J Rheum Dis. 2012;15(5):e117–9.

26. Jaben KA, Francis JH, Shoushtari AN, Abramson DH. Isolated abducens nerve palsy following Pembrolizumab. Neuroophthalmology. 2020;44(3):182–5.

27. Aaltonen T, Amerio S, Amidei D, Anastassov A, Annovi A, Antos J, et al. Measurement of the cross section for prompt isolated diphoton production using the full CDF run II data sample. Phys Rev Lett. 2013;110(10):101801.

28. Alemdar M, Iseri P, Selekler HM, Serbest AS, Komsuoglu SS. Isolated abducens nerve palsy associated with retinoic acid therapy: a case report. Strabismus. 2005;13(3):129–32.

29. Dixit G, Dhingra A, Kaushal D. Vincristine induced cranial neuropathy. J Assoc Physicians India. 2012;60:56–8.

30. Toker E, Yenice O, Ogut MS. Isolated abducens nerve palsy induced by vincristine therapy. J AAPOS. 2004;8(1):69–71.

31. Vogrig A, Muniz-Castrillo S, Joubert B, Picard G, Rogemond V, Skowron F, et al. Cranial nerve disorders associated with immune checkpoint inhibitors. Neurology. 2021;96(6):e866–e75.

32. Park JS, Kwak SJ, Gil HW, Kim SY, Hong SY. Glufosinate herbicide intoxication causing unconsciousness, convulsion, and 6th cranial nerve palsy. J Korean Med Sci. 2013;28(11):1687–9.

33. Kini YK, Kharkar VR, Kini AY. Transient diplopia with ipsilateral abducent nerve palsy and ptosis following a maxillary local anesthetic injection: a case report and review of literature. Oral Maxillofac Surg. 2012;16(4):373–5.

34. Lee RT, Oster MW, Balmaceda C, Hesdorffer CS, Vahdat LT, Papadopoulos KP. Bilateral facial nerve palsy secondary to the administration of high-dose paclitaxel. Ann Oncol. 1999;10(10):1245–7.

35. Liss GM, House RA, Wills MC. Cranial neuropathy associated with chlorinated solvents. Re: facial nerve palsy after acute exposure to dichloromethane. Am J Ind Med. 2006;49(4):310.

36. Jacubovich RM, Landau D, Bar Dayan Y, Zilberberg M, Goldstein L. Facial nerve palsy after acute exposure to dichloromethane. Am J Ind Med. 2005;48(5):389–92.

37. Snavely SR, Hodges GR. The neurotoxicity of antibacterial agents. Ann Intern Med. 1984;101(1):92–104.

38. Landier W. Ototoxicity and cancer therapy. Cancer. 2016;122(11):1647–58.

39. Brough H. Acquired auditory neuropathy spectrum disorder after malaria treated with quinine. Trop Doct. 2020;50(3):246–8.

40. Arslan E, Orzan E, Santarelli R. Global problem of drug-induced hearing loss. Ann N Y Acad Sci. 1999;884:1–14.

41. Ehyai A, Freemon FR. Progressive optic neuropathy and sensorineural hearing loss due to chronic glue sniffing. J Neurol Neurosurg Psychiatry. 1983;46(4):349–51.

42. Azzam P, Mroueh M, Francis M, Daher AA, Zeidan YH. Radiation-induced neuropathies in head and neck cancer: prevention and treatment modalities. Ecancermedicalscience. 2020;14:1133.

43. Gans RE, Rauterkus G, Research Associate. Vestibular toxicity: causes, evaluation protocols, intervention, and management. Semin Hear. 2019;40(2):144–53.

44. Prayuenyong P, Taylor JA, Pearson SE, Gomez R, Patel PM, Hall DA, et al. Vestibulotoxicity associated with platinum-based chemotherapy in survivors of cancer: a scoping review. Front Oncol. 2018;8:363.

45. Sheppard A, Hayes SH, Chen GD, Ralli M, Salvi R. Review of salicylate-induced hearing loss, neurotoxicity, tinnitus and neuropathophysiology. Acta Otorhinolaryngol Ital. 2014;34(2):79–93.

46. Papadopoulou M, Anastasakis S. Transient glossopharyngeal nerve palsy due to mandibular nerve block. BMJ Case Rep. 2022;15(7):e251033.

47. Samoon Z, Shabbir-Moosajee M. Vincristine-induced vocal cord palsy and successful re-treatment in a patient with diffuse large B cell lymphoma: a case report. BMC Res Notes. 2014;7:318.

48. Hodgson PS, Neal JM, Pollock JE, Liu SS. The neurotoxicity of drugs given intrathecally (spinal). Anesth Analg. 1999;88(4):797–809.

49. Eicher W, Neundorfer B. [Paralysis of the recurrent laryngeal nerve following a booster injection of tetanus toxoid (associated with local allergic reaction)]. Munch Med Wochenschr. 1969;111(34):1692–1695.

50. Martin F. [Side effects of drugs on the larynx]. Laryngol Rhinol Otol (Stuttg). 1986;65(9):477–479.

51. Murata K, Araki S, Yokoyama K, Sata F, Yamashita K, Ono Y. Autonomic neurotoxicity of alcohol assessed by heart rate variability. J Auton Nerv Syst. 1994;48(2):105–11.

52. Chow JCH, Cheung KM, Au KH, Zee BCY, Lee J, Ngan RKC, et al. Radiation-induced hypoglossal nerve palsy after definitive radiotherapy for nasopharyngeal carcinoma: clinical predictors and dose-toxicity relationship. Radiother Oncol. 2019;138:93–8.

53. Ray M, Marwaha RK, Trehan A. Chemotherapy related fatal neurotoxicity during induction in acute lymphoblastic leukemia. Indian J Pediatr. 2002;69(2):185–7.

54. Peter JV, Sudarsan TI, Moran JL. Clinical features of organophosphate poisoning: a review of different classification systems and approaches. Indian J Crit Care Med. 2014;18(11):735–45.

55. Worek F, Wille T, Koller M, Thiermann H. Toxicology of organophosphorus compounds in view of an increasing terrorist threat. Arch Toxicol. 2016;90(9):2131–45.

56. Winder C, Balouet JC. The toxicity of commercial jet oils. Environ Res. 2002;89(2):146–64.

57. Pall HS, Nightingale S, Clough CG, Spooner D. Progressive multiple cranial neuropathies pre-

senting as a delayed complication of radiotherapy in infancy. Postgrad Med J. 1988;64(750):303–5.

58. Pearson-Smith JN, Patel M. Antioxidant drug therapy as a neuroprotective countermeasure of nerve agent toxicity. Neurobiol Dis. 2020;133:104457.

59. Ranawaka UK, Lalloo DG, de Silva HJ. Neurotoxicity in snakebite—the limits of our knowledge. PLoS Negl Trop Dis. 2013;7(10):e2302.

60. Sithole HL. The ocular complications of an envenomous snakebite. S Afr Fam Pract. 2013;55(2):161–3.

61. Garcia C, Lagos M, Truan D, Lattes K, Vejar O, Chamorro B, et al. Human intoxication with paralytic shellfish toxins: clinical parameters and toxin analysis in plasma and urine. Biol Res. 2005;38(2–3):197–205.

62. Zhang F, Xu X, Li T, Liu Z. Shellfish toxins targeting voltage-gated sodium channels. Mar Drugs. 2013;11(12):4698–723.

63. Costa PR, Estevez P, Solino L, Castro D, Rodrigues SM, Timoteo V, et al. An update on ciguatoxins and CTX-like toxicity in fish from different trophic levels of the Selvagens Islands (NE Atlantic, Madeira, Portugal). Toxins (Basel). 2021;13(8):580.

64. Levine DZ. Ciguatera: current concepts. J Am Osteopath Assoc. 1995;95(3):193–8.

65. Rowney NC, Johnson AC, Williams RJ. Cytotoxic drugs in drinking water: a prediction and risk assessment exercise for the thames catchment in the United Kingdom. Environ Toxicol Chem. 2009;28(12):2733–43.

66. Haliga RE, Morarasu BC, Ursaru M, Irimioaia V, Sorodoc L. New insights into the organophosphate-induced intermediate syndrome. Arh Hig Rada Toksikol. 2018;69(2):191–5.

67. Mendoza A, Zonja B, Mastroianni N, Negreira N, Lopez de Alda M, Perez S, et al. Drugs of abuse, cytostatic drugs and iodinated contrast media in tap water from the Madrid region (central Spain):A case study to analyse their occurrence and human health risk characterization. Environ Int. 2016;86:107–18.

68. Moretti M, Bonfiglioli R, Feretti D, Pavanello S, Mussi F, Grollino MG, et al. A study protocol for the evaluation of occupational mutagenic/carcinogenic risks in subjects exposed to antineoplastic drugs: a multicentric project. BMC Public Health. 2011;11:195.

69. Graeve CU, McGovern PM, Alexander B, Church T, Ryan A, Polovich M. Occupational exposure to antineoplastic agents. Workplace Health Saf. 2017;65(1):9–20.

70. Thomas RJ. Neurotoxicity of antibacterial therapy. South Med J. 1994;87(9):869–74.

71. Finsterer J, Scorza FA, Scorza C, Fiorini A. COVID-19 associated cranial nerve neuropathy: a systematic review. Bosn J Basic Med Sci. 2022;22(1):39–45.

Bullet Points

- A broad range of CN pathologies can occur following chemotherapy treatment.
- Some forms of CN damage occur rarely, while ototoxicity and vocal cord paresis are more common.
- CN dysfunction can be a persistent toxicity following chemotherapy treatment.

Introduction

Chemotherapy-induced peripheral neurotoxicity (CIPN) is typically characterized by sensory or sensorimotor nerve dysfunction, but autonomic and CN pathology can occur [1]. CN manifestations are broad and include anosmia, visual loss, ototoxicity, and vocal cord paresis [2]. While some CN manifestations of CIPN are rare, other manifestations are common, affecting a substantial proportion of treated patients. Cranial neurotoxicity can occur as part of a generalized toxic peripheral neuropathy or as an isolated CN dysfunction, as described below.

Olfactory Manifestations

Chemotherapy-induced taste and smell alterations are common, but the specific mechanisms remain unclear. The mechanism of olfactory dysfunction may reflect damage to olfactory epithelial cells rather than an effect on olfactory nerve integrity [3]. An observational study of taste and smell alterations in chemotherapy-treated patients identified that taste alterations were more common in carboplatin- and docetaxel-treated patients [4]. Quantitative testing revealed objective olfactory deficits in platinum- and taxane-treated patients, with the majority of patients developing hyposmia following treatment [5].

Auditory Manifestations

Ototoxicity is a common CN manifestation of neurotoxic chemotherapy, most notably platinum-based chemotherapy [6]. Cisplatin is associated with irreversible sensorineural hearing loss, whereas other platinum analogues like carboplatin and oxaliplatin are less ototoxic [6]. Cisplatin-induced ototoxicity is dose-dependent and occurs more frequently in younger pediatric patients [7]. Sensory neuropathy, tinnitus, and hearing loss were clustered in cisplatin-treated patients and related to age and cumulative dose [8]. Depending on dose, cisplatin produces ototoxicity in 20–70% of patients [9]. However, of 1410 cisplatin-treated adult testicular cancer survivors, 35% reported

Authors of this chapter: Susanna B. Park and Matthew C. Kiernan.

subjective difficulty hearing, while 78% presented with evidence of hearing loss defined on audiometric testing [10]. Similarly, 73% of 153 cisplatin-treated pediatric cancer patients demonstrated evidence of sensorineural hearing loss [7]. Hearing loss was more common in younger patients with higher cisplatin dose per cycle [7].

Cisplatin produces outer hair cell death and leads to elevated inner ear platinum levels in mouse models compared to oxaliplatin- or carboplatin-treated mice [11]. These results suggested that cisplatin is more readily taken up into the cochlea than other platinum-based chemotherapies [11], potentially explaining the difference in relative ototoxicity. There are only rare case reports of ototoxicity of other chemotherapies, including vinca alkaloids [12] and taxanes [13].

Clinical guidelines suggest baseline assessment of auditory function (via pure-tone audiometry) prior to treatment to enable early detection of emergent ototoxicity during cisplatin treatment [14]. There is some evidence that sodium thiosulfate may be protective against ototoxicity, but this agent is not recommended due to potential effects on treatment efficacy and survival [14]. A range of other otoprotective agents have been trialled unsuccessfully. There are no established treatment strategies, but there is a potential role for assistive devices to manage hearing loss and cognitive behavioral therapy to manage tinnitus in this setting [14].

Ocular Manifestations

Ocular manifestations can occur with neurotoxic chemotherapy treatment, including corneal nerve injury [15]. There is preclinical evidence of reduced corneal nerve density in oxaliplatin-treated mice [16] and in a range of other experimental models [17]. Corneal confocal microscopy (CCM) is a technique enabling imaging of corneal nerve parameters in the clinical setting, potentially providing insights into neurotoxicity development. However, to date, there have been a lack of longitudinal studies of CCM in chemotherapy-treated patients, which would be necessary to demonstrate corneal nerve changes over time. Further, there are discrepancies between available studies in terms of methods, sample size, and results [17]. Accordingly, some studies have identified reduced corneal nerve fiber length in neurotoxic chemotherapy-treated patients [18] compared to controls, while others have not [19]. Chiang et al. [18] identified reduced average nerve fiber length and inferior whorl length in 70 paclitaxel- or oxaliplatin-treated patients who were less than 2 years post-treatment compared to controls. However, in 63 docetaxel- or oxaliplatin-treated patients who were 5 years post chemotherapy cessation, corneal nerve fiber length or density was within normal range [19]. In a mixed cohort of 95 patients treated with different chemotherapy types, there was no reduction in corneal nerve fiber length, but a change in density to tortuosity ratio [20]. In total, there is emerging evidence of corneal nerve involvement in chemotherapy neurotoxicity, but further studies are required to determine the utility of CCM in neurotoxicity assessment.

Ocular symptoms, including blurred vision, dry eye, and ocular pain, are reported following chemotherapy treatment [15]. Oculomotor nerve manifestations, including ptosis and ophthalmoplegia, have been reported with a range of chemotherapy treatments, but are typically rare. Diplopia and ptosis have been reported following immune checkpoint inhibitors [21]. Ptosis can occur following oxaliplatin treatment [22] but is rare [23]. There are multiple case reports of ptosis or ophthalmoplegia occurring with vincristine treatment [24, 25], but this is rare, with only 2 out of 103 vincristine-treated pediatric patients developing cranial neuropathy, including ptosis and vocal cord paralysis in the context of prominent autonomic, sensory, and motor neuropathy [26].

Case reports of optic neuritis developing during chemotherapy can be found for a range of chemotherapies, including cisplatin [27], oxaliplatin [28], 5-fluorouracil [29], and cabazitaxel [30]. There are also reports of optic neuritis from immune checkpoint inhibitors, including pembrolizumab and ipilimumab [31]. Overall, optic nerve dysfunction is rare. There are reports of reduced optic cup size in the optic nerve head of patients treated with tamoxifen, but only with short-term use [32]. However, a large-scale retrospective cohort study from a US health claims database of women treated with taxanes or tamoxifen found that taxane treatment was associated with an elevated risk of optic neuropathy development (hazard ratio 4.44; 95% CI 1.04–18.87) [33]. Reduced retinal nerve fiber layer thickness has also been found in patients with paclitaxel and cisplatin treatment, suggesting optic nerve involvement [34].

Vocal Manifestations

Vocal fold motion impairment and vocal cord paresis are potential consequences of chemotherapy. A systematic review of chemotherapy-related vocal fold motion impairment found that 86% of cases reported in the literature were due to vincristine administration [35]. There are multiple reports of vincristine-induced hoarseness and vocal cord paresis [24, 36] but this side effect does not occur in all patients. In a retrospective review of >1000 vincristine-treated pediatric acute lymphoblastic leukemia patients, vocal fold paralysis occurred in only 0.5% [37]. Cases have also been reported arising from paclitaxel [38] and cisplatin [39] treatment, as well as hoarseness following oxaliplatin treatment [23, 40]. In the context of chemotherapy toxicity, vocal cord paralysis was typified by dysphonia and stridor [35]. The majority of cases in the literature have been reported in children. Rarely, chemotherapy-induced vocal cord paralysis can affect airway function and require surgical intervention.

Vestibular Impairment

While there have been some reports of vestibular nerve toxicity following chemotherapy, there remains little specific evidence of vestibular nerve involvement. Symptoms including balance impairment, dizziness, and vertigo are commonly reported by chemotherapy-treated patients, but may be explained by other comorbidities, including sensory or autonomic neuropathy. Vestibulocochlear neuropathy has been reported following immune checkpoint inhibitor treatment [21]. There are some reported cases of vestibular function in cisplatin-treated patients, but only occur rarely. In some case series, 4.1% of cisplatin-treated patients displayed abnormal vestibular function [41], with other series reporting normal vestibular nerve function in all assessed cisplatin-treated patients [42].

Other Cranial Nerve Manifestations

Oxaliplatin produces an acute neurotoxicity characterized by cold-associated paresthesia, cramps, and fasciculations which occur in the first week following oxaliplatin infusion in the majority of patients [43]. Symptoms of CN dysfunction occur as part of this acute syndrome, including jaw pain (often on first bite), perioral numbness, slurred speech, transient visual field defects, and throat tightness [43]. Over 60% of 86 oxaliplatin-treated patients reported masticatory spasms, particularly on first bite, while other CN manifestations were reported in less than 20% of patients, including visual field changes, eye pain, voice changes, and ptosis [44]. However, other series report jaw spasm or stiffness in 26–34% of oxaliplatin-treated patients [23, 40]. Laryngopharyngeal spasm is reported as a rare but dramatic acute neurotoxicity manifestation in oxaliplatin-treated patients, but is not reported in all series [40].

Other CN palsies have been rarely reported in association with chemotherapy treatment, including abducens nerve palsy following immune checkpoint inhibitor treatment [21] or vincristine treatment [45]. Bilateral abducens paralysis following oxaliplatin treatment has been reported, producing diplopia [46]. Vincristine treatment has been reported to produce CN VI palsy [47] or bilateral facial palsy [48]. Although facial nerve manifestations of neurotoxic chemotherapy are rarely reported, electrophysiological assessment of facial nerve function in oxaliplatin-treated patients revealed prolonged latencies, suggesting asymptomatic involvement [49].

Conclusions

There is a spectrum of CN manifestations following chemotherapy, which remain less common than sensorimotor nerve involvement. Thorough diagnostic workup and consideration of differential diagnoses is important to rule out other causes of CN symptoms. There remains a lack of large-scale data on the prevalence of CN involvement in chemotherapy-treated patients and no consistent prevention or treatment strategies. Some forms of CN dysfunction can be persistent and produce a long-lasting impact on cancer patients, such as long-term hearing loss, which are important considerations for cancer survivorship care.

References

1. Park SB, Goldstein D, Krishnan AV, Lin CS, Friedlander ML, Cassidy J, Koltzenburg M, Kiernan MC. Chemotherapy-induced peripheral neurotoxicity: a critical analysis. CA Cancer J Clin. 2013;63(6):419–37.
2. Stone JB, DeAngelis LM. Cancer-treatment-induced neurotoxicity—focus on newer treatments. Nat Rev Clin Oncol. 2016;13(2):92–105.
3. Genter MB, Doty RL. Toxic exposures and the senses of taste and smell. Handb Clin Neurol. 2019;164:389–408.
4. Amézaga J, Alfaro B, Ríos Y, Larraioz A, Ugartemendia G, Urruticoechea A, Tueros I. Assessing taste and smell alterations in cancer patients undergoing chemotherapy according to treatment. Support Care Cancer. 2018;26(12):4077–86.
5. Riga M, Chelis L, Papazi T, Danielides V, Katotomichelakis M, Kakolyris S. Hyposmia: an underestimated and frequent adverse effect of chemotherapy. Support Care Cancer. 2015;23(10):3053–8.
6. Landier W. Ototoxicity and cancer therapy. Cancer. 2016;122(11):1647–58.
7. Camet ML, Spence A, Hayashi SS, Wu N, Henry J, Sauerburger K, Hayashi RJ. Cisplatin ototoxicity: examination of the impact of dosing, infusion times, and schedules in pediatric cancer patients. Front Oncol. 2021;11:673080.
8. Zhang X, Trendowski MR, Wilkinson E, Shahbazi M, Dinh PC, Shuey MM, Feldman DR, Hamilton RJ, Vaughn DJ, Fung C, Kollmannsberger C, Huddart R, Martin NE, Sanchez VA, Frisina RD, Einhorn LH, Cox NJ, Travis LB, Dolan ME. Pharmacogenomics of cisplatin-induced neurotoxicities: hearing loss, tinnitus, and peripheral sensory neuropathy. Cancer Med. 2022;11:2801.
9. Steyger PS. Mechanisms of ototoxicity and otoprotection. Otolaryngol Clin North Am. 2021;54(6):1101–15.
10. Ardeshirrouhanifard S, Fossa SD, Huddart R, Monahan PO, Fung C, Song Y, Dolan ME, Feldman DR, Hamilton RJ, Vaughn D, Martin NE, Kollmannsberger C, Dinh P, Einhorn L, Frisina RD, Travis LB. Ototoxicity after cisplatin-based chemotherapy: factors associated with discrepancies between patient-reported outcomes and audiometric assessments. Ear Hear. 2022;43(3):794–807.
11. Gersten BK, Fitzgerald TS, Fernandez KA, Cunningham LL. Ototoxicity and platinum uptake following cyclic administration of platinum-based chemotherapeutic agents. J Assoc Res Otolaryngol. 2020;21(4):303–21.
12. Moss PE, Hickman S, Harrison BR. Ototoxicity associated with vinblastine. Ann Pharmacother. 1999;33(4):423–5.
13. Xuan L, Sun B, Meng X, Liu C, Cong Y, Wu S. Ototoxicity in patients with invasive ductal breast cancer who were treated with docetaxel: report of two cases. Cancer Biol Ther. 2020;21(11):990–3.
14. Jordan B, Margulies A, Cardoso F, Cavaletti C, Haugnes HS, Jahn P, le Rhun E, Preusser M, Scotte F, Taphoorn MJB, Jordan K. Systemic anticancer therapy-induced peripheral and central neurotoxicity: ESMO-EONS-EANO clinical practice guidelines for diagnosis, prevention, treatment and follow-up. Ann Oncol. 2020;31(10):1306–19.
15. Chiang JCB, Zahari I, Markoulli M, Krishnan AV, Park SB, Semmler A, Goldstein D, Edwards K. The impact of anticancer drugs on the ocular surface. Ocul Surf. 2020;18(3):403–17.
16. Tyler EF, Misra SL, McGhee CNJ, Zhang J. Corneal nerve plexus changes induced by Oxaliplatin chemotherapy and Ergothioneine antioxidant supplementation. Clin Exp Ophthalmol. 2020;48(2):264–6.
17. Chiang JCB, Goldstein D, Park SB, Krishnan AV, Markoulli M. Corneal nerve changes following treatment with neurotoxic anticancer drugs. Ocul Surf. 2021a;21:221–37.
18. Chiang JCB, Goldstein D, Trinh T, Au K, Mizrahi D, Muhlmann M, Crowe P, O'Neill S, Edwards K, Park SB, Krishnan AV, Markoulli M. A cross-sectional study of sub-basal corneal nerve reduction following neurotoxic chemotherapy. Transl Vis Sci Technol. 2021b;10(1):24.
19. Bennedsgaard K, Ventzel L, Andersen NT, Themistocleous AC, Bennett DL, Jensen TS, Tankisi H, Finnerup NB. Oxaliplatin- and docetaxel-induced polyneuropathy: clinical and neurophysiological characteristics. J Peripher Nerv Syst. 2020;25(4):377–87.
20. Riva N, Bonelli F, Lasagni Vitar RM, Barbariga M, Fonteyne P, Lopez ID, Domi T, Scarpa F, Ruggeri A, Reni M, Marcatti M, Quattrini A, Agosta F, Rama P, Ferrari G. Corneal and epidermal nerve quantification in chemotherapy induced peripheral neuropathy. Front Med (Lausanne). 2022;9:832344.
21. Vogrig A, Muñiz-Castrillo S, Joubert B, Picard G, Rogemond V, Skowron F, Egri M, Desestret V,

Tilikete C, Psimaras D, Ducray F, Honnorat J. Cranial nerve disorders associated with immune checkpoint inhibitors. Neurology. 2021;96(6):e866–75.

22. Fanetti G, Ferrari LA, Pietrantonio F, Buzzoni R. Reversible bilateral blepharoptosis following oxaliplatin infusion: a case report and literature review. Tumori. 2013;99(5):e216–9.

23. Lucchetta M, Lonardi S, Bergamo F, Alberti P, Velasco R, Argyriou AA, Briani C, Bruna J, Cazzaniga M, Cortinovis D, Cavaletti G, Kalofonos HP. Incidence of atypical acute nerve hyperexcitability symptoms in oxaliplatin-treated patients with colorectal cancer. Cancer Chemother Pharmacol. 2012;70(6):899–902.

24. Bradley WG, Lassman LP, Pearce GW, Walton JN. The neuromyopathy of vincristine in man. Clinical, electrophysiological and pathological studies. J Neurol Sci. 1970;10(2):107–31.

25. Albert DM, Wong VG, Henderson ES. Ocular complications of vincristine therapy. Arch Ophthalmol. 1967;78(6):709–13.

26. Nazir HF, AlFutaisi A, Zacharia M, Elshinawy M, Mevada ST, Alrawas A, Khater D, Jaju D, Wali Y. Vincristine-induced neuropathy in pediatric patients with acute lymphoblastic leukemia in Oman: frequent autonomic and more severe cranial nerve involvement. Pediatr Blood Cancer. 2017;64(12):e26677.

27. Caraceni A, Martini C, Spatti G, Thomas A, Onofrj M. Recovering optic neuritis during systemic cisplatin and carboplatin chemotherapy. Acta Neurol Scand. 1997;96(4):260–1.

28. Beaumont W, Sustronck P, Souied EH. A case of oxaliplatin-related toxic optic neuropathy. J Fr Ophtalmol. 2021;44(7):e393–5.

29. Raina AJ, Gilbar PJ, Grewal GD, Holcombe DJ. Optic neuritis induced by 5-fluorouracil chemotherapy: case report and review of the literature. J Oncol Pharm Pract. 2020;26(2):511–6.

30. Diker S, Diker Ö. Optic atrophy after cabazitaxel treatment in a patient with castration-resistant prostate cancer: a case report. Scott Med J. 2019;64(2):71–3.

31. Sun MM, Seleme N, Chen JJ, Zekeridou A, Sechi E, Walsh RD, Beebe JD, Sabbagh O, Mejico LJ, Gratton S, Skidd PM, Bellows DA, Falardeau J, Fraser CL, Cappelen-Smith C, Haines SR, Hassanzadeh B, Seay MD, Subramanian PS, Williams Z, Gordon LK. Neuro-ophthalmic complications in patients treated with CTLA-4 and PD-1/PD-L1 checkpoint blockade. J Neuroophthalmol. 2021;41(4):519–30.

32. Eisner A, O'Malley JP, Incognito LJ, Toomey MD, Samples JR. Small optic cup sizes among women using tamoxifen: assessment with scanning laser ophthalmoscopy. Curr Eye Res. 2006;31(4):367–79.

33. Sodhi M, Yeung SN, Maberley D, Mikelberg F, Etminan M. Risk of ocular adverse events with taxane-based chemotherapy. JAMA Opthalmol. 2022;140(9):880–4.

34. Bakbak B, Gedik S, Koktekir BE, Yavuzer K, Tulek B, Kanat F, Pancar E. Assessment of ocular neurotoxicity in patients treated with systemic cancer chemotherapeutics. Cutan Ocul Toxicol. 2014;33(1):7–10.

35. Talmor G, Nguyen B, Geller MT, Hsu J, Kaye R, Caloway C. Vocal fold motion impairment following chemotherapy administration: case reports and review of the literature. Ann Otol Rhinol Laryngol. 2021;130(4):405–15.

36. Godbehere J, Payne J, Thevasagayam R. Vocal cord paralysis secondary to vincristine treatment in children: a case series of seven children and literature review. Clin Otolaryngol. 2021;46(5):1114–8.

37. Millan NC, Pastrana A, Guitter MR, Zubizarreta PA, Monges MS, Felice MS. Acute and sub-acute neurological toxicity in children treated for acute lymphoblastic leukemia. Leuk Res. 2018;65:86–93.

38. Choi BS, Robins HI. Reversible paclitaxel-induced vocal cord paralysis with later recall with vinorelbine. Cancer Chemother Pharmacol. 2008;61(2):345–6.

39. Taha H, Irfan S, Krishnamurthy M. Cisplatin induced reversible bilateral vocal cord paralysis: an undescribed complication of cisplatin. Head Neck. 1999;21(1):78–9.

40. Argyriou AA, Cavaletti G, Briani C, Velasco R, Bruna J, Campagnolo M, Alberti P, Bergamo F, Cortinovis D, Cazzaniga M, Santos C, Papadimitriou K, Kalofonos HP. Clinical pattern and associations of oxaliplatin acute neurotoxicity: a prospective study in 170 patients with colorectal cancer. Cancer. 2013;119(2):438–44.

41. Hartwig S, Pettersson U, Stahle J. cis-Diamminedichloroplatinum: a cytostatic with an ototoxic effect. ORL J Otorhinolaryngol Relat Spec. 1983;45(5):257–61.

42. Prayuenyong P, Kasbekar AV, Hall DA, Hennig I, Anand A, Baguley DM. Imbalance associated with cisplatin chemotherapy in adult cancer survivors: a clinical study. Otol Neurotol. 2021;42(6):e730–4.

43. Wilson RH, Lehky T, Thomas RR, Quinn MG, Floeter MK, Grem JL. Acute oxaliplatin-induced peripheral nerve hyperexcitability. J Clin Oncol. 2002;20(7):1767–74.

44. Leonard GD, Wright MA, Quinn MG, Fioravanti S, Harold N, Schuler B, Thomas RR, Grem JL. Survey of oxaliplatin-associated neurotoxicity using an interview-based questionnaire in patients with metastatic colorectal cancer. BMC Cancer. 2005;5:116.

45. Toker E, Yenice O, Oğüt MS. Isolated abducens nerve palsy induced by vincristine therapy. J AAPOS. 2004;8(1):69–71.

46. Winquist E, Vincent M, Stadler W. Acute bilateral abducens paralysis due to oxaliplatin. J Natl Cancer Inst. 2003;95(6):488–9.

47. Lash SC, Williams CP, Marsh CS, Crithchley C, Hodgkins PR, Mackie EJ. Acute sixth-nerve palsy after vincristine therapy. J AAPOS. 2004;8(1):67–8.

48. Sarkar S, Deb AR, Saha K, Das CS. Simultaneous isolated bilateral facial palsy: a rare vincristine-associated toxicity. Indian J Med Sci. 2009;63(8):355–8.

49. Yigit O, Kulak Kayikci ME, Temucin CM, Sarac S, Erman M, Belgin E. Electrophysiologic evaluation of facial nerve functions after oxaliplatin treatment. Cancer Chemother Pharmacol. 2019;84(3):513–20.

Introduction

CNs are often involved in diverse acquired and hereditary muscle diseases. CN involvement in myopathies ranges from eye movement abnormalities and/or ptosis, to facial weakness and bulbar muscle weakness with dysphagia, dysarthria, and/or dyspnea. In this chapter, CN involvement will be detailed further by describing a few muscle diseases as typical examples. The differential diagnoses will be summarized in the tables, which are, however, not exhaustive.

Author of this chapter: Kristl G. Claeys.

Ophthalmoplegia and/or Ptosis in Muscle Disorders

In many generalized muscle disorders, the extraocular muscles are spared. However, in some myopathies extraocular weakness resulting in ptosis and/or ophthalmoplegia is a predominant feature, such as in chronic progressive external ophthalmoplegia (CPEO) and in congenital myopathies, including centronuclear myopathies. Ptosis and/or ophthalmoparesis are also often present in myotonic dystrophy type 1 (DM1) and oculopharyngeal muscular dystrophy (OPMD).

Mitochondrial Myopathies: Chronic Progressive External Ophthalmoplegia (CPEO) and Kearns–Sayre Syndrome (KSS)

Symptoms (Fig. 24.1): Patients with CPEO present with bilateral ptosis of variable severity and a slowly progressive, painless, symmetric ophthalmoplegia, with sparing of the pupil (i.e., external ophthalmoplegia). Symptom onset often occurs in young adulthood. Patients usually do not experience diplopia because of the symmetrical muscle involvement and very slow progression. CPEO often co-occurs with other symptoms of mitochondrial dysfunction, such as proximal myopathy with or without exercise intolerance, facial weakness, and/or dysphagia (CPEO plus syndrome) [1]. KSS refers to the combination of

© The Author(s), under exclusive license to Springer Nature Switzerland AG 2023
W. Grisold et al., *The Cranial Nerves in Neurology*, https://doi.org/10.1007/978-3-031-43081-7_24

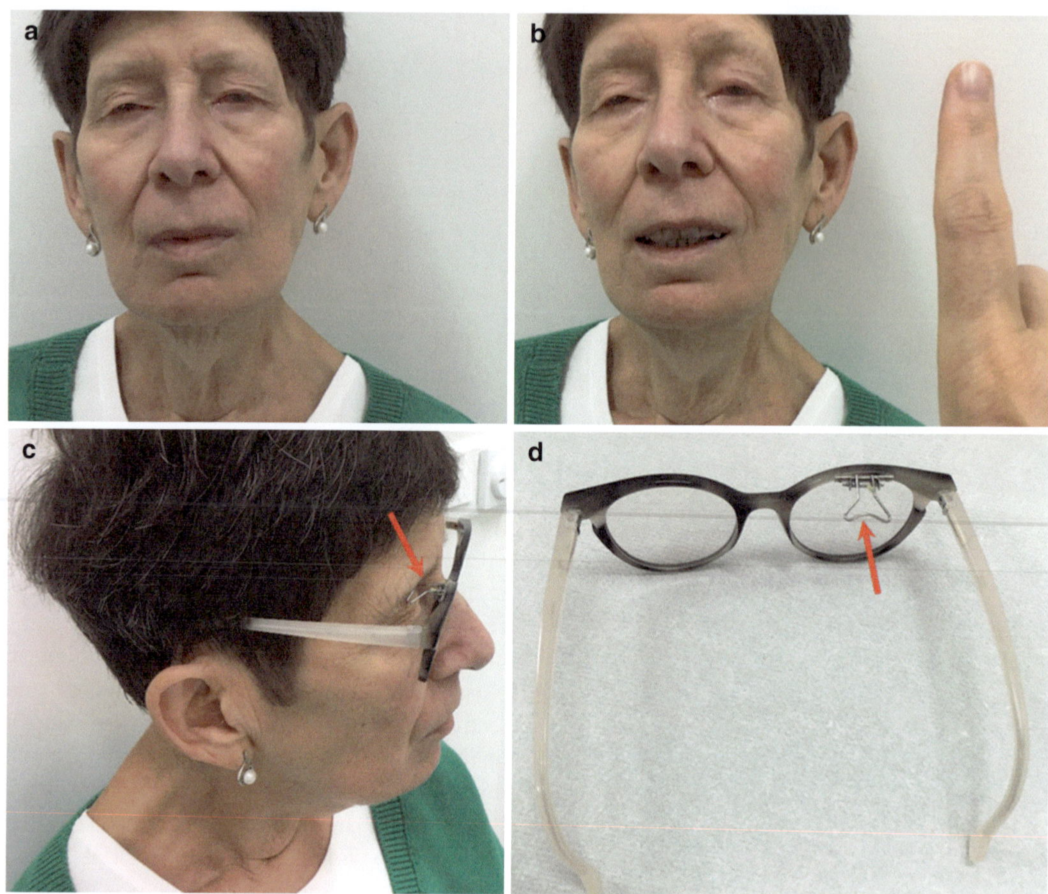

Fig. 24.1 Patient with CPEO. (**a**, **b**) Note the bilateral ptosis, inability to follow the finger of the examiner due to ophthalmoplegia, and facial weakness with horizontal smile. (**c**, **d**) Ptosis eyelid support (red arrow) attached on the glasses to reduce the ptosis

CPEO with pigmentary retinopathy and cardiac conduction defects and onset before 20 years of age [2]. KSS is usually more severe than isolated CPEO, often resulting in death by the fourth decade.

Genetics and inheritance: Inheritance of CPEO and KSS can be sporadic (50%), maternal, autosomal dominant, or autosomal recessive and caused by defects of nuclear or mitochondrial DNA (mtDNA). When sporadic, a single large de novo mtDNA deletion is often detected in muscle tissue, which is typically not transmitted to offspring [3].

Differential diagnosis: The differential diagnosis of CPEO includes OPMD, myasthenia gravis, ocular myositis, thyroid associated orbitopathy, and congenital fibrosis of the extraocular muscles (Table 24.1).

Diagnosis: Serum creatine kinase (CK) levels are usually normal or mildly elevated. Lactate in blood or CSF can sometimes be increased. Electromyography (EMG) shows nonspecific myopathic abnormalities or can be normal. Muscle biopsy can reveal signs of mitochondrial abnormalities, such as ragged-red fibers on modified Gomori trichrome staining, cytochrome-C-oxidase (COX)-negative fibers, and abnormal cristae or inclusions in the mitochondria at ultrastructural examination. Biochemical analysis may identify respiratory chain deficiencies. Confirmation of the diagnosis will result from genetic analysis, for which selec-

Table 24.1 Ptosis and/or ophthalmoplegia: muscle disorders and differential diagnoses

Hereditary muscle disorders	Acquired muscle disorders	Neuromuscular junction disorders	Central/peripheral nervous system
Chronic progressive external Ophthalmoplegia (CPEO) Other mitochondrial cytopathies Oculopharyngeal muscular dystrophy (OPMD) Myotonic dystrophy type 1 (DM1; Steinert disease) Congenital myopathies (e.g., centronuclear, myotubular, central core, nemaline myopathy) Pompe disease (glycogen storage disease type 2; GSD) Congenital fibrosis of the extraocular muscles (CFEOM)	Thyroid-associated orbitopathy Ocular myositis Giant-cell temporal arteritis Senile ptosis	Myasthenia gravis Congenital myasthenic syndromes (CMS) Lambert–Eaton myasthenic syndrome (LEMS) Botulinum toxin intoxication	Miller Fisher syndrome (MFS) Brainstem lesions Cavernous sinus lesions Ischemic CN III palsy Wernicke encephalopathy Progressive supranuclear palsy Whipple disease Neurosyphilis

tion of affected tissue will be important (e.g., skeletal muscle instead of blood to detect a single large mtDNA deletion) [4].

Treatment and management: To date, there are no curative treatments for mitochondrial diseases. Symptomatic management, such as ptosis eyelid support (Fig. 24.1c, d), ptosis surgery, cochlear implants or hearing aids, or prophylactic placement of a cardiac pacemaker, should be implemented by a multidisciplinary team.

Congenital Myopathies: Centronuclear Myopathies (CNM)

Symptoms: The severe X-linked myotubular myopathy (XLMTM) is characterized clinically by severe hypotonia and generalized muscle weakness, often leading to respiratory failure and swallowing difficulties and the presence of ophthalmoplegia. In the usually less severe dynamin-2 (*DNM2*)-related CNM, severity ranges from severely affected infant to mildly affected adults. In severe early-onset cases, infants present with generalized muscle weakness, hypotonia, and facial weakness in addition to ophthalmoplegia [5].

Genetics and inheritance: The majority of patients with CNM are boys with neonatal-onset XLMTM caused by mutations in the myotubula-

rin-1 (*MTM1*) gene. Female carriers can present a broad spectrum of clinical and pathological disease. The autosomal dominant form of CNM is caused by heterozygous mutations in the *DNM2* gene and the more rare autosomal recessive form by mutations in the amphiphysin-2 (*BIN1*) gene.

Differential diagnosis: XLMTM should be considered in the differential diagnosis of any infant who presents with hypotonia and ptosis and/or ophthalmoplegia. Similar clinical manifestations may be seen in neonatal or congenital myasthenia gravis (Table 24.1). Other congenital myopathies, such as nemaline myopathy or core myopathies, also have to be differentiated from CNM [6].

Diagnosis: In congenital myopathies, serum CK is normal to slightly elevated. EMG can show myogenic changes or can be normal. Muscle biopsy in CNM is characterized by chains of centrally placed nuclei in a large number of muscle fibers. In addition, radial rays resembling spokes on a wheel and necklace fibers can be observed. Genetic analysis will provide the causative genetic defect in many cases.

Treatment and management: Although a lot of therapeutic approaches are currently being explored in a preclinical phase, no curative therapy exists for CNM [5]. Symptomatic therapy and multidisciplinary follow-up are recommended [6].

Facial Weakness in Muscle Disorders

Facial weakness is a common symptom in several muscle diseases, including genetic myopathies (e.g., DM1 and facioscapulohumeral muscular dystrophy [FSHD]), congenital myopathies, and acquired myopathies (e.g., sporadic inclusion body myositis [sIBM] or other idiopathic inflammatory myopathies [IIM]). In more severe cases of facial weakness, the term *facies myopathica* is often used.

Myotonic Dystrophy Type 1 (DM1) or Steinert Disease

Symptoms (Fig. 24.2a): The classic form of DM1 starts in adolescence or adulthood and is characterized by progressive muscle weakness and atrophy, myalgia, percussion and action myotonia, cardiac involvement, respiratory failure, hypersomnia and excessive daytime sleepiness, frontal balding, and cataracts [7]. Muscle weakness is mainly situated in the face with facies myopathica and ptosis and in the distal limb muscles. The most severe, congenital form of DM1 occurs in infants born to mothers with Steinert disease. The neonates present with profound hypotonia, facial diplegia, feeding problems, respiratory difficulties, and skeletal deformities, such as clubfeet.

Genetics and inheritance: With a prevalence ranging from 1/7400 to 1/10700 in Europe, DM1 is the most common muscular dystrophy among adults of European ancestry. The genetic defect in DM1 is a CTG-repeat expansion in the dystrophia myotonica protein kinase (*DMPK*) gene. In DM1, the length of the CTG-repeat expansion is moderately correlated with disease severity and age of onset. DM1 is inherited in an autosomal dominant manner and there is anticipation to the next generation, meaning that the clinical phenotype becomes worse every next generation due to an increase of the length of the (unstable) CTG-repeat.

Differential diagnosis: Distal myopathies should be considered in the differential diagnosis of DM1. Important differentials of the congenital form of DM1 are XLMTM and other congenital myopathies (Table 24.2).

Diagnosis: The clinical phenotype and multisystem involvement often are very suggestive for the diagnosis of DM1, and genetic testing can be performed already as a first step, usually without the need for further examinations, such as EMG or muscle biopsy. EMG demonstrates myopathic potentials and myotonic discharges. Muscle histology reveals an increased number of internalized nuclei, type I fiber atrophy, and architectural changes, such as sarcoplasmic masses and ring fibers.

Treatment and management: To date, only symptomatic treatment is available for DM1,

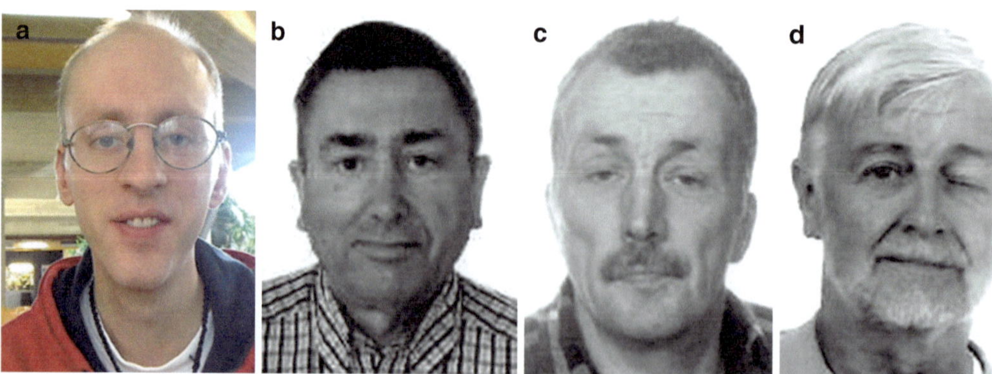

Fig. 24.2 (**a**) Patient with DM1: bilateral ptosis, facial weakness and atrophy, neck flexor atrophy, and frontal baldness. (**b**) Patient with FSHD1: asymmetrical facial weakness. (**c**) Patient with OPMD: facial weakness and bilateral ptosis (without ophthalmoplegia). (**d**) Patient with Pompe disease: asymmetrical ptosis and facial weakness

Table 24.2 Facial weakness: muscle disorders and differential diagnoses

Hereditary muscle disorders	Acquired muscle disorders	Neuromuscular junction disorders	Central/peripheral nervous system
Myotonic dystrophy type 1 (Steinert disease) Facioscapulohumeral muscular dystrophy (FSHD) Congenital myopathies and X-linked myotubular myopathy Mitochondrial diseases (including CPEO and KSS)	Sporadic inclusion body myositis (sIBM) Idiopathic inflammatory myopathies (IIM)	Myasthenia gravis Congenital myasthenic syndromes (CMS) Botulinum toxic intoxication	Guillain–Barré syndrome (GBS) and variants Chronic inflammatory demyelinating polyneuropathy (CIDP) Brainstem lesions (ischemic, tumoral, demyelinating, infection) Neurosarcoidosis Neuroborreliosis Neurosyphilis Vasculitis Idiopathic facial paresis (Bell's palsy) Moebius syndrome

such as medication against myalgia, myotonia, and excessive daytime sleepiness. Aerobic exercise should be encouraged since it effectively improves function in skeletal muscle [8]. Novel therapeutic strategies in myotonic dystrophies are currently under development [9].

Facioscapulohumeral Muscular Dystrophy (FSHD1, FSHD2)

Symptoms (Fig. 24.2b): FSHD is clinically characterized by pronounced facial weakness, scapular winging, and weakness of the elbow flexors (biceps brachii) with sparing of deltoid muscles [10]. Muscle weakness is often asymmetrical. Facial weakness presents as incomplete eyelid closure leading to sleeping with the eyes open, difficulty opposing the lips with an inability to whistle or necessitating the use of straws to drink, and a transverse smile. Weakness of ankle dorsiflexors, pectoral, and lower abdominal muscles is frequently present. Symptom onset is often in the third decade, but can vary from birth to late adulthood.

Genetics and inheritance: With an estimated prevalence from 1/8000 to 1/20,000, FSHD1 is the second most frequent hereditary muscle disease in adults. FSHD1 is caused by a heterozygous D4Z4 repeat DNA deletion on chromosome 4q and very rarely on chromosome 10qter. The gene defect in FSHD2 occurs in the structural maintenance of chromosomes flexible hinge domain containing 1 (*SMCHD1*) gene. Both FSHD1 and FSHD2 are inherited in an autosomal dominant manner.

Differential diagnosis: The main differential diagnoses of FSHD are the limb–girdle muscular dystrophies (LGMD). Additional differential diagnoses are other neuromuscular diseases presenting with facial weakness and/or scapular winging, such as Pompe disease (Fig. 24.2d), inclusion body myopathy with Paget disease of bone and frontotemporal dementia caused by a mutation in the valosin-containing protein (*VCP*) gene, late-onset endocrine myopathy, and proximal neuropathies or neuronopathies (Table 24.2).

Diagnosis: Usually the clinical presentation in FSHD patients is suggestive for the disease and genetic analysis will be performed directly. In contrast, muscle biopsy will usually not be performed in FSHD and can even be misleading because in some cases inflammatory changes can be seen.

Treatment and management: The only treatment currently available for FSHD is physiotherapy. However, new therapeutic approaches in FSHD are currently being studied both in preclinical and clinical stages [11].

Bulbar Weakness in Muscle Disorders

Both hereditary muscle diseases, such as OPMD, and acquired muscle disorders, such as sIBM, can be associated with bulbar weakness, in particular dysphagia. Interestingly, in OPMD and sIBM, dysphagia can also be the presenting symptom of the disease. Dysphagia can be very severe in some patients, necessitating surgical intervention.

Oculopharyngeal Muscular Dystrophy (OPMD)

Symptoms (Fig. 24.2c): Patients with OPMD develop progressive ptosis and dysphagia in late adulthood [12]. Additional manifestations as the disease progresses can include limitation of upward gaze, tongue atrophy and weakness, chewing difficulties, facial weakness, axial muscle weakness, and proximal weakness predominantly in the lower limbs. Swallowing difficulties increase the risk for potentially life-threatening aspiration pneumonia and cachexia and thus determine prognosis. Progressive ptosis gives rise to the so-called astrologist's posture.

Genetics and inheritance: In most cases, OPMD is transmitted in an autosomal dominant manner, caused by the abnormal expansion of the alanine-encoding (GCN)n trinucleotide repeat in exon 1 of the polyadenosine binding protein nuclear 1 (*PABPN1*) gene (11–18 repeats in OPMD instead of the normal 10 repeats) [13].

Differential diagnosis: Most important differential diagnoses of OPMD (in particular bulbar weakness and/or ptosis) include myasthenia gravis, mitochondrial disorders such as CPEO and KSS, DM1, and some congenital myopathies, such as CNM (Table 24.3).

Diagnosis: In OPMD, serum CK is normal to slightly elevated. EMG reveals nonspecific myopathic changes with the development of limb weakness. Muscle biopsy shows small rounded or angular fibers and non-consistently rimmed vacuoles in small fibers. Ultrastructurally, tubulofilamentous aggregates can be seen in approxi-mately 4% of the myonuclei [14]. Final diagnosis of OPMD is obtained by molecular genetic testing.

Treatment and management: To date, no effective treatments are available for OPMD. Therefore, symptomatic and supportive multidisciplinary therapy is important. Invalidating ptosis can be managed surgically. The initial treatment for dysphagia consists of dietary adaptations. Surgery for dysphagia should be considered in case of significant weight loss and recurrent aspiration pneumonia and when dysphagia has a significant impact on quality of life. Repetitive dilatations of the upper esophageal sphincter, cricopharyngeal myotomy, or percutaneous endoscopic gastrostomy (PEG) are possible treatments.

Sporadic Inclusion Body Myositis (sIBM)

Symptoms: Typical symptoms of patients with sIBM are swallowing difficulties or dysphagia due to bulbar muscle weakness at the upper third of the esophagus and weakness and atrophy of knee extensors, foot dorsiflexors, and finger-/wrist flexors [15]. Muscle weakness in the limbs is often asymmetrical. Mild facial weakness occurs in around 30% of the patients.

Cause: sIBM is a rare sporadic acquired muscle disease, with an inflammatory component and a degenerative component, leading to slowly progressive motor disability with a mean time to wheelchair of 14 years after symptom onset. sIBM occurs more frequently in males above the age of 50 years. Causes of death are aspiration pneumonia due to dysphagia and/or cachexia.

Differential diagnosis: The IIM, such as polymyositis and the antisynthetase syndrome, are important differentials from sIBM, because these IIM are treatable (e.g., with immunosuppressive drugs and immune modulators), whereas sIBM is not. Furthermore, the hereditary forms of IBM (hIBM) should be differentiated. hIBM patients often present with a positive family history.

Diagnosis: The clinical presentation of sIBM is often suggestive for the diagnosis and should be confirmed by muscle biopsy, which typically

Table 24.3 Bulbar weakness: muscle disorders and differential diagnoses

Hereditary muscle disorders	Acquired muscle disorders	Neuromuscular junction disorders	Central/peripheral nervous system
Oculopharyngeal muscular dystrophy (OPMD) Myotonic dystrophy type 1 (Steinert disease) Chronic progressive external ophthalmoplegia plus (CPEO+) Mitochondrial diseases Congenital and myotubular myopathy Distal myopathy with vocal cord and pharyngeal weakness (VCPDM) Myofibrillar myopathies Hereditary inclusion body myopathy (hIBM)	Sporadic inclusion body myositis (sIBM) Idiopathic inflammatory myopathies (IIM)	Myasthenia gravis Congenital myasthenic syndromes (CMS) Lambert-Eaton myasthenic syndrome (LEMS) Botulinum toxin intoxication	Brainstem lesions (ischemic, tumoral, demyelinating, inflammatory, syringobulbia) Guillain–Barré and MMiller FFisher syndrome Amyotrophic lateral sclerosis (ALS) Spinal muscular atrophy (SMA) Bulbospinal muscular atrophy (BSMA, Kennedy syndrome) Brown–Vialetto–van Laere syndrome Fazio–Londe syndrome Neuroborreliosis Neurosyphilis

shows p62-positive rimmed vacuoles and inflammatory infiltrates. Serum CK is normal to 15x the upper limit of normal. The cytosolic 5′-nucleotidase IA (NT5C1A) antibodies in serum are positive in around 50–75% of sIBM patients, but they are not specific for sIBM and can also occur in the other IIM and connective tissue diseases [16]. EMG usually shows an irritable myopathy and in some patients also a subclinical predominantly sensory polyneuropathy.

Treatment and management: To date, no curative treatment for sIBM exists. However, physiotherapy is important to maintain ambulation and independence in daily life as long as possible. Repetitive dilatations of the upper esophageal sphincter, cricopharyngeal myotomy, or percutaneous endoscopic gastrostomy (PEG) are possible treatments in cases of disabling dysphagia in sIBM patients.

References

1. McClelland C, Manousakis G, Lee MS. Progressive external ophthalmoplegia. Curr Neurol Neurosci Rep. 2016;16:53.
2. Tsang SH, Aycinena ARP, Sharma T. Mitochondrial disorder: Kearns-Sayre syndrome. Adv Exp Med Biol. 2018;1085:161–2.
3. Moraes CT, DiMauro S, Zeviani M, et al. Mitochondrial DNA deletions in progressive external ophthalmoplegia and Kearns Sayre syndrome. N Engl J Med. 1989;320:1293–9.
4. Milone M, Wong LJ. Diagnosis of mitochondrial myopathies. Mol Genet Metab. 2013;110:35–41.
5. Tasfaout H, Cowling BS, Laporte J. Centronuclear myopathies under attack: a plethora of therapeutic targets. J Neuromuscul Dis. 2018;5:387–406.
6. Claeys KG. Congenital myopathies: an update. Dev Med Child Neurol. 2020;62:297–302.
7. Johnson NE. Myotonic muscular dystrophies. Continuum (Minneap Minn). 2019;25:1682–95.
8. Mackenzie SJ, Hamel J, Thornton CA. Benefits of aerobic exercise in myotonic dystrophy type 1. J Clin Invest. 2022;132:e160229.
9. Izzo M, Battistini J, Provenzano C, Martelli F, Cardinali B, Falcone G. Molecular therapies for myotonic dystrophy type 1: from small drugs to gene editing. Int J Mol Sci. 2022;23:4622–47.
10. Sacconi S, Briand-Suleau A, Gros M, Baudoin C, Lemmers RJLF, Rondeau S, et al. FSHD1 and FSHD2 form a disease continuum. Neurology. 2019;92:e2273–85.
11. Wang LH, Tawil R. Current therapeutic approaches in FSHD. J Neuromuscul Dis. 2021;8:441–51.
12. Mirabella M, Silvestri G, de Rosa G, Di Giovanni S, Di Muzio A, Uncini A, et al. GCG genetic expansions in Italian patients with oculopharyngeal muscular dystrophy. Neurology. 2000;54:608–14.
13. Brais B, Bouchard JP, Xie YG, Rochefort DL, Chrétien N, Tomé FM, et al. Short GCG expansions in the PABP2 gene cause oculopharyngeal muscular dystrophy. Nat Genet. 1998;18:164–7.
14. Yamashita S. Recent progress in oculopharyngeal muscular dystrophy. J Clin Med. 2021;10:1375–85.
15. Machado PM, Dimachkie MM, Barohn RJ. Sporadic inclusion body myositis: new insights and potential therapy. Curr Opin Neurol. 2014;27:591–8.
16. Herbert MK, Pruijn GJ. Novel serology testing for sporadic inclusion body myositis: disease-specificity and diagnostic utility. Curr Opin Rheumatol. 2015;27:595–600.

> **Bullet Points**
> - Cranial nerve (CN) lesions represent the predominant disease manifestation in some rare genetic conditions (e.g., Leber's hereditary optic neuropathy).
> - Neurogenetic (mainly neuromuscular) disorders, such as Charcot–Marie–Tooth neuropathies, may involve the CNs as part of their complex phenotypic spectrum.
> - CN dysfunction may secondarily be caused by some multisystem disorders, such as mitochondrial diseases or neurofibromatosis.

Introduction

Over the past decade, massive parallel sequencing technologies (also referred to as next-generation sequencing [NGS]) have helped to elucidate the molecular underpinnings of numerous genetic disorders [1]. As the majority of the 20,000 genes of the human genome are actively expressed in the nervous system [2], around 40% of all monogenic conditions clinically involve either the central or the peripheral nervous system, according to the Online Mendelian Inheritance in Man (OMIM) database [3], as a consequence, it has become increasingly relevant for clinical neurologists to be familiar with the basic principles of molecular genetic testing and the phenotypes associated with certain genetic defects. In view of the enormous clinical heterogeneity of neurogenetic disorders, it is not far to seek that some of these conditions may also involve the CNs. In addition, the relationship between genetic factors and CNs is further corroborated by elaborate basic research efforts using mouse models which have led to a better molecular understanding of CN development and the related pathophysiology [4].

Defects in these genes may result in variable inborn manifestations which have been summarized as congenital cranial dysinnervation disorders (CCDDs) in the biomedical literature [5]. Generally speaking, they constitute a clinically and genetically heterogeneous group of neurogenic syndromes primarily affecting ocular muscles and facial innervation, with the responsible genes influencing the development of the brainstem and different CNs [6].

Given the wide range of genes involved in CN development and dysfunction, the spectrum of pathomechanisms associated with CN dysfunction in genetic disorders is extremely broad. Henceforth, this chapter can only serve as a brief overview. For the sake of simplicity, we here defined three subgroups with a few selected prototype disorders as relevant examples. These disease subgroups include (1) monogenic disorders

---

Author of this chapter: Martin Krenn.

in which CN lesions represent the core phenotype (mainly summarized as CCDDs), (2) neurogenetic disorders with potential CN involvement, and (3) multisystem disorders that may secondarily cause CN abnormalities, usually among other neurological manifestations.

Cranial Nerve Lesions as Primary Disease Manifestation

Moebius syndrome belongs to the abovementioned group of CCDDs, and although it may clinically involve different CNs, it invariably affects the facial nerve either unilaterally or bilaterally. As of today, its pathogenesis is currently best understood as a syndromic rhombencephalic maldevelopment which—apart from facial nerve palsy—may additionally lead to impaired ocular movements (most prominently affecting abduction), dysfunction of lower CNs, and also general motor impairment [7]. Although de novo mutations in the genes *PLXND1* and *REV3L* have already been suggested as causative, these associations have so far not been confirmed independently [8].

Second, *Duane syndrome* typically causes strabismus due to an anomalous innervation of extraocular muscles. The underlying abnormality is a paradoxical innervation of the lateral rectus muscle caused by a pathological misdirection of axons originally destined for the medial rectus muscle [9]. In the vast majority of cases without a family history, however, no specific molecular defect can be determined [10]. Yet, familial (and rarely sporadic) cases may be associated with rare genetic variation in the genes *CHN1*, *MAFB*, or *SALL4* and should therefore be considered for genetic testing [11–13].

In recent years, pathogenic mutations in collagen, type XXV, alpha 1 (*COL25A1*) have also been identified as a novel molecular cause of recessively inherited ocular CCDD phenotypes. It has been suggested that a lack of COL25A1 protein interferes with functional pathways involved in oculomotor neuron development [14].

Aside from the CCDDs, another prototype disorder primarily affecting a CN is *Leber's hereditary optic neuropathy (LHON)*, which is clinically characterized by bilateral, painless, subacute visual disturbances due to a genetically determined optic nerve degeneration. LHON usually manifests in early adulthood and is caused by maternally inherited pathogenic variants in the mitochondrial DNA (mtDNA) [15]. Idebenone, a targeted medication that reduces oxidative stress, has already been approved for the treatment of a selected subgroup of patients with LHON [16].

Cranial Nerve Lesions in Complex Neurogenetic Disorders

The spectrum of neurogenetic disorders clinically involving the CNs is broad and can further be subdivided into inherited polyneuropathies, hereditary motor neuron disorders, and also more complex neurogenetic conditions that can involve both the central and peripheral nervous systems.

First and foremost, the *inherited polyneuropathies* (also termed Charcot–Marie–Tooth disease [CMT]) exhibit a wide clinical range including motor, sensory, and autonomic abnormalities. Although the most common genetic CMT subtype (CMT1A) is usually confined to upper and lower limbs, some other genetic etiologies of CMT are specifically prone to an involvement of CNs. For instance, *MFN2*-related polyneuropathy, the most common axonal subtype, may cause optic atrophy, vocal cord palsy, and auditory impairment in some cases [17–19]. Second, mutations in the *TRPV4* gene are a major cause of inherited axonal polyneuropathies. This gene is typically associated with vocal cord palsy in the vast majority of cases (>90%), but also with hearing impairment in a smaller number of affected individuals [20]. Further, patients with pathogenic variants in *MPZ* may display optic nerve atrophy and hearing impairment [21].

Moreover, the hereditary motor neuron disorders comprise different molecular etiologies and phenotypes, some of which may also affect the lower CNs. *Spinal and bulbar muscular atrophy (SBMA)*, also referred to as *Kennedy's disease*, is an X-linked, hereditary motor neuron disorder caused by an abnormal CAG (polyglutamine) trinucleotide expansion in the gene *AR*, encoding the androgen receptor. This toxic mutational mechanism leads to a degeneration of lower motor neurons and muscle tissue, clinically causing flaccid muscle weakness, bulbar features (tongue fasciculations, dysarthria, and dysphagia), but also non-neurological (e.g., endocrine and cardiological) abnormalities [22]. At the moment, there is no specific disease-modifying treatment available, but promising targets have been identified, thus raising hope for future developments [23]. Furthermore, there are also hereditary forms of amyotrophic lateral sclerosis (ALS) that are usually associated with more severe phenotypes than SBMA. For example, *SOD1*-related ALS, the second most common hereditary subtype of ALS, may often cause bulbar involvement [24].

Eventually, there are also neurogenetic disorders that clinically extend beyond pure peripheral nervous system manifestations, but may also cause CN lesions. For instance, one complex clinical phenotype that characteristically involves the vestibular nerve is a condition termed *cerebellar ataxia, neuropathy, vestibular areflexia syndrome (CANVAS)*. Although this clinical constellation is already well known and described extensively in the literature, its exact molecular underpinnings have only been unraveled very recently. Accordingly, the condition was found to be caused by a biallelic, intronic AAGGG repeat expansion in the *RFC1* gene [25]. Individuals with CANVAS usually present with a progressive unsteadiness occurring around the sixth decade of life, which is often accompanied by sensory ataxia, cerebellar dysfunction, vestibular impairment, and spasmodic cough [26].

Cranial Nerve Lesions in Multisystem Disorders

Apart from typical neurogenetic disorders, a larger number of complex multisystem disorders may secondarily involve the peripheral and/or central nervous system and thus also the CNs. To illustrate this group of diseases, mitochondrial disorders and the different types of neurofibromatosis are used as representative examples.

Mitochondrial disorders represent one possible genetic etiology underlying secondary CN dysfunction. For example, one of the clinical hallmarks of mitochondrial disorders is sensorineural hearing loss that may either occur as an isolated clinical finding (non-syndromic) or as part of a more complex phenotype (syndromic) [27]. Moreover, there is anecdotal evidence that *POLG*-related mitochondrial disorder may cause oculomotor nerve lesions with contrast agent enhancement [28]. Similar imaging findings involving different CNs have been reported in mitochondrial neurogastrointestinal encephalomyopathy (MNGIE) [29]. The same condition may also be associated with abnormal brainstem auditory evoked responses, indicating a delayed central conduction time [30].

Besides, the three types of *neurofibromatosis*, that is, neurofibromatosis types 1 (NF1) and 2 (NF2) and schwannomatosis, are monogenic multisystem disorders causing different types of nervous system tumors, with some of them originating from the CNs. First, NF1 is an autosomal dominant multisystem disorder characterized by various neurocutaneous manifestations (café au lait spots, neurofibromas, etc.). The most common CN manifestation in NF1 is optic pathway glioma, which affects around 20% of the patients at some point during their life [31]. By contrast, peripheral nerve sheath tumors (PNST) have a much lower prevalence in NF1, but, if present, may also originate from CNs in rare cases [32]. Second, NF2 is a hereditary condition that is clinically characterized by bilateral vestibular schwannomas causing various symptoms, such as tinnitus, hearing loss, and balance dysfunction. In this context, it is worthy of note that schwannomas in NF2 are not exclusively confined to the vestibular nerve, but may also arise from other CNs, most commonly the oculomotor and the trigeminal nerve; however, neuropathies associated with these lesions are usually rare [33]. Third, schwannomatosis is another genetic condition (caused by dominantly inherited variants in *SMARCB1* or *LZTR1*) which is associated with multiple schwannomas and meningiomas that may also involve CNs [34].

Discussion

In general, CN lesions may be encountered in a broad spectrum of different monogenic disorders, either as the primary or (much more commonly) as a secondary disease manifestation. As compared to acquired or so-called idiopathic lesions, hereditary causes of CN abnormalities are relatively rare, but should be considered under specific clinical circumstances in both pediatric and adult individuals. Although there are no established guidelines for genetic testing in patients with CN dysfunction, a genetic etiology may especially be taken into consideration in cases with early-onset (or congenital) CN lesions for which no acquired cause could be established. Other red flags with regard to a genetic cause are a family history for the disease or a syndromic phenotype.

In conditions with primary CN involvement, the responsible molecular defects alter motor neuron specification or the development of motor nerves, thus highlighting the importance of the underlying pathomechanisms, such as cell signaling, cytoskeletal transport, and microtubule function for axonal growth and guidance [35]. By contrast, in disorders with secondary CN involvement, the disease mechanisms are even more heterogeneous, ranging from inherited neoplastic lesions to mitochondrial dysfunction, only to name a few.

It is also noteworthy that the phenotypes associated with genetically caused CN lesions may clinically be reminiscent of those caused by primary muscle diseases or inherited disorders of the neuromuscular junction, which therefore represent relevant differential diagnoses. Among others, this may include the board spectrum of congenital myasthenic syndromes and different myopathic disorders, such as oculopharyngeal or facioscapulohumeral muscular dystrophy, that typically involve muscles that are supplied by CNs.

As the landscape of molecular testing is constantly evolving at a rapid pace, further genetic etiologies are likely to be discovered in future years. This is particularly relevant, as a correct molecular diagnosis usually has important implications with respect to genetic counseling, family planning, and, as exemplified by LHON, in some cases even specific treatment [16]. However, for the vast majority of genetic etiologies, the currently available treatment approaches are mainly symptomatic.

Given the heterogeneity of molecular causes, the most suitable molecular testing method depends on the exact phenotype and the mode of inheritance. Although comprehensive testing such as NGS has been demonstrated as a cost-effective and useful diagnostic tool for different neurogenetic/neuromuscular disorders [36], it is usually recommended to discuss cases in interdisciplinary boards beforehand [37].

References

1. Ng SB, Turner EH, Robertson PD, Flygare SD, Bigham AW, Lee C, et al. Targeted capture and massively parallel sequencing of 12 human exomes. Nature. 2009;461(7261):272–6.
2. Negi SK, Guda C. Global gene expression profiling of healthy human brain and its application in studying neurological disorders. Sci Rep. 2017;7(1):897.
3. Rexach J, Lee H, Martinez-Agosto JA, Nemeth AH, Fogel BL. Clinical application of next-generation sequencing to the practice of neurology. Lancet Neurol. 2019;18(5):492–503.
4. Cordes SP. Molecular genetics of cranial nerve development in mouse. Nat Rev Neurosci. 2001;2(9):611–23.
5. Gutowski NJ, Bosley TM, Engle EC. 110th ENMC international workshop: the congenital cranial dysinnervation disorders (CCDDs). Naarden, the Netherlands, 25-27 October, 2002. Neuromuscul Disord. 2003;13(7–8):573–8.
6. Whitman MC. Axonal growth abnormalities underlying ocular cranial nerve disorders. Annu Rev Vis Sci. 2021;7:827–50.
7. Verzijl HT, van der Zwaag B, Cruysberg JR, Padberg GW. Mobius syndrome redefined: a syndrome of rhombencephalic maldevelopment. Neurology. 2003;61(3):327–33.
8. Tomas-Roca L, Tsaalbi-Shtylik A, Jansen JG, Singh MK, Epstein JA, Altunoglu U, et al. De novo mutations in PLXND1 and REV3L cause Mobius syndrome. Nat Commun. 2015;6:7199.
9. Gutowski NJ. Duane's syndrome. Eur J Neurol. 2000;7(2):145–9.
10. Barry BJ, Whitman MC, Hunter DG, Engle EC. Duane Syndrome. In: Adam MP, Mirzaa GM, Pagon RA, Wallace SE, Bean LJH, Gripp KW, et al., editors. GeneReviews((R)). Seattle; 1993.

11. Miyake N, Chilton J, Psatha M, Cheng L, Andrews C, Chan WM, et al. Human CHN1 mutations hyperactivate alpha2-chimaerin and cause Duane's retraction syndrome. Science. 2008;321(5890):839–43.

12. Park JG, Tischfield MA, Nugent AA, Cheng L, Di Gioia SA, Chan WM, et al. Loss of MAFB function in humans and mice causes Duane syndrome, aberrant extraocular muscle innervation, and inner-ear defects. Am J Hum Genet. 2016;98(6):1220–7.

13. Al-Baradie R, Yamada K, St Hilaire C, Chan WM, Andrews C, McIntosh N, et al. Duane radial ray syndrome (Okihiro syndrome) maps to 20q13 and results from mutations in SALL4, a new member of the SAL family. Am J Hum Genet. 2002;71(5):1195–9.

14. Shinwari JM, Khan A, Awad S, Shinwari Z, Alaiya A, Alanazi M, et al. Recessive mutations in COL25A1 are a cause of congenital cranial dysinnervation disorder. Am J Hum Genet. 2015;96(1):147–52.

15. Yu Wai-Man P, Chinnery PF. Leber hereditary optic neuropathy. In: Adam MP, Mirzaa GM, Pagon RA, Wallace SE, Bean LJH, Gripp KW, et al., editors. GeneReviews((R)). Seattle; 1993.

16. Carelli V, Carbonelli M, de Coo IF, Kawasaki A, Klopstock T, Lagreze WA, et al. International consensus statement on the clinical and therapeutic Management of Leber hereditary optic neuropathy. J Neuroophthalmol. 2017;37(4):371–81.

17. Ando M, Hashiguchi A, Okamoto Y, Yoshimura A, Hiramatsu Y, Yuan J, et al. Clinical and genetic diversities of Charcot-Marie-Tooth disease with MFN2 mutations in a large case study. J Peripher Nerv Syst. 2017;22(3):191–9.

18. Bombelli F, Stojkovic T, Dubourg O, Echaniz-Laguna A, Tardieu S, Larcher K, et al. Charcot-Marie-tooth disease type 2A: from typical to rare phenotypic and genotypic features. JAMA Neurol. 2014;71(8):1036–42.

19. Pipis M, Feely SME, Polke JM, Skorupinska M, Perez L, Shy RR, et al. Natural history of Charcot-Marie-Tooth disease type 2A: a large international multicentre study. Brain. 2020;143(12):3589–602.

20. Echaniz-Laguna A, Dubourg O, Carlier P, Carlier RY, Sabouraud P, Pereon Y, et al. Phenotypic spectrum and incidence of TRPV4 mutations in patients with inherited axonal neuropathy. Neurology. 2014;82(21):1919–26.

21. Sanmaneechai O, Feely S, Scherer SS, Herrmann DN, Burns J, Muntoni F, et al. Genotype-phenotype characteristics and baseline natural history of heritable neuropathies caused by mutations in the MPZ gene. Brain. 2015;138(Pt 11):3180–92.

22. Breza M, Koutsis G. Kennedy's disease (spinal and bulbar muscular atrophy): a clinically oriented review of a rare disease. J Neurol. 2019;266(3):565–73.

23. Hashizume A, Fischbeck KH, Pennuto M, Fratta P, Katsuno M. Disease mechanism, biomarker and therapeutics for spinal and bulbar muscular atrophy (SBMA). J Neurol Neurosurg Psychiatry. 2020;91(10):1085–91.

24. Bernard E, Pegat A, Svahn J, Bouhour F, Leblanc P, Millecamps S, et al. Clinical and molecular landscape of ALS patients with SOD1 mutations: novel pathogenic variants and novel phenotypes. A single ALS center study. Int J Mol Sci. 2020;21(18):6807.

25. Cortese A, Simone R, Sullivan R, Vandrovcova J, Tariq H, Yau WY, et al. Biallelic expansion of an intronic repeat in RFC1 is a common cause of late-onset ataxia. Nat Genet. 2019;51(4):649–58.

26. Cortese A, Tozza S, Yau WY, Rossi S, Beecroft SJ, Jaunmuktane Z, et al. Cerebellar ataxia, neuropathy, vestibular areflexia syndrome due to RFC1 repeat expansion. Brain. 2020;143(2):480–90.

27. Hutchin TP, Cortopassi GA. Mitochondrial defects and hearing loss. Cell Mol Life Sci. 2000;57(13–14):1927–37.

28. Bayat M, Yavarian Y, Bayat A, Christensen J. Enhancement of cranial nerves, conus medullaris, and nerve roots in POLG mitochondrial disease. Neurol Genet. 2019;5(5):e360.

29. Petcharunpaisan S, Castillo M. Multiple cranial nerve enhancement in mitochondrial neurogastrointestinal encephalomyopathy. J Comput Assist Tomogr. 2010;34(2):247–8.

30. Gamez J, Minoves T. Abnormal brainstem auditory evoked responses in mitochondrial neurogastrointestinal encephalomyopathy (MNGIE): evidence of delayed central conduction time. Clin Neurophysiol. 2006;117(11):2385–91.

31. Shofty B, Ben Sira L, Constantini S. Neurofibromatosis 1-associated optic pathway gliomas. Childs Nerv Syst. 2020;36(10):2351–61.

32. Newell C, Chalil A, Langdon KD, Karapetyan V, Hebb MO, Siddiqi F, et al. Cranial nerve and intramedullary spinal malignant peripheral nerve sheath tumor associated with neurofibromatosis-1. Surg Neurol Int. 2021;12:630.

33. Fisher LM, Doherty JK, Lev MH, Slattery WH 3rd. Distribution of nonvestibular cranial nerve schwannomas in neurofibromatosis 2. Otol Neurotol. 2007;28(8):1083–90.

34. Dhamija R, Plotkin S, Asthagiri A, Messiaen L, Babovic-Vuksanovic D. Schwannomatosis. In: Adam MP, Mirzaa GM, Pagon RA, Wallace SE, Bean LJH, Gripp KW, et al., editors. GeneReviews((R)). Seattle; 1993.

35. Whitman MC, Engle EC. Ocular congenital cranial dysinnervation disorders (CCDDs): insights into axon growth and guidance. Hum Mol Genet. 2017;26(R1):R37–44.

36. Krenn M, Tomschik M, Rath J, Cetin H, Grisold A, Zulehner G, et al. Genotype-guided diagnostic reassessment after exome sequencing in neuromuscular disorders: experiences with a two-step approach. Eur J Neurol. 2020;27(1):51–61.

37. Pena LDM, Jiang YH, Schoch K, Spillmann RC, Walley N, Stong N, et al. Looking beyond the exome: a phenotype-first approach to molecular diagnostic resolution in rare and undiagnosed diseases. Genet Med. 2018;20(4):464–9.

Cranial Nerves and Autoimmune Conditions

Introduction

The CNs are unique in their function and localization to serve as the interface between the central and peripheral nervous systems. Thus, it is not surprising that they are particularly prone to injury caused by autoimmune diseases targeting the central or the peripheral nervous systems. A clinical neurologist is confronted almost daily with cranial neuropathies, in which autoimmune conditions need to be considered or ruled out.

Probably the most frequent constellation is optic neuritis as part of multiple sclerosis or neuromyelitis optica spectrum diseases. Another example is bilateral facial paresis in Guillain–Barré syndrome (GBS) or sarcoidosis.

In this chapter, I will review the literature regarding frequency of CN involvement, its underlying pathogenesis, and specific treatment of autoimmune conditions in the central and peripheral nervous systems. Furthermore, I will discuss the value of specific CN deficit patterns in the differential diagnosis of autoimmune diseases.

Cranial Nerve Involvement in Autoimmune Conditions of the Central Nervous System

Multiple Sclerosis (MS) and Neuromyelitis Spectrum Disorder (NMOSD)

The most common CN involvement in MS and NMOSD is optic neuritis [1]. Acute optic neuritis has an estimated lifetime prevalence of 0.6/1000 and an annual incidence of 1–5/100,000, with a mean onset of 31–32 years [1]. It is the presenting symptom in 25% of MS patients and occurs in about 70% during the disease course. Half of MS patients with optic neuritis develops the full picture of MS by 15 years. This probability strongly relates to the presence of MS lesions in MRI of the brain [2]. In Asia, NMOSD is more common and optic neuritis is the initial manifestation of NMOSD in 42%, whereas 63% of

---

Author of this chapter: Helmar Lehmann.

W. Grisold et al., *The Cranial Nerves in Neurology*, https://doi.org/10.1007/978-3-031-43081-7_26

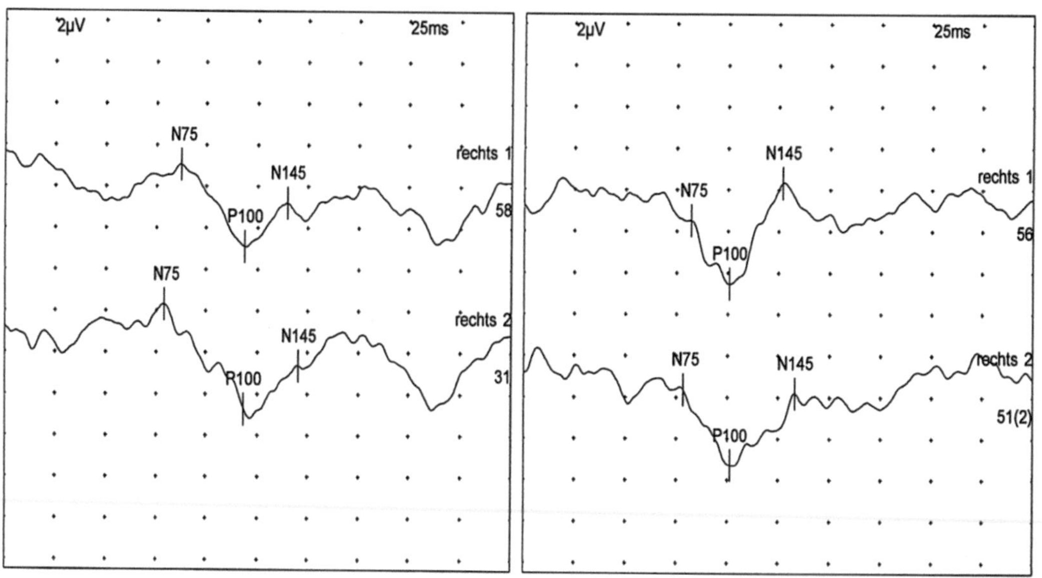

Fig. 26.1 Visual evoked potentials in a patient with optic neuritis of the right eye. P100 latency was prolonged to 119 ms on the right side, whereas on the left side it was normal (101 ms)

patients with NMOSD develop optic neuritis during the disease course [3].

Symptoms of optic neuritis are profound vision loss, optic disc edema, and painful eye movements. The diagnosis is usually established on clinical grounds and supported by abnormal visually evoked potentials (VEPs) which usually show prolonged P100 latency (Fig. 26.1). The VEP result does not necessarily correlate with the severity of the optic nerve lesion. Preserved potentials may indicate better chances of recovery; however, even in entirely absent cortical responses, recovery is possible because it reflects total conduction block due to severe demyelination rather than axonal damage [4].

Standard treatment of optic neuritis in MS and NMOSD are intravenous or oral corticosteroids in high doses [5]. Prognosis is more favorable in optic neuritis associated with MS as compared to optic neuritis as part of NMOSD [6].

Other CNs are much more rarely affected in MS. Several studies report that dysfunction of the olfactory sense occurs in a significant proportion of patients with MS, although loss of smell is seldom reported as predominant symptom [7].

CNs III–XII are also rarely affected in MS. Clinical deficits, such as oculomotor abnor-malities or sensory deficits, are usually caused by demyelinating lesions in the brainstem, thereby mimicking CN deficits. Rarely, contrast enhancement can be observed on the cisternal parts of the CNs adjacent to a demyelinating lesion (Fig. 26.2).

One study found CN enhancement in 8.2% of analyzed MS patients, most frequently in the trigeminal nerve (2.7%) and abducens nerve (2.2%) [8]. It has been debated whether this enhancement reflects a demyelinating process of the peripheral myelin in these parts of the nerves. However, the close proximity of brainstem lesions indicates that the inflammation and hence enhancement are rather caused by continuous encroachment of adjacent myelin rather than a specific autoimmune attack on peripheral myelin [9].

Giant Cell Arteritis

Giant cell arteritis, or temporal arteritis, is the most common primary vasculitis in the northern hemisphere, with an incidence of 18 per 100,000 in the USA [10] and 22.2 per 100,000 individuals 50 years of age and older in Sweden [11].

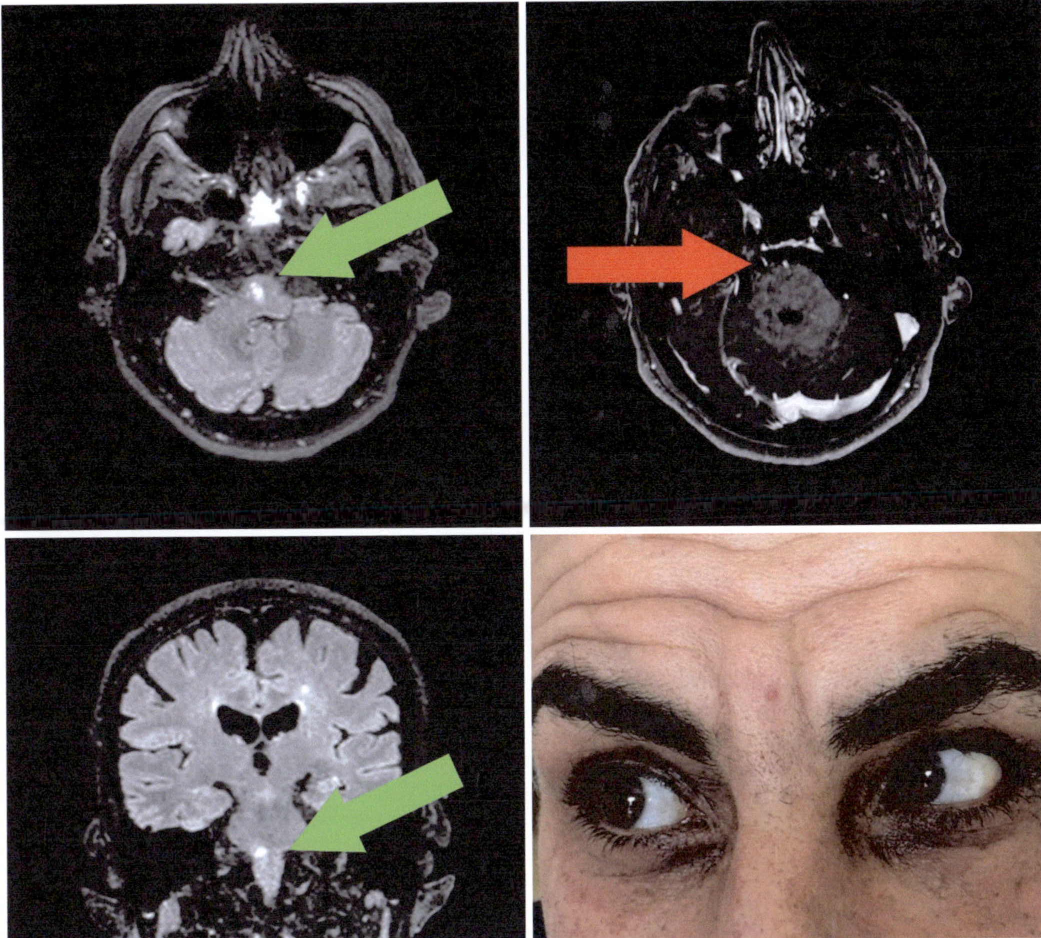

Fig. 26.2 Left upper and lower image: T2-FLAIR-weighted axial and coronal MRI showing brainstem lesion (green arrow) in a patient with multiple sclerosis. Right upper image shows gadolinium-enhanced abducens nerve adjacent to the brainstem lesion. The patient presented with diplopia and showed abductor deficit on the right eye

It usually affects patients older than 50 years, and the most common symptoms include headaches, tenderness of temporal arteries, jaw claudication, and vision loss. It is caused by inflammation of the vessel walls of the extracranial arteries, and this histopathological change (associated with giant cells) confirms the diagnosis. Rarely, other CNs can also be affected, unilaterally or bilaterally. These CN deficits are usually caused by ischemia of small vascular branches. Nerves that have been described include abducens, vestibulocochlear, and vagus nerves [12–14]. Treatment usually consists of corticosteroids, cyclophosphamide, or tocilizumab.

Neurosarcoidosis

Sarcoidosis is a multiorgan inflammatory granulomatous disease. Involvement of the nervous system is frequent, and in around 50% of patients, neurological deficits are the initial clinical manifestation. Cranial neuropathy is very common, with the facial and optic nerve most frequently involved, often bilaterally [15].

Diagnosis is often difficult, particularly if histological confirmation is not possible. Cranial and spinal MRI may show parenchymal lesions and contrast enhancement of the meninges and CNs. The most important ancillary examination, apart from neuroimaging, is analysis of the cerebrospinal fluid (CSF), which shows pleocytosis, elevated cerebrospinal protein, and oligoclonal bands in the majority of patients. CSF angiotensin-converting enzyme (ACE) levels are also elevated in nearly 50% of patients [16]. In any case, careful workup is recommended to seek out manifestations outside the nervous system, which greatly improve the diagnostic certainty in cases with suspected neurosarcoidosis. Bronchoscopic tissue collection (bronchoalveolar lavage, endobronchial biopsy, transbronchial lung biopsy, cryobiopsy, and endobronchial ultrasound fine-needle aspiration) is often used and can be performed complimentarily to increase the diagnostic yield, even in cases with normal lung function [16].

Treatment consists of corticosteroids and immunosuppressants, such as methotrexate, mycophenolate mofetil, or azathioprine. TNF-alpha antagonists are also used in the treatment of sarcoidosis, but warrants cautions since it may paradoxically lead to an inflammatory demyelinating condition in the central or peripheral nervous systems [17].

Rarer Autoimmune Conditions with Cranial Neuropathy

Cogan's syndrome: Rare conditions of presumed autoimmune origin which may affect CN function include Cogan's syndrome. Cogan's syndrome is a systemic vasculitis that affects visual and vestibulocochlear function, and thus, it is not a CN disease in the term's true sense. It is rather a vasculitis that leads histopathologically to inflammation of parts of the inner ear in addition to keratitis, uveitis, and (epi)scleritis [18].

Granulomatosis with polyangiitis: Cranial neuropathy may also occur in 2–10% of patients with granulomatosis with polyangiitis (former Wegener's granulomatosis) and involvement of the optic, the oculomotor, the trigeminal, and facial nerves was described [19].

IgG4-related disease: IgG4-related disease is rare and shares some features of an autoimmune inflammatory condition, although its pathogenesis is poorly understood [20]. It goes along with general symptoms, i.e., subacute weight loss, fatigue, and inflammatory masses mimicking malignant tumors in one or several organs, frequently in the submandibular glands, pancreas, or kidney. Central and peripheral nervous system manifestations may occur, caused by masses in the pituitary gland or meninges. CNs can be involved either by local compression or by chronic inflammatory infiltrates in the perineurium. Cranial neuropathy described in the context of IgG4-related disease includes vestibulocochlear and facial nerve palsy [20, 21]. In the case of an orbital mass, nerves emerging from the superior orbital fissure (oculomotor, trochlear, and branches of the trigeminal nerve) can be affected [21]. Also, rhinosinusitis can affect olfactory nerve function [22]. Diagnosis of IgG4-related disease is often difficult. About two-thirds of patients have elevated IgG levels in the serum. CSF can show a mild pleocytosis. Histopathological examination is recommended whenever possible, which shows IgG-positive lymphocytic infiltrates with IgG4-positive plasma cells. IgG4-related disease is treated with corticosteroids.

Systemic lupus erythematodes (SLE): SLE can rarely affect CNs. In a study of 1827 SLE patients, only 39 had cranial neuropathy, with optic, facial, and vestibulocochlear neuropathy occurring most frequently [23].

Panarteritis nodosa: In panarteritis nodosa, CN injury is reported rarely and mostly includes the oculomotor, trochlear, or abducens nerve [24, 25].

Sjögren's syndrome: In Sjögren's syndrome, the trigeminal nerve is frequently affected, leading to facial numbness. Other CNs involved are the facial and vestibulocochlear nerve, or multiple CN palsies in different combinations [26].

Cranial Nerve Involvement in Autoimmune Conditions of the Peripheral Nervous System

Cranial Nerve Involvement in Guillain–Barré Syndrome

The term GBS encompasses a spectrum of variants that were discovered in the last century and then extensively characterized (Table 26.1) [27]. The most common variant in western countries is acute inflammatory demyelinating polyneuropathy (AIDP). It refers to the "classical" GBS, with demyelinating changes in nerve conduction studies and inflammatory infiltrates in nerve roots and peripheral nerves. In Asia, axonal variants are more common. These can be further distinguished as a pure motor form (acute motor axonal neuropathy [AMAN]) and a variant where sensory and motor nerve fibers are affected (the so-called acute motor–sensory axonal neuropathy [AMSAN]). The Miller Fisher syndrome (MFS), a variant of GBS with predominantly CN involvement, is much rarer compared to the other variants. It often manifests clinically with the "triple-A-triad" of ataxia, absent eye movements, i.e., ophthalmoplegia, and areflexia [28].

Another subtype which deserves acknowledgement due to its specific clinical phenotype with predominant involvement of the facial nerve was first described by Ropper and is clinically characterized by facial diplegia with paresthesias (FDP) and absent or only minor motor deficit (Fig. 26.3). It occurs in less than 5% of all GBS cases [27].

Acute Inflammatory Demyelinating Polyneuropathy: CN involvement in AIDP occurs in 43–50% of all cases [30] and includes mostly facial weakness (31%), bulbar weakness (25%), and involvement of oculomotor nerves in 15% [31]. CNs I and II, which derive from the diencephalon and which are therefore part of the central nervous system, are usually spared in AIDP. In fact, involvement of the olfactory nerve during GBS was not reported before 2019, and the temporal sequence of olfactory dysfunction followed by GBS is thus a unique syndrome of the COVID-19 pandemic [32, 33].

Likewise, also optic nerve involvement is only rarely reported in GBS. Pathomechanisms may include inflammatory lesions in the optic nerve caused by the aberrant immune response or more likely indirect nerve damage by development of papilloedema and increased intracranial nerve pres-

Table 26.1 Clinical subtypes of Guillain–Barré syndrome

	AIDP	AMAN	AMSAN	MFS	FDP
Frequency distribution	Frequent in western countries	Rare	Rare	Rare	Rare
Symptoms	Progressive para-/ tetraparesis Sensory deficits Weak or absent reflexes	Progressive para-/ tetraparesis No sensory deficits Weak or absent reflexes	Often severe tetraparesis Severe sensory deficits Absent or reduced reflexes	Ophthalmoplegia Areflexia Ataxia	Paresthesias Absent or only minor motor deficit
Cranial nerve deficits	Frequent	Occasionally, but less frequent than in AIDP	Present	Specific pattern with absent eye movements, anisokoria, etc.	Bilateral facial weakness
Autoantibodies	None specific	GM1 IgG GD1a IgG	GM1 IgG GD1a IgG	GQ1b IgG	

AIDP acute inflammatory demyelinating polyneuropathy, *AMAN* acute motor axonal neuropathy, *AMSAN* acute motor–sensory axonal neuropathy, *FDP* facial diplegia with paresthesias, *GD1a/GM1/GQ1b* gangliosides, *IgG* immunoglobulin, *MFS* Miller Fisher syndrome

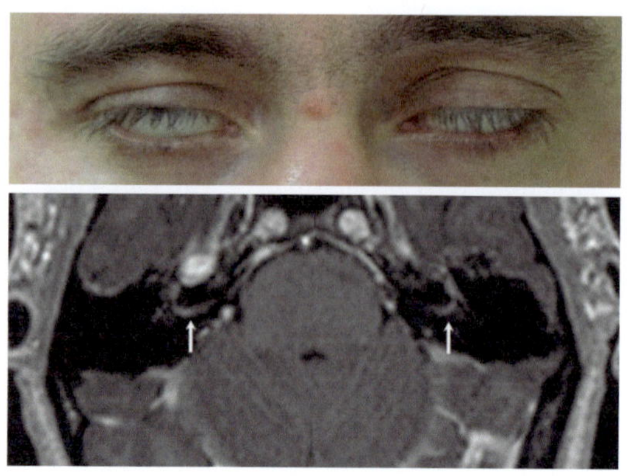

Fig. 26.3 (**a**) Bilateral Bell's palsy with inability for complete eyelid closure (bilateral lagophtalmos). (**b**) After intravenous gadolinium administration, bilateral strong enhancement of the facial nerve in its extra- and intracanalicular segments is visible (white arrows), axial T1-weighted gradient echo sequence. (Reproduced with permission from [29])

sure due to reduced CSF drainage through the inflamed spinal nerve roots [34, 35]. Oculomotor nerves are affected in up to 15% of all cases, and clinical symptoms may include diplopia, pupillary dysfunction, and accommodation deficits [36]. In comatose ventilated patients with fulminating GBS, the absent pupillary reflex may lead to the erroneous assumption of brain death [37]. Facial weakness is reported in almost every third patient with GBS, ranging from mild often asymmetric facial weakness up to facial diplegia. Overlaps with the FDP variant may occur. Facial or bulbar weakness at hospital admission is a strong predictor and indicates an almost fourfold increased odds ratio for the requirement of mechanical ventilation due to respiratory insufficiency within the first week [38].

Miller Fisher Syndrome: The few autopsy studies in MFS indicate segmental demyelination with associated macrophages and lymphocytes, prominently in the CNs, particularly CN VII, X, and XI [39]. The blink reflex, which can indicate damage to nerve fiber tracts in the trigeminal and facial nerves as well as in the brainstem, can be abnormal, occasionally in a way that is typically seen in brainstem lesions [40].

Notably, in some patients with MFS and MFS/GBS overlap, a delayed facial nerve palsy can occur [41]. The frequency has been reported to range from 6% in GBS and MFS to 8% in AIDP and 9% in AMAN patients. Prognosis is usually favorable; without any specific additional treatment, all 16 patients in the study by Tatsumoto and colleagues had resolution of facial palsy 3 weeks after developing delayed facial weakness. Another variant of GBS, termed pharyngeal–cervical–brachial weakness, is clinically characterized by progressive oropharyngeal and cervicobrachial weakness. It may also overlap with MFS. Patients with pharyngeal–cervical–brachial weakness often have anti-GT1a and anti-GQ1b IgG antibodies [42].

Cranial Neuropathy in Chronic Immune Neuropathies

Cranial neuropathy is considered to occur rarely in chronic inflammatory demyelinating polyradiculoneuropathy (CIDP). One large cohort study assessing frequency found CN deficits in only 11% of patients with typical CIDP [43]. Facial and bulbar palsy were the predominant symptoms in these patients. Subclinical involvement of trigeminal nerve fibers has been postulated based on several studies that showed reduced trigeminal nerve branches in corneal confocal microscopy in CIDP; however, this method is seldom used in clinical practice and the clinical value remains unclear [44]. In cases of rapid disease onset and relapsing disease course, CN involvement may point to a GBS with treatment-related fluctuations rather than to a CIDP with acute onset [45]. In multifocal acquired demyelinating sensory and motor neuropathy, a CIDP variant, cranial neuropathy may occur more frequently [43]. A rare syndrome within the spectrum of chronic immune neuropathies is chronic ataxic neuropathy, ophthalmoplegia, IgM paraprotein, cold agglutinins, and disialosyl antibodies (CANOMAD), which goes along with ocular and/or bulbar nerve palsies [46].

Discussion

As outlined above, a variety of autoimmune conditions must be considered in a patient with a deficit of a singular or multiple CNs. From this clinical perspective, the 12 CN pairs can be divided into three categories:

1. *CNs I and II*: CNs I and II are predominantly affected in (autoimmune) conditions of the central nervous system. An explanation for this susceptibility is that the two nerves do not emanate from the brainstem and are parts of the central rather than peripheral nerves. Histologically, the myelin sheaths are established by olfactory ensheathing glia (CN I) and oligodendrocytes (CN II), but not Schwann cells. As outlined above, exceptions to this rule may apply; however, damage to other CNs, e.g., in MS, is best explained as simply due to the close proximity of central nervous system inflammatory lesions to CN roots. Alternatively, optic nerve damage in GBS, for example, is secondary and due to increased CSF pressure.

   The myelin composition, including the quantity and localization of myelin proteins within the myelin sheaths, considerably varies in the central and peripheral nervous systems. Candidate antigens in MS, such as proteolipid protein (PLP) [47], account for over 50% of the proteins in the central nervous system and is only expressed in minor quantity in peripheral nervous system myelin [48]. Also, myelin basic protein (MBP) is expressed in much higher quantity in the central (approximately 30%) compared to peripheral myelin (5–15%) [48]. Myelin oligodendrocyte glycoprotein (MOG) can be found in the central nervous system, where it is expressed on the outer lamellae of myelin and may thus be much more accessible to autoreactive T cells or autoantibodies. In the peripheral nervous system, MOG can only be found in non-myelinating Schwann cells, but not in the myelin in vivo [49].

2. *CNs III–VII*: These nerves are often affected in autoimmune diseases of the peripheral nervous system, i.e., GBS and MFS. Candidate autoantigens in these conditions are primarily gangliosides. The most abundant gangliosides in the adult mammalian nervous system are GM1, GD1a, GD1b, and GT1b, and motor nerve terminals and nodes of Ranvier are particularly enriched with gangliosides [50]. There is some evidence that the selective neuropathy to certain CNs is caused by fine specificity of these antibodies and the ganglioside composition of CN tissue. For example, MFS is strongly associated with anti-GQ1b antibodies [27]. These antibodies bind to paranodal myelin and nodes of Ranvier and to neuromuscular junctions in extraocular and somatic muscles, thereby inducing oculomotor deficit [51]. Notably, GQ1b is twice as frequently expressed in the extraocular nerves than in other CNs [51].

3. *Caudal CNs*: The caudal CNs are rarely involved in autoimmune conditions. Whether this is caused by their localization, accessibility to immune effectors, different fiber and/or antigen composition, or simply underdiagnosis is not known.

Recommendations

In patients with cranial neuropathy, a diagnostic pathway based on case history and careful clinical examination is usually more efficacious than an unsystematic approach applying multiple lab tests to diagnose or to exclude an underlying autoimmune disease [52]. An MRI and an examination of the CSF may help exclude many differential diagnoses, particularly those that indicate systemic autoimmune, infectious, and neoplastic causes. Diagnostic recommendations that can be made to exclude autoimmune conditions in common cranial neuropathies are as follows:

- *Olfactory nerve dysfunction*: In patients with hyposmia or anosmia, COVID-19 should be excluded. The MRI should be checked for lesions that may indicate MS. Other rare autoimmune conditions that should be looked for are IgG4-related disease (thickening of the sinus mucous membrane in the MRI [22], IgG4 serum levels) and granulomatosis with polyangiitis (antineutrophil cytoplasmic auto-antibody [c-ANCA] positive) [53]. The latter may show mucosal thickening of the nasal cavity and the paranasal sinus, indicating granulomatous tissue [54].

- *Optic nerve*: The most relevant differential diagnosis is optic neuritis caused by MS and NMOSD. Thus, MRI and CSF examination is mandatory to look for signs of inflammation, disseminated in time and space. Neuroimaging of the spinal cord can be indicated to look for NMOSD typic lesions, particularly in patients with recurrent or bilateral optic neuritis. In the CSF, elevated ACE levels may indicate neuro-sarcoidosis. Laboratory test examinations should include antibodies against aquaporin-4 and MOG, and in the case of inconclusive results, serological testing for SLE and vasculitis should also be performed.

- *Oculomotor dysfunction (CNs III, IV, VI)*: The leading symptom, i.e., diplopia, can be caused by dysfunction of any of the three CNs. Ischemic or neoplastic brainstem lesions can mimic oculomotor dysfunction by cranial neuropathy (although usually more central nervous system symptoms are present) and should therefore be excluded by MRI. Myasthenia should be checked by the appropriate clinical, electrophysiological (decrement), and serological tests. In case of bilateral or multiple CN deficits, one should look for clinical signs of peripheral neuropathy, indicating GBS or MFS. Reasonable antibody testing may include GQ1b antibodies.

- *Trigeminal nerve*: In cases of trigeminal neuropathy, MRI is helpful to look for signs of MS, masses related to granulomas, or IgG4-related disease.

- *Facial nerve*: Unilateral facial nerve palsy is usually idiopathic or caused by infection with herpes virus (Ramsay–Hunt syndrome). Bilateral facial palsy is often caused by Lyme disease. Relevant autoimmune-mediated differential diagnoses for bilateral facial palsy

that should be considered and tested for are GBS, neurosarcoidosis, and SLE.

- *Vestibulocochlear nerve*: This nerve is rarely affected by autoimmune conditions, but cases of Cogan's syndrome and SLE with vestibulocochlear neuropathy have been described. Iatrogenic autoimmune neuritis may occur in cancer patients who are treated with immune checkpoint inhibitors [55].

- *Caudal CNs*: The caudal CNs are much less frequently affected in autoimmune conditions. The glossopharyngeal nerve may be affected by pharyngeal–cervical–brachial weakness; therefore, antibody testing for GQ1b and GT1a might be indicated. Likewise, the vagal nerve efferents to the heart and intestinal organs might be affected in GBS, resulting in (sometimes severe) autonomic dysfunction. The accessory nerve is basically a peripheral nerve that innervates the trapezoid and sternocleidomastoid muscle. A rare differential that may cause dysfunction of the accessory nerve includes the pharyngeal–cervical–brachial weakness variant of GBS. Notably, the spinal accessory nerve is occasionally affected in neuralgic amyotrophy [56, 57]. The function of the hypoglossal nerve might be indirectly affected by masses in association with granulomatosis with polyangiitis [58].

References

1. Toosy AT, Mason DF, Miller DH. Optic neuritis. Lancet Neurol. 2014;13:83–99.
2. Optic Neuritis Study Group. Multiple sclerosis risk after optic neuritis: final optic neuritis treatment trial follow-up. Arch Neurol. 2008;65:727–32.
3. Kim S-H, Mealy MA, Levy M, et al. Racial differences in neuromyelitis optica spectrum disorder. Neurology. 2018;91:e2089–99.
4. Leocani L, Guerrieri S, Comi G. Visual evoked potentials as a biomarker in multiple sclerosis and associated optic neuritis. J Neuroophthalmol. 2018;38:350–7.
5. Morrow SA, Fraser JA, Day C, Bowman D, Rosehart H, Kremenchutzky M, Nicolle M. Effect of treating acute optic neuritis with bioequivalent oral vs intravenous corticosteroids: a randomized clinical trial. JAMA Neurol. 2018;75:690–6.
6. Gospe SM, Chen JJ, Bhatti MT. Neuromyelitis optica spectrum disorder and myelin oligodendrocyte glycoprotein associated disorder-optic neuritis: a compre-

hensive review of diagnosis and treatment. Eye Lond Engl. 2021;35:753–68.

7. Doty RL, Li C, Mannon LJ, Yousem DM. Olfactory dysfunction in multiple sclerosis. N Engl J Med. 1997;336:1918–9.

8. Haider L, Chan W-SE, Olbert E, Mangesius S, Dal-Bianco A, Leutmezer F, Prayer D, Thurnher M. Cranial nerve enhancement in multiple sclerosis is associated with younger age at onset and more severe disease. Front Neurol. 2019;10:1085.

9. Shor N, Amador MDM, Dormont D, Lubetzki C, Bertrand A. Involvement of peripheral III nerve in multiple sclerosis patient: report of a new case and discussion of the underlying mechanism. Mult Scler Houndmills Basingstoke Engl. 2017;23:748–50.

10. Buttgereit F, Dejaco C, Matteson EL, Dasgupta B. Polymyalgia rheumatica and giant cell arteritis: a systematic review. JAMA. 2016;315:2442.

11. Petursdottir V, Johansson H, Nordborg E, Nordborg C. The epidemiology of biopsy-positive giant cell arteritis: special reference to cyclic fluctuations. Rheumatol Oxf Engl. 1999;38:1208–12.

12. Jay WM, Nazarian SM. Bilateral sixth nerve pareses with temporal arteritis and diabetes. J Clin Neuroophthalmol. 1986;6:91–5.

13. Nelson DA. Speech pathology in giant cell arteritis. Review and case report. Ann Otol Rhinol Laryngol. 1989;98:859–62.

14. Fytili C, Bournia VK, Korkou C, Pentazos G, Kokkinos A. Multiple cranial nerve palsies in giant cell arteritis and response to cyclophosphamide: a case report and review of the literature. Rheumatol Int. 2015;35:773–6.

15. Fritz D, van de Beek D, Brouwer MC. Clinical features, treatment and outcome in neurosarcoidosis: systematic review and meta-analysis. BMC Neurol. 2016;16:220.

16. Voortman M, Drent M, Baughman RP. Management of neurosarcoidosis: a clinical challenge. Curr Opin Neurol. 2019;32:475–83.

17. Nozaki K, Silver RM, Stickler DE, Abou-Fayssal NG, Giglio P, Kamen DL, Daniel R, Judson MA. Neurological deficits during treatment with tumor necrosis factor-alpha antagonists. Am J Med Sci. 2011;342:352–5.

18. Espinoza GM, Wheeler J, Temprano KK, Keller AP. Cogan's syndrome: clinical presentations and update on treatment. Curr Allergy Asthma Rep. 2020;20:46.

19. de Groot K, Schmidt DK, Arlt AC, Gross WL, Reinhold-Keller E. Standardized neurologic evaluations of 128 patients with Wegener granulomatosis. Arch Neurol. 2001;58:1215–21.

20. Wick CC, Zachariah J, Manjila S, Brown WC, Malla P, Katirji B, Cohen M, Megerian CA. IgG4-related disease causing facial nerve and optic nerve palsies: case report and literature review. Am J Otolaryngol. 2016;37:567–71.

21. AbdelRazek MA, Venna N, Stone JH. IgG4-related disease of the central and peripheral nervous systems. Lancet Neurol. 2018;17:183–92.

22. Hanaoka M, Kammisawa T, Koizumi S, Kuruma S, Chiba K, Kikuyama M, Shirakura S, Sugimoto T, Hishima T. Clinical features of IgG4-related rhinosinusitis. Adv Med Sci. 2017;62:393–7.

23. Hanly JG, Li Q, Su L, et al. Peripheral nervous system disease in systemic lupus erythematosus: results from an international inception cohort study. Arthritis Rheumatol (Hoboken, NJ). 2020;72:67–77.

24. Topaloglu R, Besbas N, Saatci U, Bakkaloglu A, Oner A. Cranial nerve involvement in childhood polyarteritis nodosa. Clin Neurol Neurosurg. 1992;94:11–3.

25. Wahezi DM, Gomes WA, Ilowite NT. Cranial nerve involvement with juvenile polyarteritis nodosa: clinical manifestations and treatment. Pediatrics. 2010;126:e719–22.

26. Perzyńska-Mazan J, Maślińska M, Gasik R. Neurological manifestations of primary Sjögren's syndrome. Reumatologia. 2018;56:99–105.

27. Shahrizaila N, Lehmann HC, Kuwabara S. Guillain-Barré syndrome. Lancet Lond Engl. 2021;397:1214–28.

28. Fisher M. An unusual variant of acute idiopathic polyneuritis (syndrome of ophthalmoplegia, ataxia and areflexia). N Engl J Med. 1956;255:57–65.

29. Lehmann HC, Macht S, Jander S, Hartung H-P, Methner A. Guillain-Barré syndrome variant with prominent facial diplegia, limb paresthesia, and brisk reflexes. J Neurol. 2012;259:370–1.

30. Song Y, Zhang Y, Yuki N, Wakerley BR, Liu C, Song J, Wang M, Feng X, Hao Y, Wang Y. Guillain-Barré syndrome in eastern China: a study of 595 patients. Eur J Neurol. 2021;28:2727–35.

31. Doets AY, Verboon C, van den Berg B, et al. Regional variation of Guillain-Barré syndrome. Brain J Neurol. 2018;141:2866–77.

32. Kajita M, Sato M, Iizuka Y, Mashimo Y, Furuta N, Kakizaki S. Guillain-Barré syndrome after SARS-CoV-2 infection. J Gen Fam Med. 2022;23:47–9.

33. Palaiodimou L, Stefanou M-I, Katsanos AH, et al. Prevalence, clinical characteristics and outcomes of Guillain-Barré syndrome spectrum associated with COVID-19: a systematic review and meta-analysis. Eur J Neurol. 2021;28:3517–29.

34. Kharbanda PS, Prabhakar S, Lal V, Das CP. Visual loss with papilledema in Guillain-Barre syndrome. Neurol India. 2002;50:528–9.

35. Gardner WJ, Spitler DK, Whitten C. Increased intracranial pressure caused by increased protein content in the cerebrospinal fluid; an explanation of papilledema in certain cases of small intracranial and intraspinal tumors, and in the Guillain-Barre syndrome. N Engl J Med. 1954;250:932–6.

36. Fausett BV, Trobe JD. Paralysis of accommodation with preserved pupillary function as the initial manifestation of Guillain-Barré syndrome. J Neuroophthalmol. 2012;32:148–9.

37. Kang B-H, Kim K-K. Fulminant Guillain-Barré syndrome mimicking cerebral death following acute viral hepatitis a. J Clin Neurol Seoul Korea. 2007;3:105–7.

38. Walgaard C, Lingsma HF, Ruts L, Drenthen J, van Koningsveld R, Garssen MJP, van Doorn PA,

Steyerberg EW, Jacobs BC. Prediction of respiratory insufficiency in Guillain-Barré syndrome. Ann Neurol. 2010;67:781–7.

39. Phillips MS, Stewart S, Anderson JR. Neuropathological findings in Miller Fisher syndrome. J Neurol Neurosurg Psychiatry. 1984;47:492–5.

40. Arányi Z, Kovács T, Sipos I, Bereczki D. Miller Fisher syndrome: brief overview and update with a focus on electrophysiological findings. Eur J Neurol. 2012;19:15–20, e1–3.

41. Tatsumoto M, Misawa S, Kokubun N, Sekiguchi Y, Hirata K, Kuwabara S, Yuki N. Delayed facial weakness in Guillain-Barré and Miller Fisher syndromes. Muscle Nerve. 2015;51:811–4.

42. Wakerley BR, Yuki N. Pharyngeal-cervical-brachial variant of Guillain-Barre syndrome. J Neurol Neurosurg Psychiatry. 2014;85:339–44.

43. Shibuya K, Tsuneyama A, Misawa S, Suichi T, Suzuki Y, Kojima Y, Nakamura K, Kano H, Prado M, Kuwabara S. Cranial nerve involvement in typical and atypical chronic inflammatory demyelinating polyneuropathies. Eur J Neurol. 2020;27:2658–61.

44. Schneider C, Bucher F, Cursiefen C, Fink GR, Heindl LM, Lehmann HC. Corneal confocal microscopy detects small fiber damage in chronic inflammatory demyelinating polyneuropathy (CIDP). J Peripher Nerv Syst JPNS. 2014;19:322–7.

45. Ruts L, Drenthen J, Jacobs BC, van Doorn PA, Dutch GBS Study Group. Distinguishing acute-onset CIDP from fluctuating Guillain-Barre syndrome: a prospective study. Neurology. 2010;74:1680–6.

46. Willison HJ, O'Leary CP, Veitch J, et al. The clinical and laboratory features of chronic sensory ataxic neuropathy with anti-disialosyl IgM antibodies. Brain J Neurol. 2001;124:1968–77.

47. Hohlfeld R, Dornmair K, Meinl E, Wekerle H. The search for the target antigens of multiple sclerosis, part 1: autoreactive CD4+ T lymphocytes as pathogenic effectors and therapeutic targets. Lancet Neurol. 2016;15:198–209.

48. Quarles RH. Comparison of CNS and PNS myelin proteins in the pathology of myelin disorders. J Neurol Sci. 2005;228:187–9.

49. Pagany M, Jagodic M, Schubart A, Pham-Dinh D, Bachelin C, Baron van Evercooren A, Lachapelle F, Olsson T, Linington C. Myelin oligodendrocyte glycoprotein is expressed in the peripheral nervous system of rodents and primates. Neurosci Lett. 2003;350:165–8.

50. Gong Y, Tagawa Y, Lunn MPT, Laroy W, Heffer-Lauc M, Li CY, Griffin JW, Schnaar RL, Sheikh KA. Localization of major gangliosides in the PNS: implications for immune neuropathies. Brain J Neurol. 2002;125:2491–506.

51. Chiba A, Kusunoki S, Obata H, Machinami R, Kanazawa I. Ganglioside composition of the human cranial nerves, with special reference to pathophysiology of Miller Fisher syndrome. Brain Res. 1997;745:32–6.

52. Carroll CG, Campbell WW. Multiple cranial neuropathies. Semin Neurol. 2009;29:53–65.

53. Fasunla JA, Hundt W, Lutz J, Förger F, Thürmel K, Steinbach S. Evaluation of smell and taste in patients with Wegener's granulomatosis. Eur Arch Otorhinolaryngol. 2012;269:179–86.

54. Muhle C, Reinhold-Keller E, Richter C, Duncker G, Beigel A, Brinkmann G, Gross WL, Heller M. MRI of the nasal cavity, the paranasal sinuses and orbits in Wegener's granulomatosis. Eur Radiol. 1997;7:566–70.

55. Vogrig A, Muñiz-Castrillo S, Joubert B, et al. Cranial nerve disorders associated with immune checkpoint inhibitors. Neurology. 2021;96:e866–75.

56. van Alfen N, van Engelen BGM. The clinical spectrum of neuralgic amyotrophy in 246 cases. Brain J Neurol. 2006;129:438–50.

57. Favero KJ, Hawkins RH, Jones MW. Neuralgic amyotrophy. J Bone Joint Surg Br. 1987;69:195–8.

58. Finley JC, Bloom DC, Thiringer JK. Wegener granulomatosis presenting as an infiltrative retropharyngeal mass with syncope and hypoglossal paresis. Arch Otolaryngol Head Neck Surg. 2004;130:361–5.

Introduction

The autonomic nervous system controls all inner organs and ensures homeostasis. The autonomic nervous system is involved in several central nervous system structures. Peripheral autonomic fibers travel with several cranial nerves (V, VII, IX, X), depicted in more detail below. Those fibers originate from central autonomic network structures. Of central importance are the Edinger–Westphal nucleus, the superior salivatory nucleus, and the dorsal motor nucleus. Specific to mammals is a distinct innervation of the heart through the nucleus ambiguus in addition to parasympathetic innervation through cranial nerves, forming a "face–heart" connection that is important for complex social engagement and interaction [1].

Origins and Pathways

Parasympathetic preganglionic origins:

- Oculomotor nerve fibers originate from the Edinger–Westphal nucleus.
- The facial nerve transports fibers originating from the superior salivatory nucleus.
- The glossopharyngeal nerve carries innervation from the inferior salivatory nucleus.
- The vagal nerve fibers conduct output of the dorsal motor nucleus, sending efferent signals to the heart, respiratory tract, gastrointestinal tract, liver, gallbladder, and pancreas. In addition and specific to mammals, they also conduct output of the area surrounding the nucleus ambiguus to the heart.

Parasympathetic postganglionic neurons: Postganglionic neurons are organized in a plexus formed of ganglia located near the target organs (e.g., pulmonary, cardiac plexus in the mediastinum, myenteric and submucosal plexus in the enteric nervous system).

Sympathetic pathways to cranial effectors: Primarily T1–T2 segments provide sympathetic output fibers to the superior cervical ganglion neurons. Postganglionic fibers follow vascular structures and include innervation of brain vessels [2].

Author of this chapter: Walter Struhal.

© The Author(s), under exclusive license to Springer Nature Switzerland AG 2023

W. Grisold et al., *The Cranial Nerves in Neurology*, https://doi.org/10.1007/978-3-031-43081-7_27

Autonomic Symptoms

The leading function of the cranial nerve parasympathetic system is providing secretomotor functions (dysfunction causing xerophthalmia, xerostomia, burning tongue, cracking lips, and oral infections). After injury, improper innervation may occur and lead to innervation prevailing sympathetic innervation. One example is gustatory facial sweating after parotid gland surgery, where the parasympathetic secretomotor innervation aberrantly innervates facial sweat glands. Aberrant facial innervation may also lead to innervation of lacrimal glands, causing lacrimation in meals ("crocodile tears").

Autonomic Nervous System Fiber Involvement in Cranial Nerves

Trigeminal nerve (V): The trigeminal nerve does not contain autonomic fibers when leaving the pons [3]. Postganglionic peripheral parasympathetic fibers travel together with trigeminal nerve branches to reach the sublingual, lacrimal, parotid, and submandibular glands [4]. That explains why parasympathetic innervations stay intact even in central trigeminal nuclear damage (Fig. 27.1).

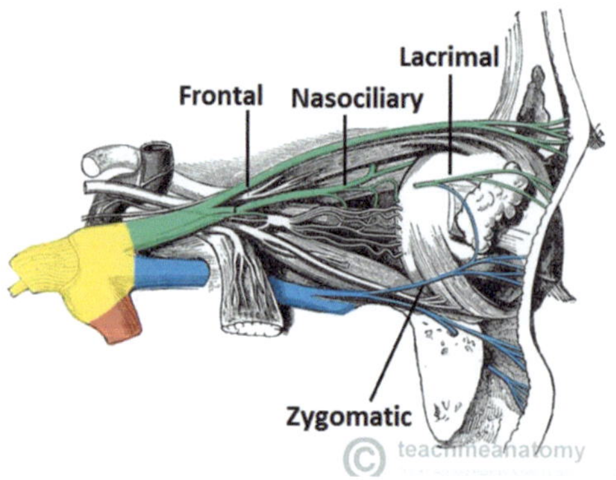

Fig. 27.1 Parasympathetic fibers from the facialis travel with the trigeminal nerve to lacrimal effector organs. (Reproduced with kind permission from Dr. Oliver Jones, TeachMeAnatomy)

Facial nerve (VII): The facial nerve contains motor and autonomic fibers, with minor somatosensory components. Efferents form the nervus intermedius, which is responsible for parasympathetic innervation of the glands and mucosa of the face [5]. Taste fibers from the anterior two-thirds of the tongue through the chorda tympani travel central to the geniculate ganglion and synapse further to the solitary nucleus [4].

Glossopharyngeal nerve (IX): The glossopharyngeal nerve provides visceral efferent innervation to the parotid [6]. It tethers to the internal carotid artery and provides afferents from the carotid body and sinus, representing an important part of the baroreceptor arc. The glossopharyngeal nerve provides taste afferents through the lingual branch of the posterior third of the tongue [7].

Vagal nerve (X): The vagal nerve serves as a hub for the parasympathetic nervous system and incorporates parasympathetic efferent fibers from the dorsal vagal nucleus to many thoracic and abdominal target structures up to the left colon flexure [8]. The current description focuses on the cranial area, and an in-depth description may be found elsewhere [9]. Of major importance for cardiovascular control is the baroreceptor reflex (Fig. 27.2). Fibers carry visceral cranial afferents and efferents to the pharynx, larynx, esophagus, aorta, and many thoracic and abdominal viscera.

Cranial nerve 0: Cranial nerve 0 is referred to as the nervus terminalis. It is present in invertebrates and vertebrates, including humans. It is rostral to the other 12 cranial nerves and is associated with gonadotropin release and may have a role in human reproductive functions and behaviors. While it was also discussed to play a role in pheromone detection for mate selection, this may not have relevance in human brain functioning since the vomeronasal organ, which processes pheromone signals in animals, has ceased its function during human evolution [10, 11].

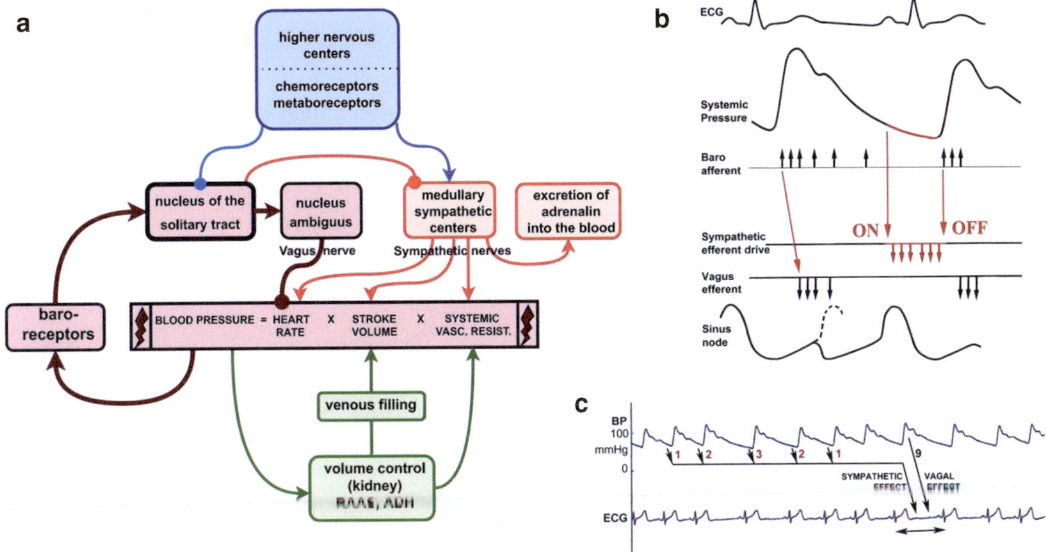

Fig. 27.2 Scheme of the human baroreceptor reflex controlling blood pressure. Glossopharyngeal nerve fibers form the afferents to the nucleus of the solitary tract, while the vagus nerve carries efferent fibers of the nucleus vagus. (Reproduced with kind permission from Biol Psychol, 172, "The multibranched nerve: vagal function beyond heart rate variability." (**a**) innervation scheme, (**b**) biosignals of blood pressure and heart rate as well as physiologic influences, (**c**) interrelation of blood pressure and heart rate. Page 108378. Copyright Elsevier [8])

Effector Organs

Autonomic cranial effectors are controlled by sympathetic, parasympathetic, and trigeminal sensorimotor fibers [9].

Pupil: Fibers to the pupil follow the internal carotid artery into the cavernous sinus to enter the superior orbital fissure. Sympathetic output elicits pupil dilatation through adrenergic innervation to the iris dilatator muscle. The ciliary ganglion innervates the pupil via short ciliary nerves and elicits pupil constriction and contraction of the ciliary muscles [12].

Superior tarsal muscle: Innervated by superior cervical ganglion neurons, this muscle is tonically active during wakefulness [13].

Facial skin: Fibers follow the external carotid artery and innervate the constrictor as well as dilate the cutaneous vasculature of the face during stress/emotions/heat. Sympathetic fibers elicit vasodilation of the facial veins via adrenergic receptors. Sweating is provided by the superior cervical ganglion (cholinergic innervation). Parasympathetic innervation is usually not innervating sweat glands, but postganglionic parasympathetic fibers may form functional connections to sweat glands as aberrant innervation in response to sympathetic nerve lesions causing pathologic sweating.

Glands (lacrimal, parotid, submaxillary): Parasympathetic output innervates secretory cells. Those cells are also innervated through sympathetic output.

Vessels: Sympathetic innervation throughout the body constricts vessels. Dural and cortical surface vessels are dilated by trigeminal fibers via release of substance P, neurokinins, and calcitonin gene-related peptide [14].

Selected Autonomic Syndromes and Signs in Cranial Nerves Based on Autonomic Dysfunction

Horner's Syndrome

One of the most referred syndromes of cranial nerves in context with the autonomic nervous system is the Horner's syndrome [15]. This syndrome is caused by an interruption of sympathetic ocular innervation. In short, denervation of the superior tarsal muscle results in incomplete ptosis, sympathetic denervation of the inner eye causes myosis based on parasympathetic predominance, and sympathetic denervation of forehead/face or ipsilateral arm leads to hypohidrosis of the skin [16, 17].

The original description depicted enophthalmos in association with Horner's syndrome. Enophthalmos per se is only rarely present and often mimicked by ptosis. Therefore, usually the following triad of symptoms is regarded to be Horner's syndrome: ptosis, myosis, and hypohidrosis.

Hypohidrosis may only occur if the fibers are not compromised distal of the bifurcation, since the sympathetic forehead fibers follow the external carotid artery. Horner's syndrome may show a lower lid elevation ("reverse ptosis sign") caused by smooth muscle paresis to the inferior tarsal plate.

Important hints to determine the lesion site in Horner's syndrome are depicted in Fig. 27.3. Management is dependent on the suspected lesion site.

Harlequin Syndrome

The leading sign of Harlequin syndrome is unilateral dysfunction of the facial sympathetic system, causing ipsilateral flushing and hyperhidrosis and contralateral hypohidrosis or anhidrosis and paleness [18]. This may lead to a reddish hemifacial skin discoloration dependent on the current state of hemodynamic homeostasis.

Harlequin syndrome may be observed in rare cases of Adie's syndrome, which is characterized by tonic pupils and muscular hyporeflexia, and Ross syndrome, which involves tonic pupils, muscular hyporeflexia, and segmental anhidrosis [19]. Both syndromes are often observed with a more widespread involvement of the autonomic nervous system.

Flynn Phenomenon

Flynn phenomenon is diagnosed in patients showing paradoxical constriction of the pupils to darkness. It may occur in congenital achromatopsia, optic atrophy, old bilateral optic neuritis, strabismus, and congenital nystagmus, among others. For those who have not had the chance to see a patient showing this phenomenon, the following video may be of interest [20].

Hypolacrimation

Hypolacrimation may be caused by keratoconjunctivitis sicca, causing conjunctival injection, discomfort, and photophobia. This condition may be challenging to diagnose based on reflex tearing, as many patients report excessive lacrimation. Hypolacrimation may be seen in peripheral facial palsy with ipsilateral loss of tearing in proximal lesions. If the fibers are interrupted near the brain stem, cranial nerve VIII involvement may be present. Management includes artificial tears and lid hygiene [21].

Another cause may be lesions of the sphenopalatine ganglion. Patients often report pain and hypesthesia in the V/2 area. Lesions in the zygomaticotemporal nerve, a branch of the zygomatic nerve, may be depicted by hypolacrimation and headaches [22].

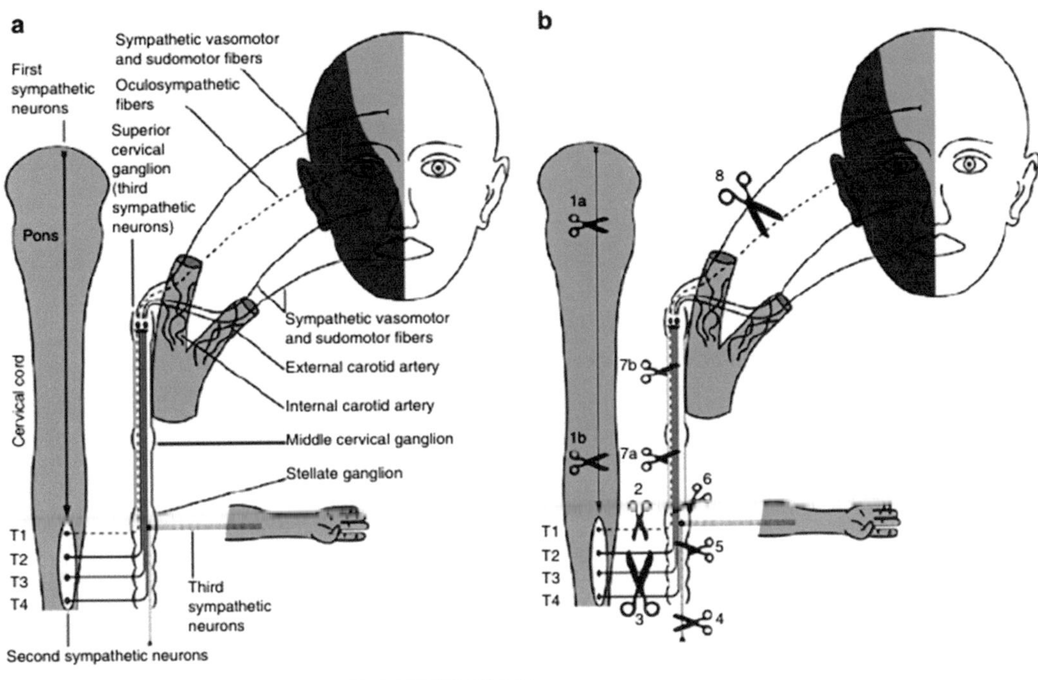

lesion site	DF	Arm	Horners Syndrome
1	HF	-	central
2	0	=	preganglionic
3	HF	=	0
2+3	HF	=	preganglionic
4	0	-	0
5	HF	-	0
6	HF	-	preganglionic
7	HF	=	preganglionic
8	MFHN	=	postganglionic

Fig. 27.3 Schematic sketch and table helping to diagnose the location of a sympathetic lesion often including Horner's syndrome. DF, areas of disturbed facial flushing; arm, sympathetic arm innervation; hf, hemifacial; *, medial forehead and nose (**a**) illustration of preganglionic and postganglionic sympathetic innervation of face and arm, (**b**) possible lesion sites numbered and clinical presentation outlined in the table. (Reproduced with kind permission from Springer)

Autonomic Function Tests of Cranial Nerves

The following focuses on autonomic function tests that are widely available without dedicated autonomic equipment.

Deep breathing:
- Test: Deep breaths (inhale 5 s and exhale 5 s)
- Afferent cranial nerve: Vagus
- Central structure: Nucleus of tractus solitarius
- Efferent cranial nerve: Vagus
- Normal response: HR increase during inspiration, HR decrease during expiration

Facial immersion:
- Test: Facial ice water immersion
- Afferent: Vagus
- Central structure: Medullary centers
- Efferent: Vagus, sympathetic
- Normal response: Bradycardia and vasoconstriction

Coughing:
- Test: Three deep coughs
- Afferent: Cranial nerve IX
- Central structure: Nucleus of tractus solitarius
- Efferent: Vagus, sympathetic
- Normal response: HR increase and then fall in heart rate; vasoconstriction

Pupil cycle time:
- Test: Lighting the edge of pupil
- Afferent: Optic nerve
- Central structure: Edinger–Westphal nucleus
- Efferent: Cranial nerve III
- Normal response: Cycles of dilation–constriction

Mental arithmetic:
- Test: Calculation—7 for 2 min
- No afferent
- Central structure: Cortex
- Efferent: Sympathetic efferents, cardiac vagus
- Normal result: Rise in blood pressure and HR

Startle:
- Test: Sudden loud noise
- Afferent: Cochlear nerve
- Central: Auditory cortex and hypothalamus
- Efferent: Sympathetic efferents, vagus
- Normal result: Rise in blood pressure and HR

Recommendations for Further Reading

Physiology and Pathophysiology of the Autonomic Nervous System [21].

Bedside Approach to Autonomic Disorders [15].

References

1. Porges SW. The polyvagal theory: new insights into adaptive reactions of the autonomic nervous system. Cleve Clin J Med. 2009;76(Suppl 2):S86–90. https://doi.org/10.3949/ccjm.76.s2.17.
2. Goadsby PJ. Autonomic nervous system control of the cerebral circulation. Handb Clin Neurol. 2013;117:193–201. https://doi.org/10.1016/B978-0-444-53491-0.00016-X.
3. Angeles Fernández-Gil M, Palacios-Bote R, Leo-Barahona M, Mora-Encinas JP. Anatomy of the brainstem: a gaze into the stem of life. Semin Ultrasound CT MR. 2010;31(3):196–219. https://doi.org/10.1053/j.sult.2010.03.006.
4. Diamond M, Wartmann CT, Tubbs RS, Shoja MM, Cohen-Gadol AA, Loukas M. Peripheral facial nerve communications and their clinical implications. Clin Anat (NY). 2011;24(1):10–8. https://doi.org/10.1002/ca.21072.
5. Mavrikakis I. Facial nerve palsy: anatomy, etiology, evaluation, and management. Orbit (Amst Neth). 2008;27(6):466–74. https://doi.org/10.1080/01676830802352543.
6. Ong CK, Chong VFH. The glossopharyngeal, vagus and spinal accessory nerves. Eur J Radiol. 2010;74(2):359–67. https://doi.org/10.1016/j.ejrad.2009.05.064.
7. García Santos JM, Sánchez Jiménez S, Tovar Pérez M, Moreno Cascales M, Lailhacar Marty J, Fernández-Villacañas Marín MA. Tracking the glossopharyngeal nerve pathway through anatomical references in cross-sectional imaging techniques: a pictorial review. Insights Imaging. 2018;9(4):559–69. https://doi.org/10.1007/s13244-018-0630-5.
8. Karemaker JM. The multibranched nerve: vagal function beyond heart rate variability. Biol Psychol. 2022;172:108378. https://doi.org/10.1016/j.biopsycho.2022.108378.
9. Low AL, Benarroch E. Clinical autonomic disorders. 3rd ed. LWW; 2008.
10. Sonne J, Reddy V, Lopez-Ojeda W. Neuroanatomy, cranial nerve 0 (terminal nerve). Treasure Island, FL: StatPearls Publishing; 2022. Online. http://europepmc.org/books/NBK459159.
11. Verhaeghe J, Gheysen R, Enzlin P. Pheromones and their effect on women's mood and sexuality. Facts Views Vis Obgyn. 2013;5:189–95.
12. McDougal DH, Gamlin PD. Autonomic control of the eye. Compr Physiol. 2015;5(1):439–73. https://doi.org/10.1002/cphy.c140014.
13. Nielsen TA, et al. Palpebral fissure response to phenylephrine indicates autonomic dysfunction in patients with type 1 diabetes and polyneuropathy. Invest Ophthalmol Vis Sci. 2022;63(9):21. https://doi.org/10.1167/iovs.63.9.21.
14. Brennan KC, Charles A. An update on the blood vessel in migraine. Curr Opin Neurol. 2010;23(3):266–74. https://doi.org/10.1097/WCO.0b013e32833821c1.
15. Struhal W, editor. Bedside approach to autonomic disorders. Cham: Springer; 2017.
16. Martin TJ. Horner syndrome: a clinical review. ACS Chem Neurosci. 2018;9(2):177–86. https://doi.org/10.1021/acschemneuro.7b00405.
17. Gross JR, McClelland CM, Lee MS. An approach to anisocoria. Curr Opin Ophthalmol. 2016;27(6):486–92. https://doi.org/10.1097/ICU.0000000000000316.
18. Korbi M, Boumaiza S, Achour A, Belhadjali H, Zili J. Harlequin syndrome: an asymmetric face. Clin Case

Rep. 2022;10(5):e05833. https://doi.org/10.1002/ccr3.5833.

19. Joshi H, Packiasabapathy S. Harlequin syndrome. In: StatPearls. Treasure Island, FL: StatPearls Publishing; 2022.

20. Flynn syndrome. Zugegriffen. 3 Nov 2022 [Online Video]. Available at: https://youtu.be/epx4q-71X-o.

21. Benarroch EE. Physiology and pathophysiology of the autonomic nervous system. Continuum (Minneap Minn). 2020;26(1):12–24. https://doi.org/10.1212/CON.0000000000000817.

22. Karl HW, Trescot AM. Nerve entrapment headaches at the Temple: zygomaticotemporal and/or auriculotemporal nerve? Pain Physician. 2019;22(1):E15–36.

Introduction

Neoplasms arising from the cranial nerves, which account for 8% of all intracranial tumors, often lead to significant morbidity and impairment of quality of life through functional disruption of the cranial nerve of origin, as well as adjacent cranial nerves. Tumors can originate from the Schwann cells (schwannoma/neurofibroma), glia (optic nerve glioma), or sensory epithelium (esthesioneuroblastomas). In addition, meningiomas are often intimately associated with cranial nerves; however, these tumors do not directly arise from neural structures and instead originate from arachnoidal cap cells in the dura. A multidisciplinary team is often required to determine the best approach to management to reduce the morbidity associated with both the natural history of the tumor and the treatment. Ultimately, there is a major need for novel drugs that target vulnerable oncogenic pathways of these cranial nerve tumors, which become possible with advancements in our understanding of the biology.

Clinical Presentation

Clinical manifestation of these cranial nerve tumors can vary greatly depending on important factors, such as the cranial nerve of origin, tumor size, and tumor growth rate. Typically, the first sign of a tumor is neurological deficits associated with the nerve from which the tumor develops. As the tumor grows larger in size, it can also compromise adjacent cranial nerves leading to more complex cranial neuropathies, as well as symptoms associated with compression of the brainstem including headaches, nausea/vomiting, and hydrocephalus.

Authors of this chapter: Suganth Suppiah, Yosef Ellenbogen, and Gelareh Zadeh.

Certain tumors have predisposition for specific cranial nerves. Esthesioneuroblastomas develop from the olfactory nerve (CN I) and present with nasal obstruction or epistaxis. Less commonly, these tumors present with hyposmia. Optic nerve gliomas affect the optic nerve (CN II), as the name suggests, and often cause progressive visual impairment, proptosis, and hormonal problems secondary to hypothalamic dysfunction. Schwannomas are more common along the trigeminal nerve (CN V) and vestibulocochlear nerve (CN VIII). These tumors tend to present with hearing loss, vertigo, tinnitus, and facial neuropathy. Schwannomas arising from the lower cranial nerves lead to dysphagia, dysarthria, and dysphonia. Involvement with the vagal nerve (CN X) can cause carotid sinus reflex dysfunction resulting in bradycardia, hypotension, and recurrent syncopal episodes.

Epidemiology and Natural History

Schwannomas are slow-growing, benign, Schwann cell-derived tumors that represent the most common neoplasm of the cranial nerves. The overall incidence of vestibular schwannomas is estimated at 1.51 per 100,000 [1, 2]. Almost 2/3 of all schwannomas develop on the vestibular nerve, with only 15% developing along other cranial nerves [1]. These encapsulated tumors develop sporadically in 90% of cases, with the remaining occurring in the context of hereditary tumor predispositions syndromes, such as neurofibromatosis type 2 (NF2), schwannomatosis, and Carney complex. Similarly, neurofibromas are Schwann-cell derived tumors that represent a quarter of all nerve sheath tumors [1]. Unlike schwannomas, neurofibromas tend be unencapsulated and grow in an intrafascicular pattern. Neurofibromas along cranial nerves tend to occur in the context of neurofibromatosis type 1 (NF1) and harbor a risk of malignant transformation into a malignant peripheral nerve sheath tumor (MPNST). Development of an MPNST along a cranial nerve is quite rare, but it predominantly occurs along the trigeminal nerve or vestibular nerve, which are also the cranial nerves most afflicted by schwannomas or neurofibromas.

Optic nerve gliomas are low-grade neoplasms that account for 3–5% of all pediatric brain tumors [3]. Ninety percent of optic nerve gliomas occur within the first two decades of life. These tumors can involve the optic nerve, optic chiasm, optic tracts, optic radiations, or the hypothalamus. Optic nerve gliomas also occur commonly in the setting of NF1, with 15–20% of the NF1 population developing tumors along their optic tract [4]. Notably, only 30–50% of these patients with optic nerve gliomas become symptomatic. At time of diagnosis, optic nerve gliomas are confined to the optic nerve alone in 25% of cases. When the optic nerve glioma involves the optic chiasm as well, 40% of these patients will eventually develop hormonal dysfunction from involvement of the hypothalamus or third ventricle [5].

Esthesioneuroblastomas are uncommon neoplasms that arise from the specialized sensory neuroepithelial olfactory cells and represent 3–6% of all nasal cavity tumors [6]. These tumors have a bimodal distribution, with a tendency to occur around the second and sixth decade of life, and an overall incidence of 0.4 per million of population [6]. These tumors are locally aggressive and metastasize through hematogenous and lymphatic routes.

Radiographical Features

Neuroimaging with contrast-enhanced MRI and CT techniques is an important diagnostic tool to characterize a lesion noninvasively and to guide therapeutic management plans [7]. Differential diagnosis for these cranial nerve tumors is based on the specific cranial nerve involved and the imaging features. For example, the differential diagnosis for an optic nerve glioma would include schwannoma, neurosarcoidosis, cavernous hemangioma, dermoid, meningioma, and metastases. On MRI sequences, optic nerve gliomas appear isointense or slightly hypointense on T1 sequences and hypertense on T2 sequences, compared to normal optic nerve (Fig. 28.1). The affected optic nerve is often enlarged and demonstrates mild to moderate contrast enhancement. Calcifications in optic

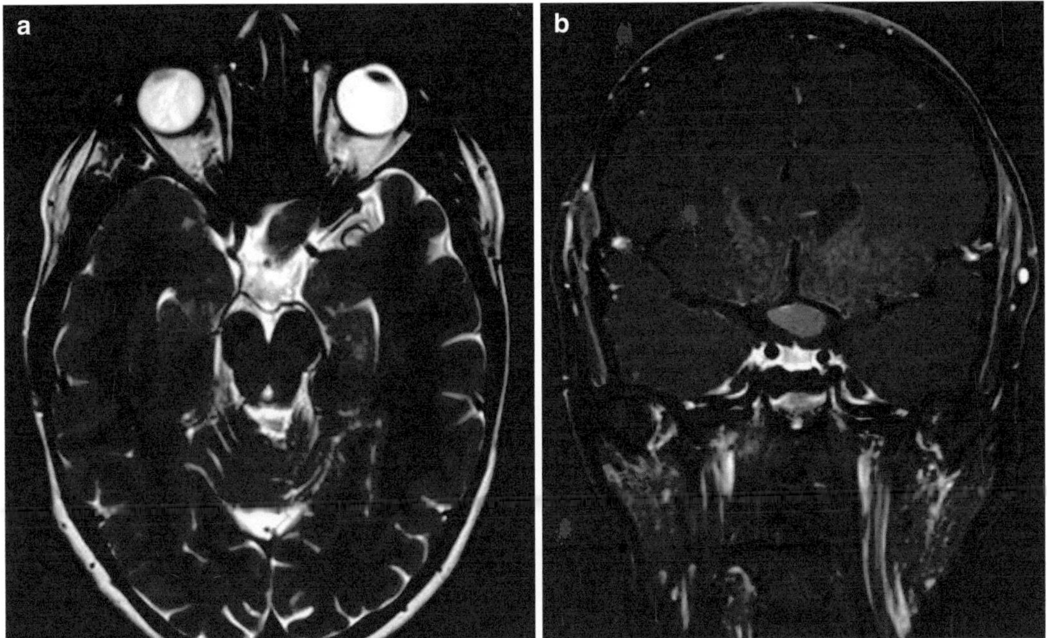

Fig. 28.1 Axial T2 (**a**), T1+ gadolinium (fat sat) coronal (**b**) MRI of right optic pathway glioma in an NF1 patient

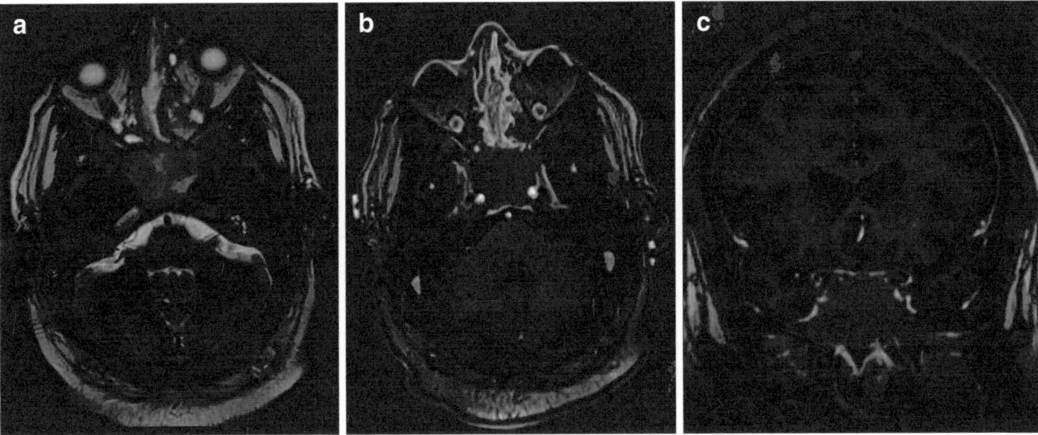

Fig. 28.2 Axial T2 (**a**), T1+ gadolinium axial (**b**), and coronal (**c**) MRI of esthesioneuroblastoma

pathway gliomas is uncommon but may be seen in rare cases.

Esthesioneuroblastomas commonly demonstrate sinus disease and bony erosions on CT scans, with a typical dumbbell-shaped mass extending across the cribriform plate. Esthesioneuroblastomas can mimic olfactory groove meningiomas on imaging and, therefore, need to be evaluated carefully. On MRI, esthesioneuroblastomas are hypointense on T1 sequences, with significant contrast enhancement (Fig. 28.2) [6]. These tumors can appear isointense or hyperintense on T2 sequences. A characteristic imaging feature of esthesioneuroblastomas is the presence of peritumoral cysts at the interface with the brain. Imaging is important for staging, as the Kadish classification is based on the anatomical extension of the tumor into nasal cavity, paranasal sinuses, intracranial/intraorbital space, and cervical lymph nodes [8].

Vestibular schwannomas present as a solid nodular lesion with an intracanalicular component within a widened internal acoustic canal. These tumors can be confined within the internal acoustic canal or protrude into the cerebellar pontine cistern as they grow larger. These tumors appear isointense on T1 sequences, with avid contrast enhancement (Fig. 28.3) [9]. On T2 sequences, schwannomas appear as heterogeneously hyperintense, with larger tumors demonstrating cystic degeneration or hemorrhagic areas [10]. Differential diagnosis of tumors for vestibular schwannomas includes other lesions that arise in the cerebellar pontine angle, including meningiomas, neurofibromas, metastases, and vascular lesions. It is often difficult to distinguish between schwannomas and neurofibromas with imaging alone. Furthermore, the presence of bilateral vestibular schwannomas is pathognomonic for NF2 syndrome.

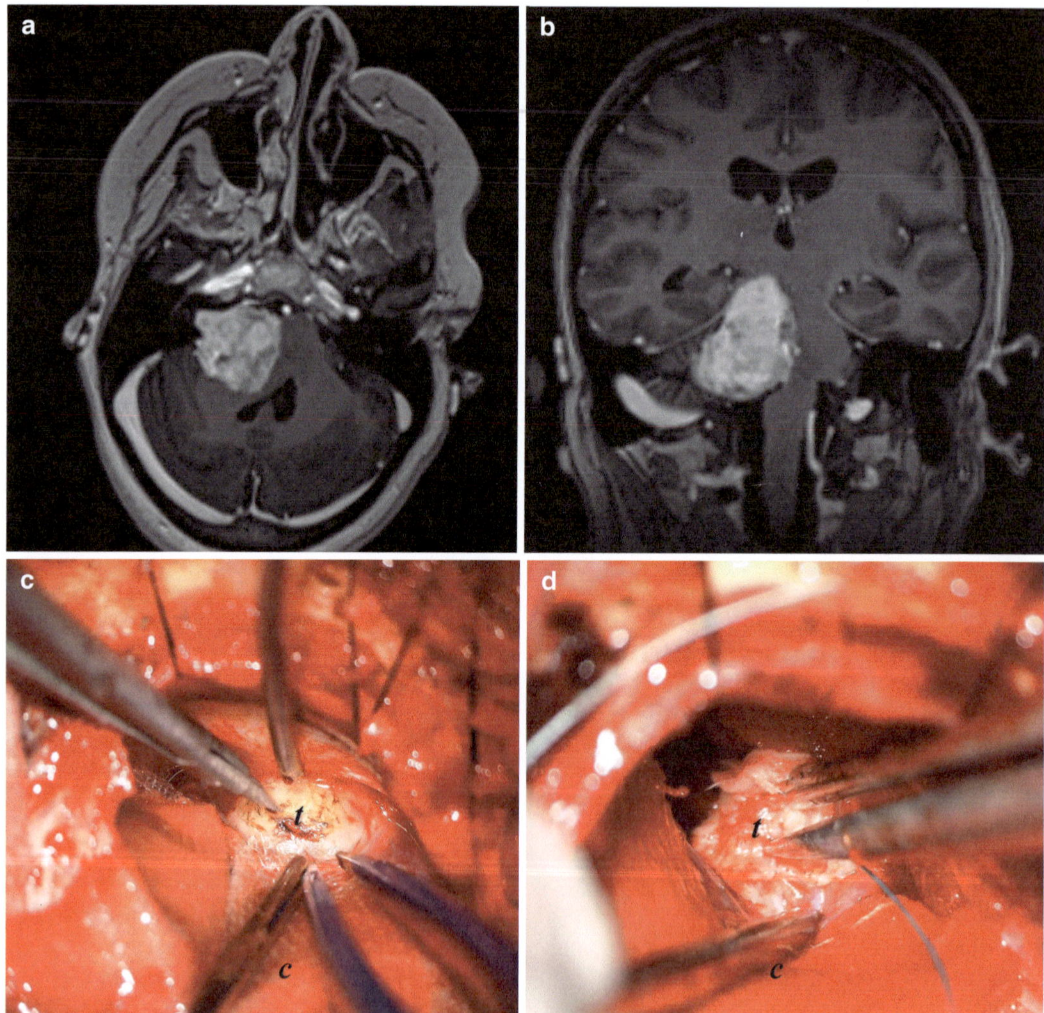

Fig. 28.3 Axial (**a**) and coronal (**b**) MRI of right vestibular schwannoma, (**c**, **d**) intraoperative photo of vestibular schwannoma approached with a retrosigmoid craniotomy. *t* tumor, *c* cerebellum

Management

Treatment options for cranial nerve tumors is highly specific for the suspected tumor pathology. For benign tumors (schwannomas, neurofibromas, and meningiomas), the options include serial observation, microsurgery, radiosurgery, and fractionated radiation therapy.

Typically, vestibular schwannomas are slow-growing tumors but do not grow continuously or at a constant rate. It appears that vestibular schwannomas tend to have higher growth rates at younger ages or in the context of NF2. In many patients, there are long periods of very slow growth rate or even growth arrest. As a result of the heterogenous growth patterns, the optimal timing of any therapeutic intervention for vestibular schwannoma often requires careful discussion with the patient. Microsurgical resection and radiation therapy are available for vestibular schwannomas [11].

Multiple operative corridors have been developed to safely access vestibular schwannomas. A translabyrinthine approach is ideal for small tumors confined to the internal acoustic canal with ipsilateral deafness. If hearing is intact, a subtemporal approach is recommended for intracanalicular tumors, while a suboccipital–retrosigmoid approach is recommended for larger tumors with significant tumor in the cerebellar pontine angle. In large tumors with significant adhesions to the facial nerve or brainstem, a planned partial resection is appropriate to preserve neurological function. The mortality rate with all surgical approaches is around 1%. With the advancements of microsurgical techniques, the rate of postoperative facial nerve deficit is 3%, with a majority of patients demonstrating partial functional recovery in long-term follow-up. Rates of postoperative facial nerve palsy are higher in reoperation procedures. The changes of postoperative hearing preservation have also increased with modern surgical techniques, with rates as high as 60% in small- and medium-sized vestibular schwannomas. Hearing preservation rates are dependent on the preoperative hearing level, size of tumor, anatomical extension of tumor, and surgical approach.

Radiosurgery with marginal dose of 12–13 Gy is also an effective treatment strategy to suppress tumor growth while also preserving neurological function [12]. Several studies have demonstrated that stereotactic radiosurgery is superior to microsurgery for vestibular schwannomas less than 3 cm in size, with five-year tumor control rates of 90–99% [11]. In addition, radiosurgery resulted in hearing preservation and facial nerve preservation rates of 41–79% and 95–99%, respectively [11].

Similarly, non-vestibular schwannomas have very tailored management options based on the nerve of origin. Intraorbital optic nerve schwannomas should be surgically removed without delay since the surgical outcomes are excellent. Similarly, gross total resection of trigeminal schwannomas is the preferred option when treatment is required. Stereotactic radiosurgery is often useful for small tumors only, while fractionated radiation therapy is restricted for inoperable tumors that are too large for radiosurgery.

A multidisciplinary team of neuro-ophthalmologists, oncologists, and surgeons are required to treat optic nerve gliomas [13]. In majority of patients, there is an initial phase of visual decline followed by stabilization. NF1-associated optic nerve gliomas are thought to have better prognosis than sporadic tumors. Optic nerve gliomas will rarely progress to the chiasm or damage contralateral fibers. Thus, patients followed conservatively with no intervention have demonstrated good long-term survival. Surgical en bloc resection is the treatment of choice for optic nerve gliomas that are the purely intraorbital with progressive growth, vision loss, and severe proptosis. Surgical resection will always lead to blindness of the ipsilateral side. As a result, optic nerve gliomas that involve the chiasm are treated with chemotherapy (<10 years of age) or a combination of chemotherapy and radiation therapy (>10 years of age) [5, 13].

Combined surgery, radiation therapy, and chemotherapy have been shown to be the best approach for esthesioneuroblastomas [14]. The best results are achieved with complete gross total resection with negative margins. Both open approaches and endoscopic endonasal approaches are currently used for the treatment of esthesioneuroblastomas, although more recent studies suggest that endoscopic approaches may provide better long-term outcomes [6]. Addition of chemotherapy and radiation therapy has been shown to significantly improve local recurrence and systemic metastatic rates. With a multimodal approach, the 5-year survival ranges from 65% to 75%.

Development of Systemic Treatment Options

Over the past few decades, there has been significant advances in our understanding of the biology of cranial nerve tumors. These advances have driven the development of systemic treatments that target key molecular oncogenic pathways and provide additional tools in the armamentarium for clinicians to use in the treatment of these difficult tumors.

Bevacizumab has become a potential treatment option for NF2 patients with progressive vestibular schwannomas [15]. In phase II studies, bevacizumab treatment induced hearing improvement in 20% of NF2 patients and volume reduction of >20% in 41% of NF2 patients [16]. Several other targeted therapies (AKT inhibitors, mTORC1 inhibitors, CXCR4 inhibitors) have shown promise in the preclinical studies but are in various stages of clinical translation. Everolimus, an mTORC1 inhibitor, is one such drug that is currently being studied, with one study showing that it is ineffective in the treatment of NF2 vestibular schwannomas, while another study demonstrated reduction in the median annual tumor growth rate [17].

Similarly, MEK inhibitors (selumetinib, refametinib, trametinib, and cobimetinib) have recently been assessed in the treatment of optic nerve gliomas and other low-grade gliomas in children [18]. Treatment with these drugs have improved the 2-year progression-free survival up to 69%, but are associated with adverse ocular events optic neuropathy, retinal vein occlusion, and retinopathy [13]. Bevacizumab has also shown promise in the treatment of optic nerve gliomas, with improvement of visual symptoms in up to 86% of refractory cases. Treatment that combined bevacizumab and irinotecan improved 2-year progression-free survival to 48% [13].

As our understanding of the molecular classification of each tumor subtype improves, we will get closer towards implementing a personalized approach towards treatment of each tumor based on its biology. Further work needs to be done at the basic science level to understand the tumor biology and translational medicine level to understand how these molecular subclasses affect the clinical behavior and response to treatment.

Conclusions

Cranial nerve tumors represent a complex set of pathologies that require multidisciplinary teams to develop effective treatment strategies that not only treat the tumor at hand but also preserve neurological function and improve quality of life. Basic science, translational, and clinical research is integral in developing novel treatment paradigms to better tackle these tumors and improve the lives of patients afflicted with this pathology.

References

1. Ostrom QT, Cioffi G, Waite K, Kruchko C, Barnholtz-Sloan JS. CBTRUS statistical report: primary brain and other central nervous system tumors diagnosed in the United States in 2014–2018. Neuro Oncol. 2021;23:iii1–iii105.
2. Carlson ML, Link MJ. Vestibular schwannomas. N Engl J Med. 2021;384:1335–48.
3. Hill CS, et al. Neurosurgical experience of managing optic pathway gliomas. Childs Nerv Syst. 2021;37:1917–29.
4. Campen CJ, Gutmann DH. Optic pathway gliomas in neurofibromatosis type 1. J Child Neurol. 2018;33:73–81. https://journals.sagepub.com/doi/full/10.1177/0883073817739509?casa_token=wmv0RWT6UI4AAAAA%3AvNA3IFtTmN3_ijCpdbT6WsRuSO96g-goHKMstIZ1_wBaQjEI6JXpTU3AYLqWdmf8HtT-2WPSyGsI.
5. Huang M, Patel J, Patel BC. Optic nerve glioma. In: StatPearls. StatPearls Publishing; 2022.
6. Fiani B, et al. Esthesioneuroblastoma: a comprehensive review of diagnosis, management,

and current treatment options. World Neurosurg. 2019;126:194–211.

7. Borges A, Casselman J. Imaging the cranial nerves: part II: primary and secondary neoplastic conditions and neurovascular conflicts. Eur Radiol. 2007;17:2332–44.

8. Arnold MA, Farnoosh S, Gore MR. Comparing Kadish and modified Dulguerov staging systems for olfactory neuroblastoma: an individual participant data meta-analysis. Otolaryngol Head Neck Surg. 2020. https://journals.sagepub.com/doi/full/10.1177/0194599820915487?casa_token=7r-27XTMMLgAAAAA%3ADjokhaSUT62Jp7x_moOC7AKp_IKXxrXkkP3wczxBsQFfvO9Al5RxPfI1VJHC_7T9amyewCYp7RtV.

9. Connor SEJ. Imaging of the vestibular schwannoma: diagnosis, monitoring, and treatment planning. Neuroimaging Clin. 2021;31:451–71.

10. Forgues M, et al. Non-contrast magnetic resonance imaging for monitoring patients with acoustic neuroma. J Laryngol Otol. 2018;132:780–5.

11. Goldbrunner R, et al. EANO guideline on the diagnosis and treatment of vestibular schwannoma. Neuro Oncol. 2020;22:31–45.

12. Buss EJ, Wang TJC, Sisti MB. Stereotactic radiosurgery for management of vestibular schwannoma: a short review. Neurosurg Rev. 2021;44:901–4.

13. Farazdaghi MK, Katowitz WR, Avery RA. Current treatment of optic nerve gliomas. Curr Opin Ophthalmol. 2019;30:356–63.

14. Safi C, et al. Treatment strategies and outcomes of pediatric esthesioneuroblastoma: a systematic review. Front Oncol. 2020;10:1247. https://www.frontiersin.org/articles/10.3389/fonc.2020.01247/full.

15. Gupta VK, Thakker A, Gupta KK. Vestibular schwannoma: what we know and where we are heading. Head Neck Pathol. 2020;14:1058–66.

16. Lu VM, et al. Efficacy and safety of bevacizumab for vestibular schwannoma in neurofibromatosis type 2: a systematic review and meta-analysis of treatment outcomes. J Neuro-Oncol. 2019;144:239–48.

17. Tamura R, Toda M. A critical overview of targeted therapies for vestibular schwannoma. Int J Mol Sci. 2022;23:5462.

18. Hill CS, Devesa SC, Ince W, Borg A, Aquilina K. A systematic review of ongoing clinical trials in optic pathway gliomas. Childs Nerv Syst. 2020;36:1869–86.

Bullet Points
- Nerve repair
- Nerve graft
- Nerve fiber transfer
- Cranial nerve repair treatment algorithm

Introduction

Physical interruption of a cranial nerve, like in all peripheral nerves, not only disrupts its course and denervates the target organ, but also causes a loss of cortical representation of the region represented by the nerve. Depending on the quality of the nerve involved, i.e., motor, sensory, or mixed, cortical representations can be abruptly absent after injury and potentially reorganize and degenerate with time. Reconstructing the involved traumatized extracranial nerve aims at maintaining not only muscular and somatosensory integrity, but also reestablishing the afferent and efferent brain interaction.

Open nerve lesions can be generally subdivided into lesions with preserved nerve continuity and nerve injuries with a loss of continuity [1].

Closed nerve lesions could be perioperatively overlooked, are challenging, and are profoundly based on thorough experience of the peripheral nerve surgeon in order to develop a surgical strategy.

Appropriate treatment algorithms are clearly defined and should be followed with consideration of the individual aspects of each case [2–4].

Primary repair, which represents a microsurgical repair, should be performed within 7 days after nerve injury. Best-case scenario represents a clean, sharp nerve transection with no or minimal crush components and adequate soft tissue conditions. Short-term reinnervation of the target organ ensures central neuron reorganization and minimizes apoptosis of neurons [3]. A secondary nerve repair should be carried out if primary repair is not possible. Frequent reasons for a secondary repair are initial clinically undetected nerve lesions, severe wound contamination, local infections, bone and soft tissue defects, and a general critical condition of the patient. High-resolution ultrasound (HRUS), MRI, and electrophysiology are supportive diagnostic measures.

Fundamental well-trained microsurgical technical expertise, along with appropriate magnification of a minimum of 3.5-fold, microsurgical instruments, and suture material of a minimum of 8.0 (0.4 Ph.Eur.) monofilament permanent suture, is a requirement for a promising nerve repair approach [5].

Authors of this chapter: Robert Schmidhammer and Savas Tsolakidis.

Analysis

The surgical approach and choice of technique depend on several factors, e.g., nerve defect distance, available proximal and distal nerve stumps, available nerve donors, muscle atrophy, and the surgical goal of innervation. The time elapsed since the trauma also plays a key role in decision making [3, 4]. When aiming for reintegration of cortico–central–peripheral nerve connections, the best results can be obtained when the nerve pathway is reconstructed within 6 months. However, in the authors' opinion and surgical experience, moderate to good results are still possible 12–18 months after trauma depending on individual factors, e.g., age and comorbidities of the patient. Developing a surgical plan demands a detailed analysis of the existing situation, and based on experience a strategy is designed that should be reviewed beforehand, be based on a thorough clinical examination, and be substantiated by electrophysiological and MRI findings. Double crush lesions, which are lesions of the same nerve on different levels during its course, should not be missed. Due to perioperative findings and anatomical variations, the initially established surgical plan in some cases has to be adapted. This requires not only microsurgical skills, but profound expertise in peripheral nerve surgery and reconstruction.

Microsurgical Methods of Cranial Nerve Repair

Direct Nerve Repair

Microsurgical end-to-end coaptation of a proximal and distal nerve stump should be performed in an appropriate fashion, meaning both stumps should rest in a well-vascularized tissue environment with no or minimal tension [3]. Tension causes a reduction of vascular support, resulting in nerve ischemia with significant reduction of blood perfusion [6, 7]. The tolerance for tension mainly depends on the individual elastic retraction of the affected nerve. Ignoring these retraction properties leads to nerve fibrosis and thus results in functional impairment. Moreover, microsutures under tension are prone to rupture and/or developing scar tissue at the repair site. The best possible trauma case would be a clearly transected nerve with clean, distinguishable nerve ends and fascicular pattern and without nerve tissue loss in a clean, well-vascularized tissue environment. Care should be taken to avoid suturing both nerve ends in a tight manner by performing epineurial single stitches. In addition, the authors always prefer to secure the stitching with fibrin glue. Direct nerve repair keeps the time of functional cortical reorganization to a minimum and thus leads to the best functional results.

Nerve Autografting

In cases where a modest tension or tension-free nerve end coaptation is not feasible and a segmental loss is present, autologous nerve grafting should be considered as the gold standard microsurgical procedure. According to the dogma of Millesi [2, 3], nerve restoration with interfascicular nerve grafts for a segmental nerve reconstruction is preferable to the alternative of extensive tissue mobilization of both nerve stumps and/or bone reduction procedures by osteotomies in order to reduce the nerve gap distance for a primary repair. By utilizing autologous nerve grafts, a perfect scaffold, partly lined with Schwann cell basal laminae, neurotrophic factors, and adhesion molecules, is provided to facilitate nerve fiber ingrowth. In addition, an intact and vascularized wound bed provides primary nutrition for survival of isolated autologous nerve grafts. In general, 15% of original nerve fiber counts are mandatory to regain some motor function. Limiting factors are target organ atrophy and the availability of autologous nerve grafts. Grafts known as cable grafts should be avoided and instead replaced by single nerve grafts aligned individually in a good vascularized wound bed, respecting proper fascicular pattern, and sutured in an interfascicular grafting technique [3, 4]. Following the pattern of the vasa nervorum of the epineurium and paraneurium is helpful in supporting the correct alignment of the fascicles. Additionally, the intraneural topography of the motor and sensory fascicular patterns must be respected to achieve the best functional outcome.

Figure 29.1 demonstrates damaged facial nerve branches, while Fig. 29.2 reveals sural nerve grafts interpositioned for defect bridging. Figure 29.3 illustrates a clinical patient case where sural nerve grafts were put under tension and finally resulted in suture rupture and neuroma formation in the accessory nerve.

In cases of facial nerve lesions where no proximal nerve stump is available, cross facial nerve grafting should be considered. In this case, the

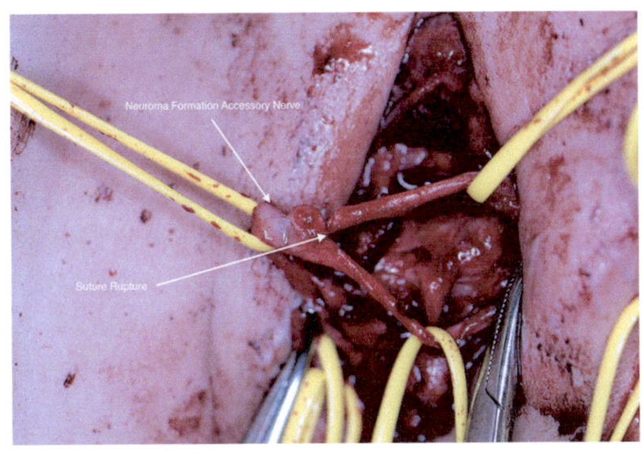

Fig. 29.3 Accessory nerve repair with sural nerve grafts after iatrogenic accessory nerve lesion. Postoperative suture rupture and neuroma formation at the coaptation site

best functional results are achieved when selecting nerve donors with equivalent function.

The authors prefer the following autologous nerve grafts in descending order, considering the acceptable morbidity after harvest and the individual circumstances of the patient:

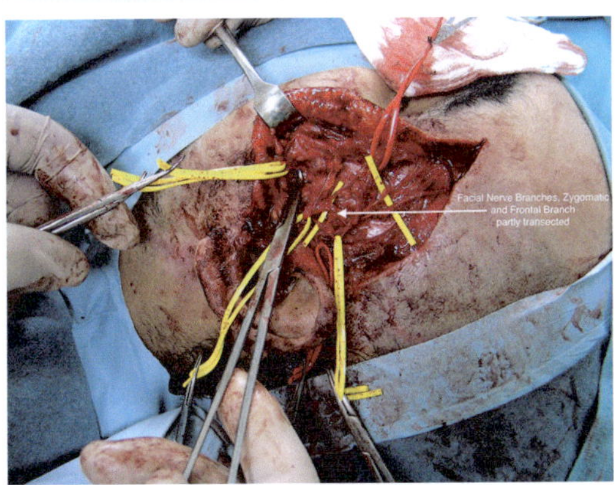

Fig. 29.1 Traumatic lesion to the left-sided facial nerve in a female patient, where the main branches of the facial nerve have been dissected

- *Sural nerve graft*: This is the preferred graft when longer and/or multiple nerve gaps have to be bridged, based on the minimal morbidity after harvest, small nerve caliber, and interneural nutrient vessels. Sequelae after harvest consist of latent, permanent numbness, dysesthesia, or hyposensitivity on the lateral border of the foot in 87.2% of cases, pain in 25.6% of cases, or cold sensitivity in 22.2% of cases. It should be highlighted that risk of neuroma formation can be significantly reduced when the proximal nerve stump after nerve graft harvest is surgically buried under the deep thigh fascia [8].

- *Saphenous nerve graft*: Sequelae after harvest consist of latent, permanent numbness, dysesthesia, or hyposensitivity on the medial thigh, the patellar region, and the upper third of the medial lower leg in most cases.

- *Anterior division of the medial antebrachial and brachial cutaneous nerve*: Sequelae after harvest consist of latent, permanent numbness or hyposensitivity on the medial side of the forearm and/or the upper arm in most cases.

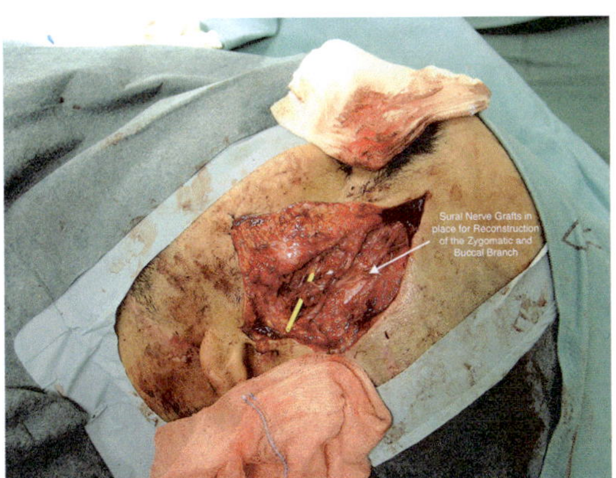

Fig. 29.2 Sural nerve grafts interpositioned for defect bridging. Sural nerve grafts have been interpositioned for reconstruction of zygomatic and buccal branches. See also Fig. 29.1

- *Lateral cutaneous nerve of the forearm*: Sequelae after harvest consist of latent, permanent numbness or hyposensitivity on the lateral side of the forearm in most cases.
- *Great auricular nerve (C2, C3)*: This nerve is ideal for defects up to 10 cm in the vicinity of the facial nerve with a very good size match. Sequelae after harvest consist of numbness in the mastoid process region, the auricle, and the skin over the parotid gland in most cases.

Microsurgical techniques for the following nerve repair methods remain equal to direct nerve repair, with the fundamental premise being focused on minimal tension or tension-free coaptation.

Nerve Allografting and Nerve Conduits

Processed allografts, which can be used for motor, sensory, and mixed nerve reconstructions, represent, in selected cases, an alternative to autologous nerve grafts. Restrictions at present are the maximal available length of 50 mm, starting with a minimum of 5 mm length. Due to the specific processing of the nerve grafts, immunogenicity has been nullified and thus does not require immunosuppression regimens [9]. Conduits consist of either fibers or an aligned matrix in the absence of any exogenous factor and are effective for small nerve defects up to 6 cm. They can be subdivided into biological conduits, consisting mostly of veins and arteries and artificial, tissue-engineered conduits for nerve defects up to 3 cm. The authors have rarely utilized nerve allografts in their last 20 years of microsurgical peripheral nerve surgery experience [10].

Nerve Fiber Transfer

As an invaluable adjunct in the armamentarium for peripheral nerve microsurgeons, nerve fiber transfers represent a useful additional axon source in cases where proximal nerve stumps are not available. With the availability and advances of perioperative neurostimulation and refined stimulation instruments, promising possibilities have emerged to identify specific fascicles responsible for particular muscle targets and divert them to a specific

acceptor nerve and/or nerve fascicle [4, 11]. In general, proximal nerve fiber transfers, where the donor and receiving fascicles are at a proximal level of its course, can be distinguished from distal ones where the target zone lies at a peripheral level in proximity of the target organ. The authors prefer in most cases to include in their surgical reconstructive strategy both nerve grafting and peripheral nerve fiber transfer if a proximal and distal nerve stump is still available and the reconstructed cranial nerve is located a long distance from the target muscle. With this combination, faster reinnervation of the target muscle is achieved, and muscular atrophy is reduced.

End-to-Side Coaptation Technique

By rerouting a denervated distal nerve stump to the side of an intact local nerve, collateral sprouting is induced after merely creating an epineurial window while completely preserving the donor nerve function [12]. This microsurgical method represents a valuable alternative for cases where a proximal nerve stump of the injured nerve is absent, although literature has substantiated that the number of axons sprouting to the injured distal nerve stump is significantly reduced in end-to-side nerve coaptations compared to an end-to-end approach. Attention should focus on the use of the homogenous function of the donor nerve for better results.

Microsurgical Neurolysis

Various gliding tissue components of the cranial nerves are mandatory for proper nerve function. The paraneurium represents the gliding tissue of the external nerve component, which interacts with the surrounding tissues and moves in harmony with various movements of different body parts. At the interfascicular level, gliding tissues are responsible for an immaculate gliding of the fascicles. Posttraumatic inflammation, remodeling, and scarring can lead to severe impairment of the gliding tissues and thus functional loss. Microsurgical neurolysis as a surgical procedure aims to reestablish appropriate nerve gliding by decompressing the fascicles [13].

It is eminent to understand the different levels of these important nerve components to perform a microsurgical release in a stepwise procedure. Ideally, a stepwise decompression of the fascicles of cranial nerves should be performed within 14 days after trauma.

Muscle–Tendon Transfers

Muscle–tendon transfers are a viable reconstructive method in cases where over a year has passed since a nerve trauma and function of denervated muscles must be replaced [14].

Figures 29.4 and 29.5 demonstrate a reconstructive procedure for achieving scapula control in a patient with a winging scapula. Figure 29.6 reveals a reconstructive muscle/tendon procedure for animating eyelid closure, elevating the mouth corner, and achieving a smile in a patient with a long-term facial nerve paralysis.

Table 29.1 shows and overview of the cranial nerves and their extracranial potential for nerve repair.

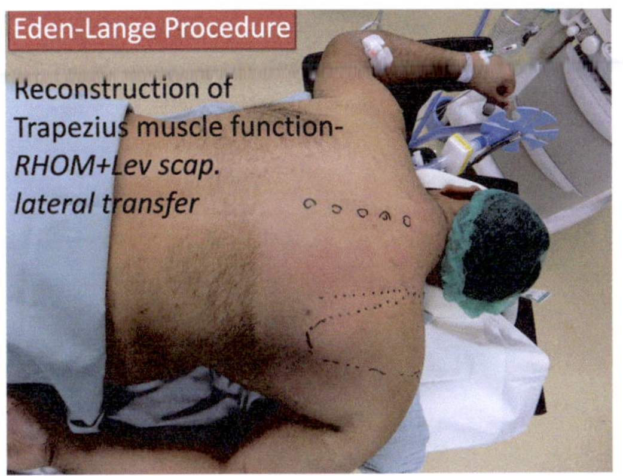

Fig. 29.4 Stabilization procedure (Eden–Lange procedure) for scapula control and reduction of scapula winging as a secondary reconstructive procedure

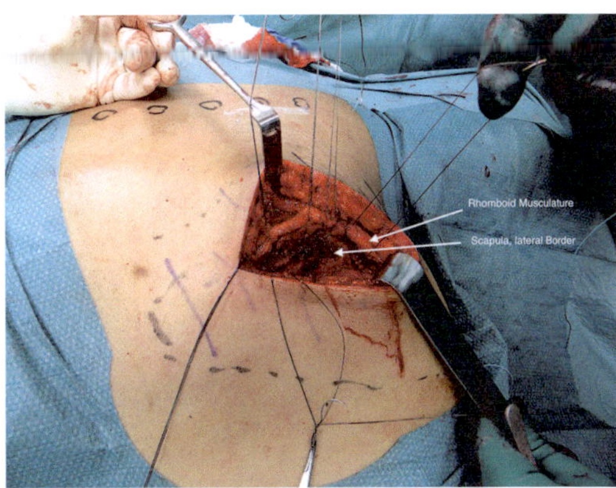

Fig. 29.5 Intraoperative setting. Definition of the rhomboid musculature for constraining the scapula and thus reducing winging. See also Fig. 29.4

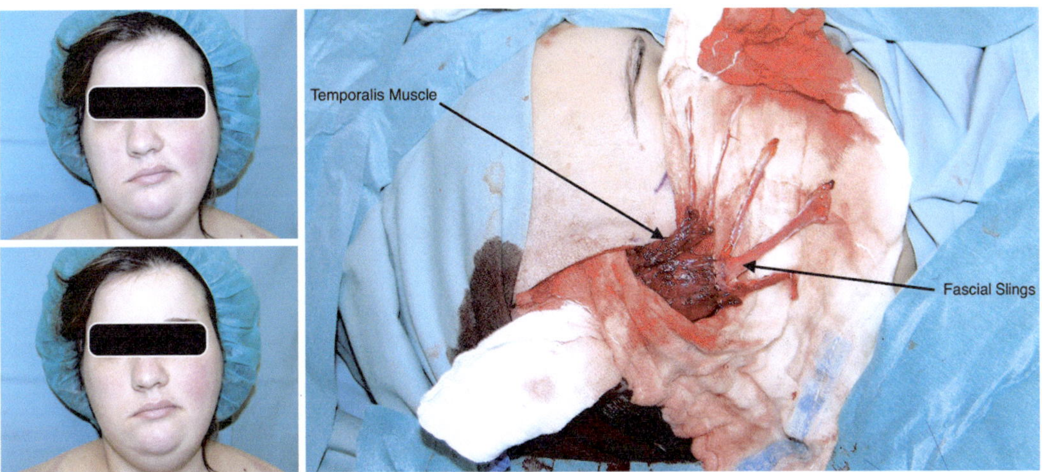

Fig. 29.6 Functional muscle transfer of fascial slings of the temporalis muscle for functional reconstruction of eyelid closure (2 slings) and mouth corner elevation and smile (3 slings) as a secondary reconstructive procedure in a prolonged facial nerve paralysis patient

Table 29.1 Overview of the cranial nerves, including extracranial potential for nerve repair

Cranial nerve	Term	Type	Type of injury with high risk of nerve involvement	Possible clinical findings	Extra-cranial trauma access for nerve repair	Prioritized nerve parts for reconstruction	Prioritized nerve grafts
I	Olfactory nerve	Sensory	Head–brain injury	Anosmia, parosmia, rhinoliquorrhoe	✗		
II	Optic nerve	Sensory	Head–brain injury	Blindness, bitemporal hemianopsia	✗[a]		
III	Oculomotor nerve	Motor Parasympathetic	Head–brain injury	Inability to turn the affected eye inwards – up and down – diplopia, ptosis	✗		
IV	Trochlear nerve	Motor	Closed head trauma	Inability to turn the affected eye downwards, strabismus, diplopia	✗		
V	Trigeminal nerve	Sensory Motor	Maxillary orbital injury	Neuralgia, hyposensitivity, hypersensitivity	✓		
VI	Abducens nerve	Motor	Head trauma	Inability to turn the affected eye laterally	✗		
VII	Facial nerve	Sensory Motor Parasympathetic	Blunt trauma, vehicle accidents, gunshots, blast injuries, falls	Residual function: waiting is acceptable for 3 months Immediate onset – complete paralysis: surgical action needed, best achieved within 72 hours post-trauma Recovery rates >90% when repaired within 14 days	✓	Zygomatic Buccal	Greater auricular nerve, cervical plexus, sural nerve
VIII	Vestibulocochlear nerve	Sensory		Hearing reduction or loss, vertigo, tinnitus	✓		
IX	Glossopharyngeal nerve	Sensory Motor Parasympathetic	Penetrating neck injuries, closed head injuries	Velopharyngeal insufficiency, dysphagia, penetrating sharp pain in the throat, neck, or ear triggered by swallowing	✓		
X	Vagal nerve	Sensory Motor Parasympathetic	Penetrating neck injuries, closed head injuries	Hoarseness, stridor, pharyngeal and palatal weakness, dysphagia, aspiration	✓		Ansa cervicalis, hypoglossal nerve
XI	Accessory nerve	Motor	Penetrating injuries, fractures involving the jugular foramen,	Shoulder weakness, pain	✓		Primary repair, nerve grafting, nerve fiber transfer
XII	Hypoglossal nerve	Motor	Penetrating injuries	Dysarthria, tongue deviation to the affected side	✓		Primary repair, grafting

✗, interventions not possible; ✓, interventions possible

[a] In rare cases, a microsurgical neurolysis of the optic nerve has been described during boney reconstructive procedures

Discussion

The armamentarium in peripheral nerve surgery has expanded over the last decade with the development of much more refined microsurgical and super-microsurgical instruments. Super-magnifying microscopes further offer three-dimensional exposure and super-detailed displays of soft tissues, nerves, and surrounding vessels, as well as the ability to additionally highlight specific tissue components via fluorescence markers.

Moreover, microsurgical technical advances like nerve fiber transfers have become a worthwhile adjunct in specific cases when no proximal nerve stump is available and/or a high nerve lesion is present. This technique harnesses a healthy dispensable donor nerve to provide the damaged nerve with intact axons to reach the target in a rapid way.

Still, in cases of nerve gaps, nerve grafting with autologous nerve grafts remains the microsurgical gold standard. Whenever possible and reasonable, direct nerve repair should be pursued. End-to-side nerve repair could represent a viable surgical strategy, although an end-to-end repair provides a much higher number of axons and thus leads to more efficient nerve regeneration. Nerve allografts and conduits, which are restricted to shorter nerve grafts, are decellularized and do not need concomitant immunosuppression therapy. In the authors' opinion, allografts and conduits should be carefully selected only in specific patient cases, e.g., no available reasonable autologous donor nerves, and/or explicit request of the patient or the patient's parents for underage individuals to not harvest autologous nerve grafts. Moreover, a deeper understanding of the constant interplay of the central nervous system with its periphery has led to more efficient rehabilitative options for the patients during their postoperative care. Despite all the technical progress and advances in microsurgical reconstructive methods, however, time and age of the patient still play a key role and represent a crucial and decisive factor in establishing an individualized strategic surgical plan. Further, human studies are needed to adequately evaluate additional treatment-supporting factors, such as stem cell therapy or pharmacologic agents to avoid neuron apoptosis and decelerate muscle atrophy.

Recommendation

Despite massive progress in the field of nerve microsurgery and super-microsurgery, the key factors for cranial nerve repair remain the same and are based on the principles of peripheral nerve repair. Several reconstructive methods exist and should be individually selected and combined. Still, time plays a key role in the development of a microsurgical strategy, and the best results are often obtained within 3–6 months after trauma. Moreover, the level of nerve trauma is an important factor, with reconstructive options for neurorestoration not only at the level of the trauma, but in the vicinity of the muscle target via peripheral nerve fiber transfers as well. Microsurgical appliances should be paired with surgical expertise, appropriate microsurgical training, and individual experience and thus in its entirety represent essential pillars to obtaining high patient satisfaction scores.

References

1. Campbell WW. Evaluation and management of peripheral nerve injury. Clin Neurophysiol. 2008;119:1951–65.
2. Millesi H. Nerve transplantation for reconstruction of peripheral nerves injured by the use of the microsurgical technique. Minerva Chir. 1967;22:950–1.
3. Millesi H. Indications and techniques of nerve grafting. In: Gelberman RH, editor. Operative nerve repair and reconstruction, vol. 1. Philadelphia: JB Lippincott; 1991. p. 525–43.
4. Dvali L, Mackinnon S. Nerve repair, grafting, and nerve transfers. Clin Plast Surg. 2003;30:203–21.
5. Ghanem A, Kearns M, Ballestin A, Froschauer S, Akelina Y, Shurey S, Legagneux J, et al. International microsurgery simulation society (IMSS) consensus statement on the minimum standards for a basic microsurgery course, requirements for a microsurgical anastomosis global rating scale and minimum thresholds or training. Injury. 2020;51(Suppl 4):S126–30.
6. Schmidhammer R, Zandieh S, Hopf R, Hausner T, Pelinka LE, Kroepfl A, Redl H. Effects of

alleviated tension at the nerve repair site using biodegradable tubular conduit: histological, electrophysiological and functional results in a rat model. Eur Surg. 2005;37(4):213–9.

7. Kline DG, Hackett ER, Davis GD, Myers MB. Effect of mobilization on the blood supply and regeneration of injured nerves. J Surg Res. 1972;12:254–66.

8. Bamba R, Loewenstein SN, Adkinson JM. Donor site morbidity after sural nerve grafting: a systematic review. J Plast Reconstr Aesthet Surg. 2021;74(11):3055–60.

9. Brooks DN, Weber RV, Chao JD, Rinker BD, Zoldos J, Robichaux MR, Ruggeri SB, Anderson KA, Bonatz EE, Wisotsky SM, Cho MS, Wilson C, Cooper EO, Ingari JV, Safa B, Parrett BM, Buncke GM. Processed nerve allografts for peripheral nerve reconstruction: a multicenter study of utilization and outcomes in sensory, mixed, and motor nerve reconstructions. Microsurgery. 2012;32(1):1–14.

10. Strauch B. Use of nerve conduits in peripheral nerve repair. Hand Clin. 2000;16:123–30.

11. Schmidhammer R, Nógrádi A, Szabó A, Redl H, Hausner T, van der Nest DG, Millesi H. Synergistic motor nerve fiber transfer between different nerves through the use of end-to-side coaptation. Exp Neurol. 2009;217(2):388–94.

12. Millesi H, Tsolakidis S. End-to-side coaptation: an important tool in peripheral nerve surgery. Eur Surg. 2005;37(4):228–33.

13. Millesi H, Rath T, Reihsner R, Zoch G. Microsurgical neurolysis: its anatomical and physiological basis and its classification. Microsurgery. 1993;14(7):430–9.

14. Rubin LR, Lee GW, Simpson RL. Reanimation of the long-standing partial facial paralysis. Plast Reconstr Surg. 1986;77(1):41–9.

Pathological Conditions Affecting Cranial Nerves at the Skull Base and Neurosurgical Intervention Strategies

---

Bullet Points

- Cranial nerves can be affected by skull base lesions in many ways.
- Each pathology has a predominance depending on patient's age.
- Cranial nerves may be affected singularly or in groups.
- Clinical presentation may help in locating the pathology before further diagnostics are performed.

Introduction

Causes for cranial nerve lesions can be classified as vascular, traumatic, iatrogenic, immunological, infectious, metabolic, genetic, nutritional, degenerative, or neoplastic [1]. This chapter focuses on pathological lesions within the skull base. Cranial nerves can be affected by skull base lesions in many ways:

1. *Entrapment of nerves caused by skull base lesions.* This can be the case in pathological conditions like osseous or cartilaginous tumors, metastasis, or specific skull base bone diseases, including but not limited to aneurysmatic bone cyst, cholesterol granulomas, chondrosarcomas, chordomas, fibrous dysplasia, metastasis, Paget's disease, plasmocytomas, or osteosarcomas [1, 2]. In addition, inflammatory lesions of the osseous skull base, like chronic skull base osteomyelitis or sinusitis of the perinasal sinuses, can lead to cranial nerve affection.

2. *Entrapment or compression caused by dural lesions.* Meningiomas are the most common primary tumor of the central nervous system and originate from the dural cap cells. Not uncommonly, they arise from dural sleeves at skull base regions [3, 4]. Other pathologies affecting cranial nerves at their dural sleeves are inflammatory pachymeningitis or Lyme disease.

3. *Neurinomas originating directly from cranial nerves.* In the case of skull base anatomy, this can include vestibular schwannomas, glossopharyngeal schwannomas, and less commonly trigeminal or facial schwannomas [5].

4. *Direct or indirect compression in the vicinity or within the cavernous sinus by arteries or venous congestion.* This is most often observed in A. communicans posterior aneurysms resulting in third nerve palsy. Other vascular pathologies include carotid cavernous fistulas, cisternal arterial loops of the superior cerebellar artery, or variations of posterior inferior cerebellar artery or vertebral artery courses resulting in oph-

---

Authors of this chapter: Fabian Winter and Karl Roessler.

thalmoplegia, trigeminal neuralgia, or hemifacial spasms [1, 6].

5. *Lesions in and around the sellar region.* Pathologies in this region most commonly affect cranial nerves within the suprasellar cisterns or indirectly by infiltrating the cavernous sinus and the skull base. Pituitary adenomas and craniopharyngiomas are the leading causes [7].

Etiological Outline

Tumorous and inflammatory skull base lesions seem to be the most common diseases leading to cranial nerve symptoms. These include primary skull base bone or cartilage tumors or benign bone tumors or metastatic disease of the skull base (often seen in prostatic cancer or breast cancer) (Table 30.1).

Table 30.1 Frequency of associations: different pathologies causing cranial nerve affection at the skull base and the basal cisterns

Pathology	Incidence
Osteosarcomas	~100 cases in the literature [8]
Chondrosarcomas	0.019 per 100,000 [9]
Chordomas	0.089 per 100,000 [10]
Fibrous dysplasia	10 per 100,000 [11]
Paget's disease	2 per 100,000 [12]
Cholesterol granulomas	0.06 per 100,000 [13]
Skull base osteomyelitis	Up to 12.7% [14]
Meningiomas	97.5 per 100,000 [15]
Lyme disease	206 per 100,000 [16]
Vestibular schwannomas	1.09 per 100,000 [5]
Glossopharyngeal schwannomas	~40 cases in the literature [1]
Aneurysm of the artery communicans posterior	0.5 per 100,000 [17]
Carotid cavernous fistula	800 per 100,000 [18]
Pituitary adenomas	16.7% [19]
Craniopharyngiomas	13 per 100,000 [20]
Metastasis	9–17% [21]

Incidence of cranial nerve affection is dependent on localization of pathology

Analysis, Symptoms, and Diagnostics

The neurological examination has excellent localization value and can differentiate among the specific presenting impairments. It is more common for multiple cranial nerves to be affected by an underlying pathology rather than a single cranial nerve alone (Table 30.2). Petroclival meningiomas are a good example of a lesion affecting multiple cranial nerves at the same time, making a topographical and ethological diagnosis possible even before getting MR images. They may affect nearly all cranial nerves, from cranial nerve II to XII, with neurological symptoms including but not limited to blurred vision, visual field reduction, double vision, facial numbness, facial pain, facial palsy, reduced hearing, tinnitus, hoarseness, swallowing problems, and dysarthria (Fig. 30.1). The same clinical situation may occur for skull base osteomyelitis, plasmacytoma, or metastatic disease of the skull base. Specific symptoms for lower cranial nerve affections include impaired speech, deglutition, sensory functions, alterations in taste, autonomic dysfunction, neuralgic pain, dysphagia, head or neck pain, and cardiac or gastrointestinal compromise, as well as dysfunction or weakness of the tongue, trapezius muscle, or sternocleidomastoid muscle [1]. For diagnosis, computed tomography (CT) and magnetic resonance imaging (MRI) play complementary roles, as both findings can often narrow the differential diagnosis [29, 30].

Table 30.2 Cranial nerve syndromes at the skull base [1, 22–28]

Syndrome	Cranial nerve affected	Pathology	Treatment
Avellis	X	Injury to nucleus ambiguous disturbing signals being sent to cranial nerve X	High-dose prednisolone, cyclosporin, resection of lesion compressing the jugular foramen
Vernet	IX, X, XI	Malignant tumor, aneurysm (ICA), otitis media, giant cell arteritis, or fracture	Depending on pathology: resection vs antibiotics
Collet–Sicard	IX, X, XI, XII	Malignant lesions, Jefferson fracture, occipital condyle fractures	Resection vs rehabilitation
Tapia	X, XII	Iatrogenic, compression by endotracheal tube during surgery	Airway endoscopy, rehabilitation
Villaret	IX, X, XI, XII	Malignant tumor in retroparotid space, osteomyelitis, aneurysm (ICA)	Depending on pathology
Jackson	X, XI, XII	Tumors (epidermoid), iatrogenic through surgical complication	Resection of tumor mass
Schmidt	X, XI	Malignant tumor, fractures, ICA pathology (aneurysms or dissection)	Depending on pathology

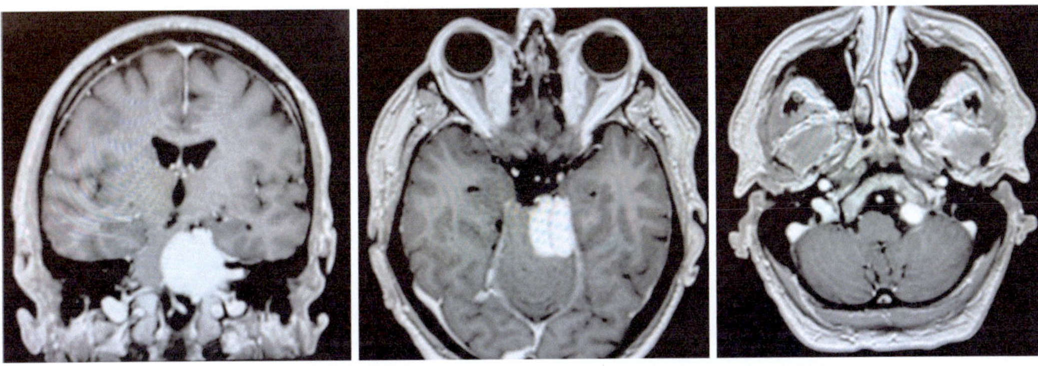

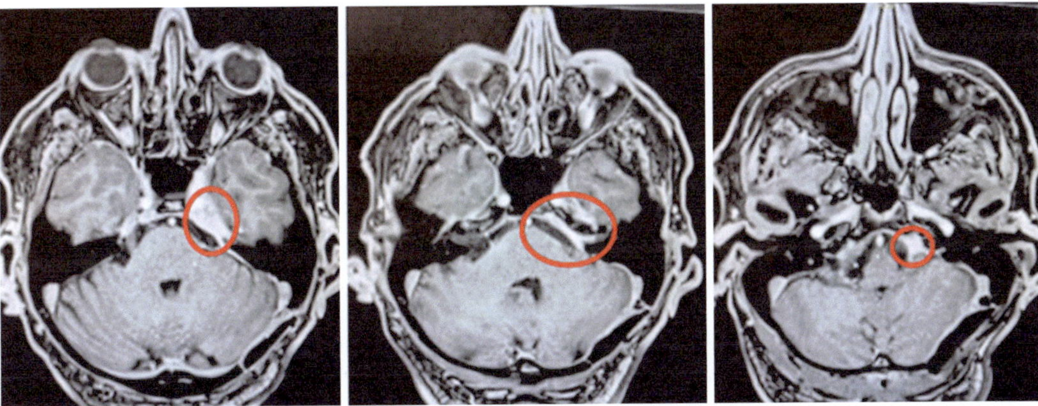

Fig. 30.1 A 45-year-old male presented with left-sided chronic CN symptoms: double vision, numbness on the left face, diminished hearing, vertigo, horsiness, swallowing problems. A large left-sided petroclival meningioma expanding from the tentorial incision down to the jugular foramen was diagnosed. Gross total resection was achieved. All symptoms disappeared. Small residuals at the dura were diagnosed at the 3-month follow-up MRI. Wait and scan was recommended. In case of recurrence, Gamma Knife irradiation can be applied

Discussion and Neurosurgical Treatment Strategies

Effective treatments are available for several pathologies, but a precondition for complete recovery is a correct and swift diagnosis. The surgeon familiar with the site of origin of each common pathology has a considerable advantage when undertaking a function-sparing procedure. In recent years, advances in interdisciplinary fields, such as imaging, radiation therapy, and progressive surgical techniques, have allowed more aggressive approaches and improved outcomes [29]. Primary skull base lesions, if space-occupying and compressing nervous tissue, are subjected to surgical resection. Specific skull base approaches, including transcranial and transsphenoidal, are used singly or in combination to remove underlying pathologies and to decompress cranial nerves. Inflammatory lesions are mostly treated by long-term antibiotics, plasmocytomas, and metastatic infiltration by chemoradiation or antihormone or targeted medication.

In vascular pathologies, endovascular interventions are also within the neurosurgical therapeutical spectrum. For embolizing aneurysms or dural arteriovenous fistulas at the cavernous sinus and within the intracranial basal cisterns, implanting intracranial stents or flow diverters induce shrinkage of the vascular lesion leading to nerve decompression.

Pituitary adenomas are the third most common primary intracranial tumors, besides meningiomas and gliomas, and thus comprise a large field of microsurgical interventions, mainly via the transsphenoidal route [7]. Nowadays, mainly endoscopic transsphenoidal surgery is performed for hormone-active and hormone-inactive (nonfunctioning) tumors. Prolactinomas, which tend to diffusely infiltrate the skull base, are a domain of primarily medical therapy using dopamine agonists like cabergoline.

Meningiomas originating from the tuberculum sellae are not rare and have been described to affect cranial nerves at the skull base in 84% [2]. However, unlike convexity meningiomas, it is not recommended to achieve a total resection at the skull base as this is associated with significantly greater postoperative cranial nerve morbidity compared with less aggressive tumor excision and postoperative one-stage precision radiation of residual dural tumor remnants using LINACs, Gamma Knife, or Cyberknife for long-term stabilization [2, 6, 31].

In patients with malignant skull base tumors at the parotid gland or cerebellopontine angle, there is also a tremendous risk to the facial nerve. When possible, the facial nerve is preserved, which may involve extensive exposure, mobilization, or even rerouting the nerve. In cases of nerve sacrifice, primary neurorrhaphy or interposition grafting may be used [5, 21].

References

1. Gutierrez S, Warner T, McCormack E, Werner C, Mathkour M, Iwanaga J, et al. Lower cranial nerve syndromes: a review. Neurosurg Rev. 2021;44(3):1345–55.
2. Schneider M, Schuss P, Güresir Á, Wach J, Hamed M, Vatter H, et al. Cranial nerve outcomes after surgery for frontal skull base meningiomas: the eternal quest of the maximum-safe resection with the lowest morbidity. World Neurosurg. 2019;125:e790–6.
3. Preusser M, Brastianos PK, Mawrin C. Advances in meningioma genetics: novel therapeutic opportunities. Nat Rev Neurol. 2018;14:106–15.
4. Mathiesen T, Lindquist C, Kihlstrom L, Karlsson B. Recurrence of cranial base meningiomas. Neurosurgery. 1996;39(1):2–9.
5. Moffat DA, Parker RA, Hardy DG, Macfarlane R. Factors affecting final facial nerve outcome following vestibular schwannoma surgery. J Laryngol Otol. 2014;128(5):406–15.
6. Westerlund U, Linderoth B, Mathiesen T. Trigeminal complications arising after surgery of cranial base meningiomas. Neurosurg Rev. 2012;35(2):203–10.
7. Hashimoto N, Kikuchi H. Transsphenoidal approach to infrasellar tumors involving the cavernous sinus. J Neurosurg. 1990;73(4):513–7.
8. Fernandes GL, Ricardo M, Natal C, Nascif RL, Tsuno MY. Primary osteosarcoma of the cranial vault. Radiol Bras. 2017;50:263.
9. Dibas M, Doheim MF, Ghozy S, Ros MH, El-Helw GO, Reda A. Incidence and survival rates and trends of skull base chondrosarcoma: a population-based study. Clin Neurol Neurosurg. 2020;198:106153.
10. Chambers KJ, Lin DT, Meier J, Remenschneider A, Herr M, Gray ST. Incidence and survival patterns of cranial chordoma in the United States. Laryngoscope. 2014;124(5):1097–102.

11. Yang L, Wu H, Lu J, Teng L. Prevalence of different forms and involved bones of craniofacial fibrous dysplasia. J Craniofac Surg. 2017;28(1):21–5.

12. Cook MJ, Pye SR, Lunt M, Dixon WG, Ashcroft DM, O'Neill TW. Incidence of Paget's disease of bone in the UK: evidence of a continuing decline. Rheumatology (Oxford). 2021;60(12):5668–76.

13. Tabet P, Saydy N, Saliba I. Cholesterol granulomas: a comparative meta-analysis of endonasal endoscopic versus open approaches to the petrous apex. J Int Adv Otol. 2019;15(2):193–9.

14. Khan MA, Quadri SAQ, Kazmi AS, Farooqui M. A comprehensive review of skull base osteomyelitis: diagnostic and therapeutic challenges among various presentations. Asian J Neurosurg. 2018;13:959–70.

15. Wiemels J, Wrensch M, Claus EB. Epidemiology and etiology of meningioma. J Neurooncol. 2010;99:307–14.

16. States U, Kugeler KJ, Schwartz AM, Delorey MJ, Mead PS, Hinckley AF. Estimating the frequency of Lyme disease diagnoses, United States, 2010–2018. Emerg Infect Dis. 2021;27(2):616.

17. Asaithambi G, Adil MM, Chaudhry SA, Qureshi AI. Incidences of unruptured intracranial aneurysms and subarachnoid hemorrhage: results of a statewide study. J Vasc Interv Neurol. 2014;7:8–11.

18. Signorelli F, Della Pepa GM, Sabatino G, Marchese E, Maira G, Puca A, et al. Diagnosis and management of dural arteriovenous fistulas: a 10 years single-center experience. Clin Neurol Neurosurg. 2015;128:123–9.

19. Ezzat S, Asa SL, Couldwell WT, Barr CE, Dodge WE, Vance ML, et al. The prevalence of pituitary adenomas: a systematic review. Cancer. 2004;101(3):613–9.

20. Bunin GR, Surawicz TS, Witman PA, Preston-Martin S, Davis F, Bruner JM. The descriptive epidemiology of craniopharyngioma. J Neurosurg. 1998;89(4):547–51.

21. Christopher LH, Slattery WH, Smith EJ, Larian B, Azizzadeh B. Facial nerve management in patients with malignant skull base tumors. J Neuro-Oncol. 2020;150(3):493–500.

22. Krasnianski M, Neudecker S, Schlüter A, Zierz S. [Avellis' syndrome in brainstem infarctions]. Fortschr Neurol Psychiatr. 2003;71(12):650–3.

23. Fox SL, West GBJ. Syndrome of Avellis; a review of the literature and report of one case. Arch Otolaryngol. 1947;46(6):773–8.

24. Jo YR, Chung CW, Lee JS, Park HJ. Vernet syndrome by varicella-zoster virus. Ann Rehabil Med. 2013;37(3):449–52.

25. Gout O, Viala K, Lyon-Caen O. Giant cell arteritis and Vernet's syndrome. Neurology. 1998;50(6):1862–4.

26. Amano M, Ishikawa E, Kujiraoka Y, Watanabe S, Ashizawa K, Oguni E, et al. Vernet's syndrome caused by large mycotic aneurysm of the extracranial internal carotid artery after acute otitis media—case report. Neurol Med Chir (Tokyo). 2010;50(1):45–8.

27. Domenicucci M, Mancarella C, Dugoni ED, Ciappetta P, Paolo M. Post-traumatic Collet-Sicard syndrome: personal observation and review of the pertinent literature with clinical, radiologic and anatomic considerations. Eur Spine J. 2015;24(4):663–70.

28. Cariati P, Cabello A, Galvez PP, Sanchez Lopez D, Garcia MB. Tapia's syndrome: pathogenetic mechanisms, diagnostic management, and proper treatment: a case series. J Med Case Rep. 2016;10:23.

29. Kelly HR, Curtin HD. Imaging of skull base lesions. Handb Clin Neurol. 2016;135:637–57.

30. Klimaj Z, Klein JP, Szatmary G. Cranial nerve imaging and pathology. Neurol Clin. 2020;38(1):115–47.

31. Sughrue ME, Kane AJ, Shangari G, Rutkowski MJ, McDermott MW, Berger MS, et al. The relevance of Simpson Grade I and II resection in modern neurosurgical treatment of World Health Organization Grade I meningiomas. J Neurosurg. 2010;113(5):1029–35.

Bullet Points
- Infectious agents, including viruses, bacteria, fungi, and parasites, can affect cranial nerves.
- Regional variations in the prevalence of the infective agent exist.
- A detailed history and clinical examination coupled with appropriate laboratory tests and neuroimaging help accurate diagnosis and treatment.

Introduction

A wide variety of infectious agents affect the cranial nerves (CNs). These cranial neuropathies may be seen in isolation, or as a part of wider involvements. Infections can directly damage the CNs, or CN damage may be a secondary consequence of the immune response resulting from the infections. This manuscript will review various aspects of infections of the CNs.

Viruses

Coronavirus Disease

The severe acute respiratory syndrome coronavirus 2 (SARS-CoV-2) resulting in the coronavirus disease 2019 (COVID-19) is a neurotrophic virus, CN involvements are reported in patients infected with COVID-19 [1]. The virus reaches the central nervous system via the neuroepithelium of the olfactory nerve and olfactory bulb and travels by neuronal retrograde transmission or by hematological spread. The virus enters the cells of the central and peripheral nervous systems using angiotensin-converting enzyme 2 (ACE-2) receptors. CN involvement reflects the neurovirulence of the virus; indeed, anosmia affects up to 50% of infected patients. The present literature contains reports of all CN involvements in patients with COVID-19. Some CNs are affected in the early period (loss of taste and smell), while others (ophthalmoparesis, dysphagia, loss of vision, and hearing loss) occur later in the course of the illness. A recent systemic review noted that CNs III, VI, and VII are commonly involved [2]. Evidence for autoimmunity in CN involvement in COVID-19 is gathering steadily, similar to that of Guillain–Barré syndrome (GBS). In a proportion of COVID-19-GBS patients, the virus was absent in acellular cerebrospinal fluid (CSF), implying no direct root infection or intrathecal viral replication. The anti-GD1b ganglioside antibodies seen in the Miller Fischer syndrome occurring in relation to COVID-19 imply novel mechanisms, as the antibodies differ from those seen in Miller Fischer syndrome unassociated with COVID-19. Uncommon case reports of post COVID-19 vaccine exist, but as of yet no direct causation has been established [3].

Authors of this chapter: Satish V. Khadilkar and Riddhi Patel.

Herpesviridae

Eight viruses of the *Herpesviridae* family infect humans, and almost all adult populations are infected with at least one of these. Herpes simplex virus (HSV) type 1 and 2, Epstein–Barr virus (EBV), cytomegalovirus, and varicella zoster virus (VZV) are the important ones. In addition, there are human herpes virus types 6–8. HSV 1 and 2 and VZV reside latently in the sensory nerve and CN ganglia.

- Herpes zoster (shingles) is an acute, cutaneous viral infection caused by the reactivation of VZV. It presents with neuralgic pain and a characteristic vesicular rash that follows a dermatomal distribution [4]. There is a 10–20% lifetime risk of developing herpes zoster infection [5].
- A broad spectrum of CN palsies result from the VZV infection. Ramsay Hunt syndrome, the most common VZV-related CN palsy, is characterized by facial palsy, vesicular eruptions (Fig. 31.1) on the auricle, and possible vestibulocochlear nerve palsy.
- VZV reactivation commonly affects the trigeminal and facial nerves. Uncommonly, the glossopharyngeal, vagus, oculomotor, trochlear, and abducens nerves are involved [6, 7].

Herpes zoster ophthalmicus, which involves the V_1 segment of the trigeminal nerve, is an ophthalmological emergency and is treated vigorously.

- The herpes simplex virus may be a causative agent in some patients with trigeminal neuralgia.
- Ocular HSV is one of the leading causes of blindness. Vestibular neuronitis, ocular neuritis, oculomotor nerve palsy, and facial palsy are reported with HSV.
- Cytomegalovirus and HSV infections have been associated with anti-GM2 antibodies and GBS variants with severe sensory loss and CN involvement.
- EBV is known to affect multiple cranial nerves.

Human Immunodeficiency Virus (HIV)

HIV is an RNA virus belonging to the family of human retroviruses (Retroviridae) and the subfamily of lentiviruses. HIV (type 1 more than 2) is reported with various cranial mononeuropathies as well as multiple neuropathies. These are seen in association with opportunistic infections and lymphoma. Rare cases have been attributed to HIV-1 itself [8, 9].

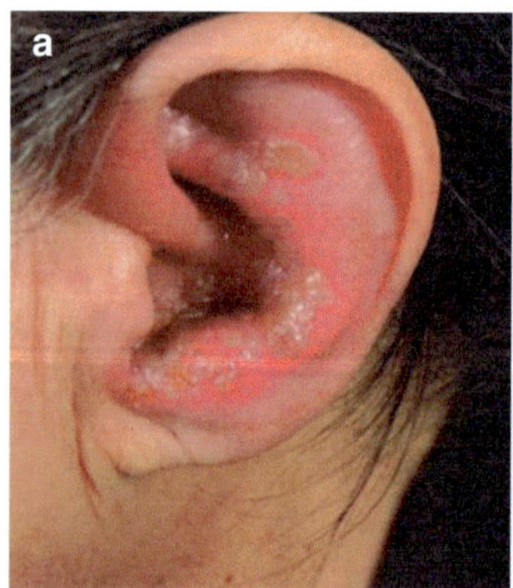
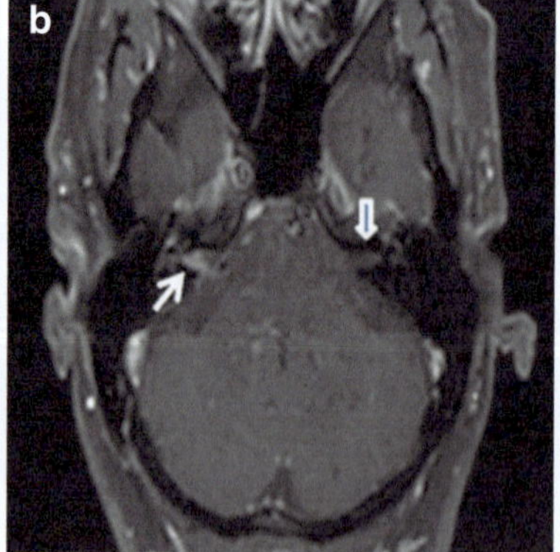
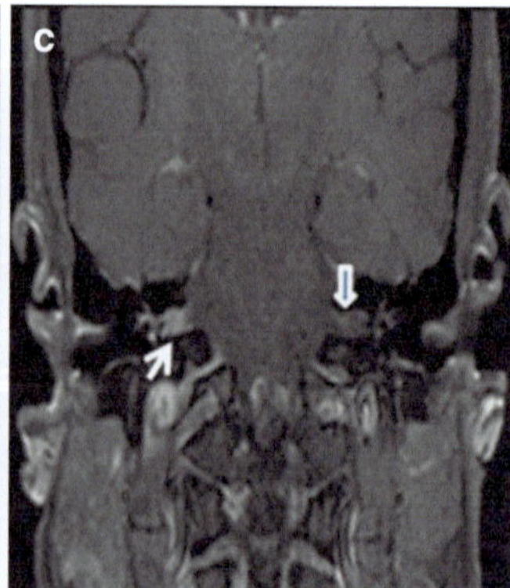

Fig. 31.1 (**a**) Vesicles on external pinna, (**b**) axial and (**c**) coronal postcontrast fat-saturated T_1-weighted imaging revealed abnormal right seventh and eighth nerve complex (shown by a solid white arrow on the right side) in the internal auditory canal as well as enhancement of the cochlea and semicircular canal compared to the left side in a patient with Ramsay Hunt syndrome. (Courtesy: (**a**) Dr. Vaidik Chauhan, ENT surgeon, Ahmedabad, Gujarat, India, and (**b**, **c**) Dr. Jaggi S, Department of Radiology, Bombay Hospital Institute of Medical Sciences, Mumbai, India)

Poliovirus

Poliovirus belongs to a family of picornaviruses (single-stranded RNA) and is an enterovirus. Ten to 15% of paralytic polio is bulbar, with the reticular formation most severely affected. CNs are affected very commonly, and CNs VII, IX, and X are most often involved. Patients have difficulty breathing or swallowing. After development and distribution of the effective vaccine, polio has become of historical importance only [10].

Other Viruses

Rabies, enteroviruses, and arboviruses (Japanese encephalitis, dengue, chikungunya) are known to lead to cranial neuropathies.

Bacteria

Tuberculosis

Central nervous system tuberculosis is prevalent in many parts of the world and is the most severe form of extrapulmonary tuberculosis. CN involvement in tuberculous meningoencephalitis (TBME) is seen in up to 45% of patients, and TBME indeed is one of the common causes of multiple CN involvement in tropical countries. In a large series, commonly involved CNs were CN II, VII, III, and VIII, in isolation and in various combinations [11]. Most of the cranial neuropathies improved without any sequelae. Optic nerve involvement in tuberculosis can be due to antituberculous treatment, hydrocephalus, optochiasmatic arachnoiditis, or papilloedema, so vision loss needs to be evaluated carefully and treatments will differ [12]. CSF mycobacterium tuberculosis (MTB) detection by multiplex polymerase chain reaction, pyrosequencing, and brain MRI with contrast are helpful in the diagnosis (Fig. 31.2). Ophthalmological evaluation is also valuable in the diagnostic process by demonstrating tubercles (Fig. 31.3).

Lyme Disease

Lyme disease is a vector-borne disease caused by *Borrelia burgdorferi* and *Borrelia mayonii*, which are spread by *Ixodes* ticks. Neurologic abnormalities are seen in about 15% of patients, often after many weeks or months into the illness [13]. Unilateral or bilateral weakness of the CN VII is common, and the optic nerve, lower CNs, and vestibulocochlear nerves can be affected. Multiple cranial neuropathies have been reported [14].

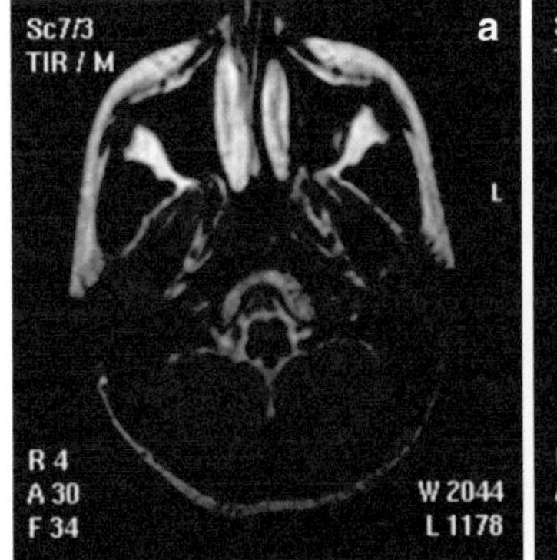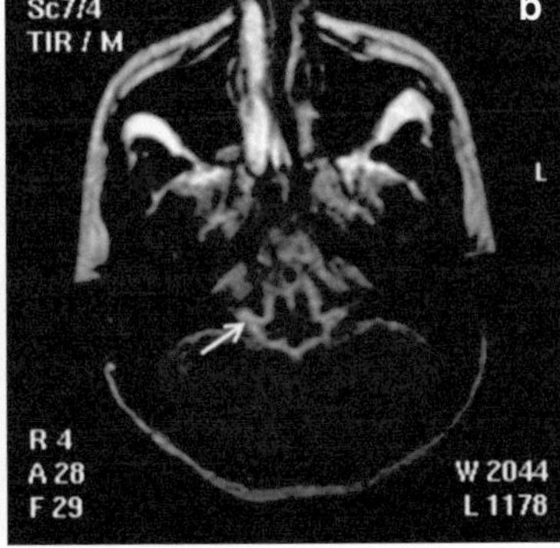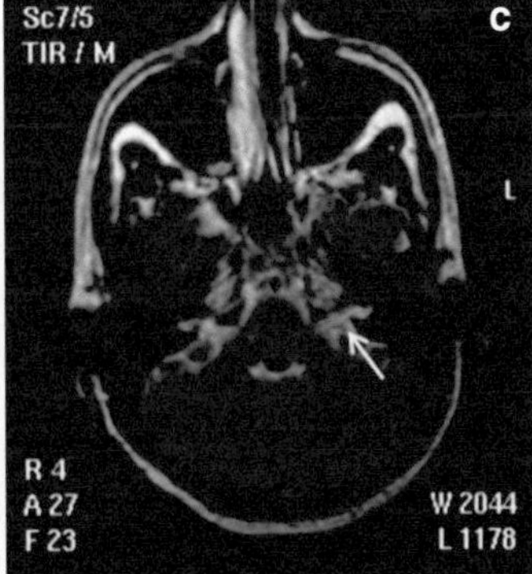

Fig. 31.2 Post-contrast FLAIR images showing diffuse enhancing exudates along the brainstem (**a**) and lower CNs (shown by white arrows) (**b, c**) in a case of TBME. (Courtesy (**a–c**): Dr Jaggi S, Department of Radiology, Bombay Hospital Institute of Medical Sciences, Mumbai, India)

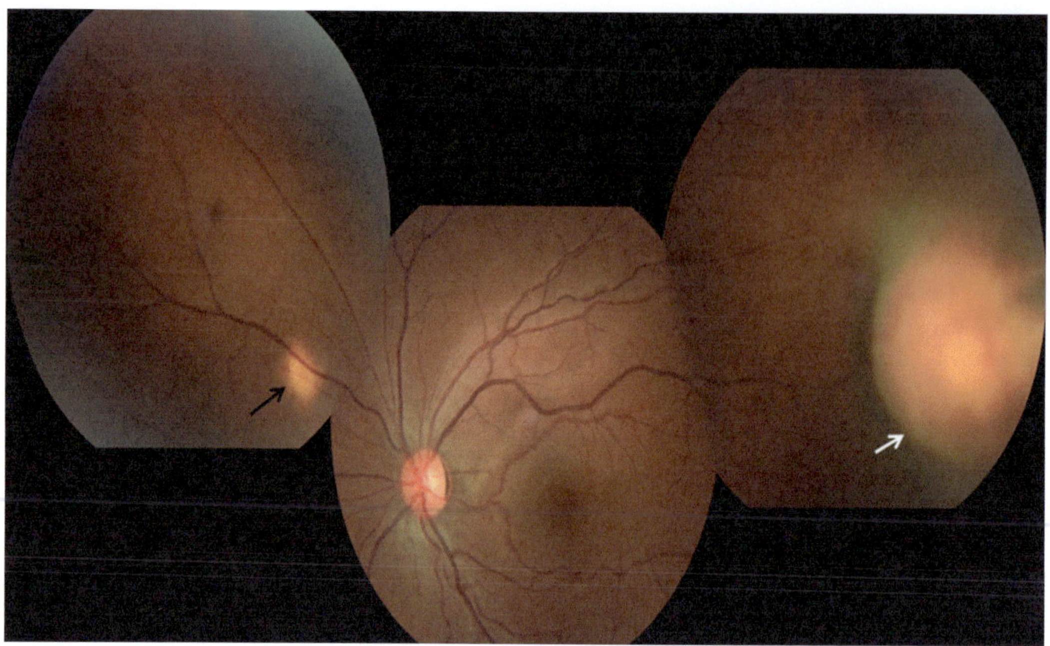

Fig. 31.3 Montage fundus photograph of the left eye of a patient with disseminated tuberculosis. The photograph shows a nasal healed choroidal tubercle (black arrow) and a large active temporal choroidal tubercle (white arrow).

(Courtesy: Dr. Morekar M, Department of Ophthalmology, Bombay Hospital Institute of Medical Sciences, Mumbai, India)

Leprosy

Leprosy, a chronic infectious disease caused by *Mycobacterium leprae*, is a common, treatable neuropathy in some parts of the world. CN paralysis in leprosy generally occurs along with peripheral neuropathy, but may also be an isolated feature. Cranial neuropathies are seen more frequently in the lepromatous type. Among various sensory modalities, temperature sense is most severely involved, and facial, trigeminal, and olfactory nerves tend to be affected [15]. Oculomotor, auditory, glossopharyngeal, vagus, spinal accessory, and hypoglossal nerves are also involved in some patients [16]. Partial paralysis of a nerve is characteristic of leprosy, and the zygomatic branch of the facial nerve which supplies the orbicularis oculi muscle is the most frequently affected [17, 18] (Fig. 31.4). There is sensory impairment, or hypopigmented and hypoesthetic patch as well, in the territory of the trigeminal nerve, especially over the maxillary branch in most cases of leprosy with facial nerve involvement. It has been postulated that the mycobacterial infection enters the malar skin through sensory fibers and progresses in such a way that it involves the peripheral motor branches of the facial nerve in the area [19].

Lepra reactions are associated with cranial neuropathies. Sensorineural hearing loss is more frequent in lepromatous leprosy with erythema nodosum leprosum reaction. Appearance of type 1 reaction puts a patient at risk of nerve damage and secondary deformities [20]. The presence of significant facial patch around the eyes or over the malar region together with type 1 lepra reaction is a risk factor for the development of lagophthalmos and paralysis of other facial muscles [21, 22]. Early recognition and medical treatment of early nerve damage with anti-leprosy medications and corticosteroids tend to result in restoration of nerve function to a large extent.

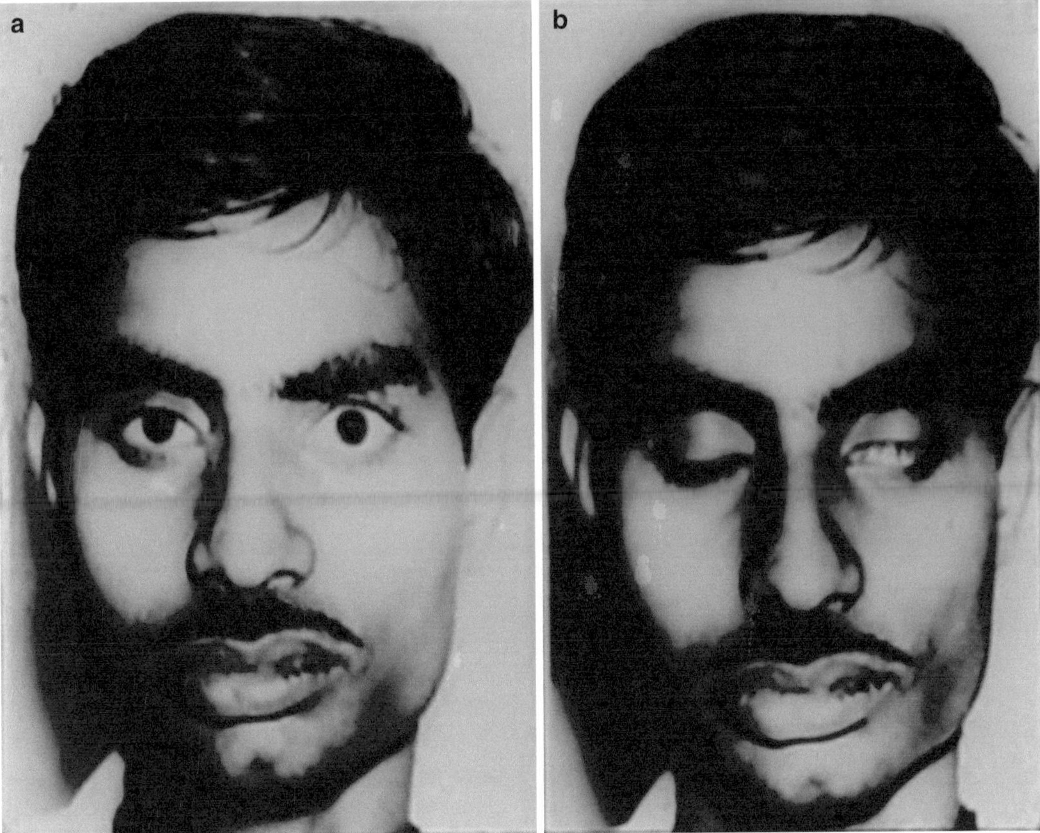

Fig. 31.4 Left-sided lagopthalmos (isolated eye closure weakness) with sparing of the lower face due to patchy facial nerve involvement in leprosy (**a, b**). (Courtesy (**a, b**): Dr Mistry N and Dr. Shetty V, Foundation for Medical Research, Mumbai, India)

Syphilis

CNs VII and VIII are most frequently involved in syphilitic basilar meningitis. Involvement of the optic [23], oculomotor, and abducens nerves has been reported [24]. Argyll Robertson pupils are characteristic of neurosyphilis. The light reflex is lost but the accommodation reflex is preserved.

Neurobrucellosis

Brucellosis is a zoonotic disease transmitted by unpasteurized milk of cows, goats, and camels. Approximately 2–5% of brucellosis sufferers will develop neurological features, referred to as neurobrucellosis [25], and CN involvement occurs in up to 25% of such patients. CN VI and VIII are particularly involved, and rarely optic neuritis has also been reported [26, 27]. Figure 31.5 shows enhancement of CNs VII, VIII, and III in a case of brucellosis.

Botulism

Botulism is caused by neurotoxin-producing *Clostridium* species. Botulinum neurotoxins are classified into 7 types, A–G [28]. Toxin types A, B, and E cause human botulism. These result in bilateral, symmetric CN palsies and flaccid limb paralysis. Early symptoms include blurry vision, diplopia, expressionless face, dysphagia, and dysarthria

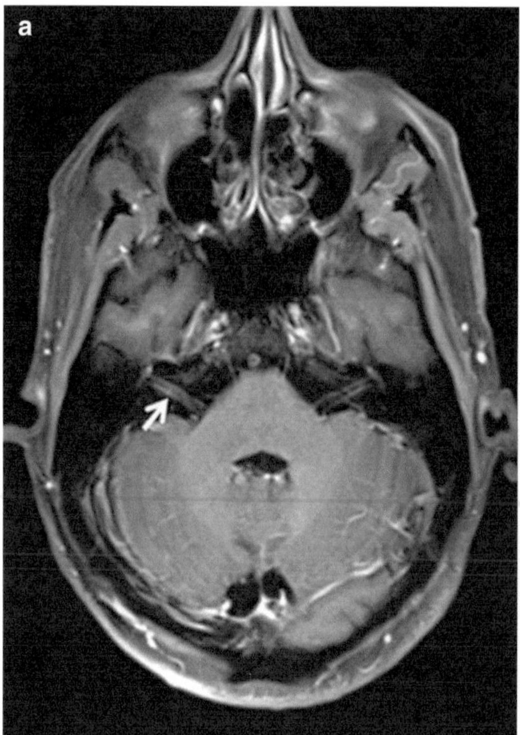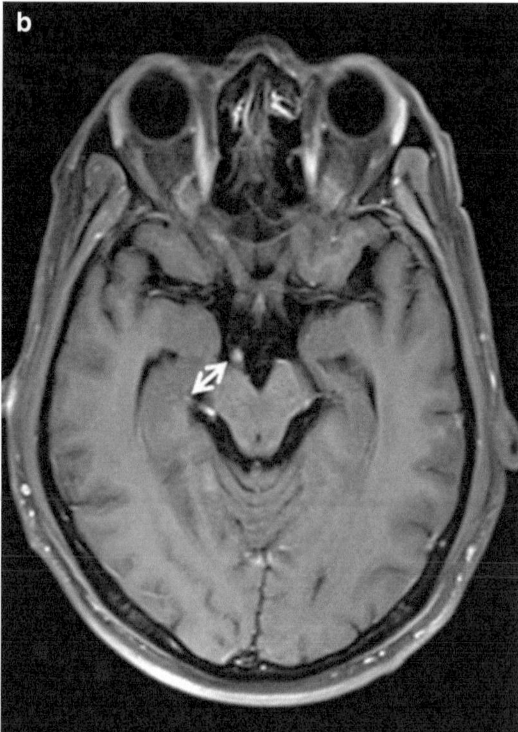

Fig. 31.5 Mild postcontrast enhancement in bilateral CN VII and VIII complex (white arrow) (**a**) and nodular post-contrast enhancement of the right CN III (white double arrow) (**b**) in neurobrucellosis. (Courtesy: Dr. Jaggi S, Department of Radiology, Bombay Hospital Institute of Medical Sciences, Mumbai, India)

followed by limb paralysis and respiratory compromise. Ocular, facial, and glossopharyngeal nerves are commonly involved.

Listeria

Listeria monocytogenes (LM) is an intracellular, facultative anaerobic gram-positive bacillus. Patients present with progressive brainstem deficits, including CN palsy (facial paresis, diplopia, dysphagia, paretic soft palate, dysarthria, and paresthesias in the trigeminal region) and cerebellar dysfunction/ataxia. CN palsy involves the oculomotor, trochlear, trigeminal, abducens, facial, glossopharyngeal, and vagus nerves. The literature shows facial and trigeminal nerve involvement very frequently [29].

Other Bacteria

Bacterial meningitis caused by *Haemophilus I influenzae*, *Streptococcus pneumoniae*, and *Neisseria meningitidis* are known to involve CN VIII. Cephalic tetanus, although a rare form of tetanus, may present with various CN palsies.

Fungi

Mucormycosis

Mucormycosis is seen in the setting of diabetes, other immunocompromised states, and, recently, in association with COVID-19. Rhino-cerebral mucormycosis is often fulminant. Black eschar may be visible on the nasal or palatine mucosa.

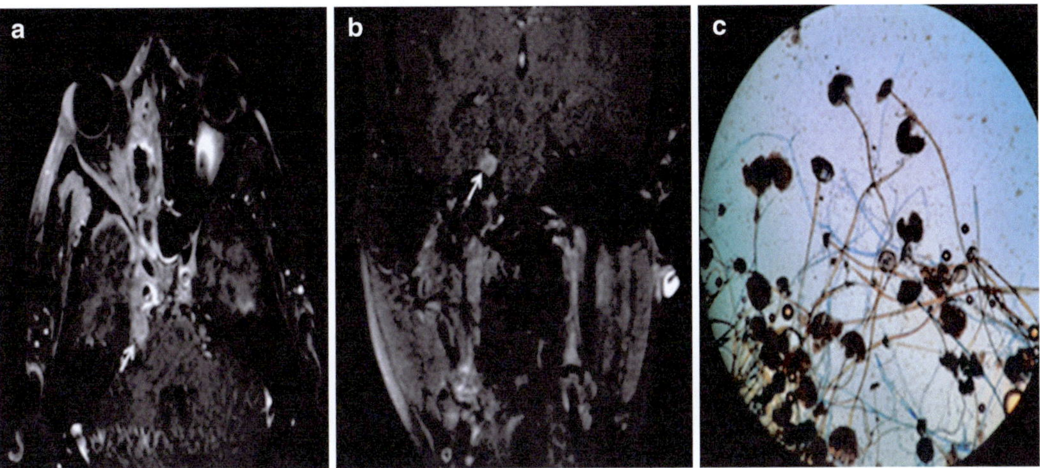

Fig. 31.6 T-weighted FLAIR axial (**a**) and coronal (**b**) images showing continuous involvement from the right trigeminal nerve (white arrow) from the right cavernous sinus to the cerebellopontine cistern. It shows diffuse thickening and post-contrast enhancement. Lactophenol cotton blue mount of mucor species (**c**) showing broad septate hyphae with mature sporangia-releasing sporangiospores. (Courtesy (**a, b**): Dr Jaggi S, Department of Radiology, Bombay Hospital Institute of Medical Sciences, Mumbai, India and (**c**) Dr Sakle A, Department of Microbiology, Bombay Hospital Institute of Medical Sciences, Mumbai, India)es, Mumbai, India)

Palatal ulceration and nasal bleeds are common. Proptosis is the most common orbital sign followed by ophthalmoplegia and visual loss. Neurological examination may reveal palsies of CNs II–VII, in addition to cerebral signs resulting from vascular compromise. A recent review of mucormycosis with COVID-19 noted that hypoxia, low immunity, hyperglycemia, and prolonged stay at the hospital may increase the risk of the development of mucor infection [30]. Imaging and staining of the mucor species are very important in diagnosis and seeing the extent (Fig. 31.6).

Cryptococcus neoformans

Cryptococcus neoformans meningitis is characterized by optic neuropathy. Necrosis of the optic nerve and chiasm by cryptococcal organisms have been described [31].

Other Fungi

Fungi like *Aspergillus* [32] and *Candida* are known to affect multiple CNs.

Parasites

Neurocysticercosis

Neurocysticercosis is the most common parasitic disease of the human central nervous system and is caused by *Taenia solium*. Seizure is the most common presentation of cerebral cysticercosis. Meningeal involvement is seen in some patients. In such patients, entrapment of CNs resulting in paralysis of extraocular muscles, hearing loss, facial nerve palsy, trigeminal neuralgia, and focal neurological symptoms related to brainstem compromise are seen in a small proportion of patients [33, 34].

Neuroschistosomiasis

Cranial neuroschistosomiasis, less common than the spinal form, is characterized by a granulomatous reaction that leads to an increase of intracranial pressure and focal neurologic signs.

Other Parasites

CN palsies in patients with toxoplasmosis are uncommon, and CN VI has been reported as a result of the mass effect. Cerebral malaria patients have been reported, with CN II, V, and VI involvement [35].

Conclusions

A wide variety of infectious agents cause CN compromise directly or indirectly. History and clinical examination can provide useful pointers to the etiology, and neuroimaging and microbiological investigations are further helpful for early recognition and effective management of these conditions. Correct diagnosis and prompt treatment are cornerstones of a good outcome.

References

1. Costello F, Dalakas MC. Cranial neuropathies and COVID-19: neurotropism and autoimmunity. Neurology. 2020;95(5):195–6 [cited 2023 Jan 30]. Available from: https://pubmed.ncbi.nlm.nih. gov/32487714/.
2. Finsterer J, Scorza FA, Scorza CA, Fiorini AC. COVID-19 associated cranial nerve neuropathy: a systematic review. Bosn J Basic Med Sci. 2022;22(1):39 [cited 2023 Jan 30]. Available from: https://www.ncbi.nlm.nih.gov/pmc/articles/ PMC8860318/.
3. Garg RK, Paliwal VK. Spectrum of neurological complications following COVID-19 vaccination. Neurol Sci. 2022;43(1):3–40 [cited 2023 Jan 30]. Available from: https://pubmed.ncbi.nlm.nih. gov/34719776/.
4. Sanjay S, Huang P, Lavanya R. Herpes zoster ophthalmicus. Curr Treat Options Neurol. 2011;13(1):79–91 [cited 2023 Jan 30]. Available from: https://pubmed. ncbi.nlm.nih.gov/21063920/.
5. Dworkin RH, Johnson RW, Breuer J, Gnann JW, Levin MJ, Backonja M, et al. Recommendations for the management of herpes zoster. Clin Infect Dis. 2007;44(Suppl 1) [cited 2023 Jan 30]. Available from: https://pubmed.ncbi.nlm.nih.gov/17143845/.
6. Tsau PW, Liao MF, Hsu JL, Hsu HC, Peng CH, Lin YC, et al. Clinical presentations and outcome studies of cranial nerve involvement in herpes zoster infection: a retrospective single-center analysis. J Clin Med. 2020;9(4) [cited 2023 Jan 30]. Available from: https://pubmed.ncbi.nlm.nih.gov/32235469/.
7. Yeh CF, Liao WH. Multiple cranial nerve palsies caused by varicella zoster virus in the absence of rash. Neurol Asia. 2016;21(1):93–5.
8. Robinson-Papp J, Simpson DM, Stucky S. Neuromuscular diseases associated with HIV-1 infection. Muscle Nerve. 2009;40(6):1043 [cited 2023 Jan 30]. Available from: https://www.ncbi.nlm. nih.gov/pmc/articles/PMC2916755/.
9. Sugimoto H, Konno S, Takamiya K, Nemoto H, Wakata N, Kurihara T. [A case of primary HIV infection presenting as mononeuritis multiplex]. Rinsho Shinkeigaku. 2006 [cited 2023 Jan 30]. Available from: https://pubmed.ncbi.nlm.nih. gov/17154036/.
10. Wasserstrom R, Mamourian AC, McGary CT, Miller G. Bulbar poliomyelitis: MR findings with pathologic correlation. AJNR Am J Neuroradiol. 1992 [cited 2023 Jan 30]. Available from: https://pubmed.ncbi. nlm.nih.gov/1595477/
11. Li X, Ma L, Zhang L, Wu X, Chen H, Gao M. Clinical characteristics of tuberculous meningitis combined with cranial nerve palsy. Clin Neurol Neurosurg. 2019;184 [cited 2023 Jan 30]. Available from: https:// pubmed.ncbi.nlm.nih.gov/31336359/.
12. Garg RK. Tuberculosis of the central nervous system. Postgrad Med J. 1999;75(881):133–40 [cited 2023 Jan 30]. Available from: https://pubmed.ncbi.nlm.nih. gov/10448488/.
13. Hildenbrand P, Craven DE, Jones R, Nemeskal P. Lyme neuroborreliosis: manifestations of a rapidly emerging zoonosis. AJNR Am J Neuroradiol. 2009;30(6):1079–87 [cited 2023 Jan 30]. Available from: https://pubmed.ncbi.nlm.nih.gov/19346313/.
14. Chaturvedi A, Baker K, Jeanmonod D, Jeanmonod R. Lyme disease presenting with multiple cranial nerve deficits: report of a case. Case rep. Emerg Med. 2016;2016:1–3 [cited 2023 Jan 30]. Available from: https://www.ncbi.nlm.nih.gov/pmc/articles/ PMC5011200/.
15. Gopinath DV, Thappa DM, Jaishankar TJ. A clinical study of the involvement of cranial nerves in leprosy. Indian J Lepr. 2004;76(1):1–9 [cited 2023 Jan 30]. Available from: https://europepmc.org/article/ med/15527054.
16. Kumar S. Cranial nerve involvement in leprosy. Indian J Lepr. 2005;77(2):177–8.
17. Khadilkar SV, Patil SB, Shetty VP. Neuropathies of leprosy. J Neurol Sci 2021;420 [cited 2023 Jan 30]. Available from: https://pubmed.ncbi.nlm.nih. gov/33360424/.
18. Reichart PA, Srisuwan S, Metah D. Lesions of the facial and trigeminal nerve in leprosy. An evaluation of 43 cases. Int J Oral Surg. 1982;11(1):14–20 [cited 2023 Jan 30]. Available from: https://pubmed.ncbi. nlm.nih.gov/6811452/.
19. Dastur DK. Pathology and pathogenesis of predilective sites of nerve damage in leprous neuritis. Nerves in the arm and the face. Neurosurg Rev. 1983;6(3):139–52 [cited 2023 Jan 30]. Available from: https://pubmed.ncbi.nlm.nih.gov/6371592/.

20. Shah PM, Dhakre VW, Prasad A, Samdani P. Multiple cranial nerve palsies secondary to a recurrence of Hansen's disease. BMJ Case Rep. 2018;2018 https://doi.org/10.1136/bcr-2017-223427.

21. de Freitas MRG, Said G. Leprous neuropathy. Handb Clin Neurol. 2013;115:499–514.

22. Kumar S, Alexander M, Gnanamuthu C. Cranial nerve involvement in patients with leprous neuropathy. Neurol India. 2006;54(3):283 [cited 2023 Jan 30]. Available from: https://www.neurologyindia.com/article.asp?issn=0028-3886;year=2006;volume=54;issue=3;spage=283;epage=285;aulast=kumar.

23. Kiss S, Damico FM, Young LH. Ocular manifestations and treatment of syphilis. Semin Ophthalmol. 2005;20(3):161–7 [cited 2023 Jan 30]. Available from: https://pubmed.ncbi.nlm.nih.gov/16282150/.

24. Musher DM. Syphilis, neurosyphilis, penicillin, and AIDS. J Infect Dis. 1991;163(6 [cited 2023 Jan 30]):1201–6. Available from: https://pubmed.ncbi.nlm.nih.gov/2037785/.

25. Bahemuka M, Rahman Shemena A, Panayiotopoulos CP, Al-Aska AK, Obeid T, Daif AK. Neurological syndromes of brucellosis. J Neurol Neurosurg Psychiatry. 1988;51(8):1017–21 [cited 2023 Jan 30]. Available from: https://pubmed.ncbi.nlm.nih.gov/3145961/.

26. Shakir RA, Al-din ASN, Araj GF, Lulu AR, Mousa AR, Saadah MA. Clinical categories of neurobrucellosis. A report on 19 cases. Brain. 1987;110(Pt 1):213–23 [cited 2023 Jan 30]. Available from: https://pubmed.ncbi.nlm.nih.gov/3801851/.

27. Bodur H, Erbay A, Akinci E, Çolpan A, Çevik MA, Balaban N. Neurobrucellosis in an endemic area of brucellosis. Scand J Infect Dis. 2003;35(2):94–7 [cited 2023 Jan 30]. Available from: https://pubmed.ncbi.nlm.nih.gov/12693557/.

28. CDC Botulism | Diagnosis and Laboratory Guidance for Clinicians. [cited 2023 Jan 30]. Available from: https://emergency.cdc.gov/agent/botulism/clinicians/diagnosis.asp.

29. Arslan F, Ertan G, Emecen AN, Fillatre P, Mert A, Vahaboglu H. Clinical presentation and cranial MRI findings of Listeria monocytogenes encephalitis: a literature review of case series. Neurologist. 2018;23(6):198–203 [cited 2023 Jan 30]. Available from: https://pubmed.ncbi.nlm.nih.gov/30379745/.

30. Singh AK, Singh R, Joshi SR, Misra A. Mucormycosis in COVID-19: a systematic review of cases reported worldwide and in India. Diabetes Metab Syndr. 2021;15(4) [cited 2023 Jan 30]. Available from: https://pubmed.ncbi.nlm.nih.gov/34192610/.

31. Merkler AE, Gaines N, Simpson SA, Dinkin MJ, Baradaran H, Schuetz AN, et al. Direct invasion of the optic nerves, chiasm, and tracts by Cryptococcus neoformans in an immunocompetent host. Neurohospitalist. 2015;5(4):217 [cited 2023 Jan 30]. Available from: https://www.ncbi.nlm.nih.gov/pmc/articles/PMC4572381/.

32. Nadkarni T, Goel A. Aspergilloma of the brain: an overview. J Postgrad Med. 2005;51(5):S37.

33. Garcia HH, Nash TE, del Brutto OH. Clinical symptoms, diagnosis, and treatment of neurocysticercosis. Lancet Neurol. 2014;13(12):1202–15 [cited 2023 Jan 30]. Available from: http://www.thelancet.com/article/S1474442214700948/fulltext.

34. García HH, Evans CAW, Nash TE, Takayanagui OM, White AC, Botero D, et al. Current consensus guidelines for treatment of neurocysticercosis. Clin Microbiol Rev. 2002;15(4):747 [cited 2023 Jan 30]. Available from: https://www.ncbi.nlm.nih.gov/pmc/articles/PMC126865/.

35. Shikani HJ, Freeman BD, Lisanti MP, Weiss LM, Tanowitz HB, Desruisseaux MS. Cerebral malaria: we have come a long way. Am J Pathol. 2012;181(5):1484–92 [cited 2023 Jan 30]. Available from: https://pubmed.ncbi.nlm.nih.gov/23021981/.

Bullet Points

- In head trauma, injuries of the cranial nerves should be suspected.
- Early recognition and treatment of cranial nerve lesions are important to avoid severe disability.

Introduction

Cranial nerve lesions are often seen in cranial trauma. They must be recognized since their sequelae can be disabling (e.g., hearing or vision loss, facial asymmetry).

Suggestive findings include nasal and ear bleeds, cerebrospinal fluid rhinorrhea or otorrhea, pupillary asymmetry, alteration of light reflex, proptosis, absent corneal reflex, and asymmetry of eye closure and facial muscles. In cooperating patients, finger counting, ocular movements, diplopia, hearing impairment, swallowing difficulties, and dysarthria can be assessed rapidly.

In studies and case series, the incidence of cranial nerve lesions in head trauma shows a high variability, from 5% to 23% in one study [1] to 1% in another large 2021 study based on the Register of the German Trauma Society [2], in

moderate to severe traumatic brain injury. Even minor head trauma is associated with cranial nerve lesions in 0.3% of cases [3].

Causes

The major causes of traumatic cranial nerve injuries are traffic-related accidents and falls. Aggression (gunshot, stabbing, blows) is much less frequent. Wartime injuries cause extensive bony and soft tissue disruption with high risk of cranial nerve lesions. Approximately 97% of cases are caused by blunt trauma, with only 3% occurring from penetrating injuries [2].

The incidence of cranial nerve injury is higher in cases with facial lesions, damage to the eye and ear, and orbital and skull base fractures [4].

Multiple mechanisms are involved in traumatic lesions of the cranial nerves, including shearing forces, bone lesions with nerve compression/transection or skull base fractures, direct or penetrating injuries, and secondary injuries from compression by hematoma or edema [5].

Posttraumatic cranial nerve lesions may also appear in combinations:

- Cranial nerves II, III, IV and VI – lesion in superior orbital fissure
- Cranial nerves I and II—in orbital fractures
- Cranial nerves VII and VIII—fractures of the temporal bone

Authors of this chapter: Tudor Lupescu and Doriana Lupescu.

The lower cranial nerves IX, X, XI, and XII are rarely injured, and if they are, injuries are almost never individually but in combination. Such injuries are seen in more severe cases, with higher mortality rates. In a study of 23 patients with Glasgow Coma Scale scores of 3–5, 21 had injuries of cranial nerves IX–XII [6].

Individual Cranial Nerve Lesions

Cranial Nerve I

Head trauma is the most common cause of olfactory nerve lesion, and anosmia is the most common manifestation of cranial nerve injury following trauma [5].

Different mechanisms are involved [7]:

- Stretching, shearing, or avulsion of the nerve in occipital or lateral head trauma, with contrecoup lesion (acceleration/deceleration forces).
- Direct tearing of the nerve filaments in a skull base fracture involving the lamina cribrosa.
- Edema, hematoma, or ischemia secondary to a craniocerebral trauma.

Cranial Nerve II

A traumatic impact on the brow region can cause a downward displacement of the orbital wall. The intraorbital content oscillates, causing stretching of the optic nerve and injury to the intraneural microvasculature and nerve fibers [8]. The nerve can be directly impacted by a bone fragment; fractures involving the optic canal can cause nerve contusion or laceration. An initial testing of visual acuity is important as a reference when vision seems to fade. Retinal damage is assessed structurally by ocular coherence tomography and functionally by electroretinography. MRI evaluates the integrity of the nerve, while visual evoked potentials assess optic nerve function [9]. Computed tomography (CT) can show bony lesions that compress the optic nerve.

There is no definite consensus on the management of cranial nerve II lesions. Controversial approaches include the use of corticosteroids and the timing of surgical decompression. Some studies recommend corticosteroids initially in all patients, whether treated conservatively or surgically [9, 10]. Nerve decompression is urgent in retrobulbar hematoma or compressive bony fragments. With preserved vision that improves, visual evoked potentials can monitor the evolution. When amelioration continues, the outcome is favorable. In patients with an initial slight recovery, which does not progress further, surgery is considered. Recent studies suggest better outcomes occur with surgery when visual acuity decreases sharply or is completely lost in a conscious patient, or with continuing alteration of vision on conservative therapy. Surgery is recommended to be done within 3 days [6].

Cranial Nerve III

In head trauma, recognizing oculomotor nerve dysfunction is important since it may account for life-threatening conditions. Proptosis and periorbital swelling limit the examination. Examination should focus on signs of dysfunction of other cranial nerves, associated neurological findings, and the level of consciousness. Imaging studies further contribute to a better diagnosis.

Important situations:

- Hemispheric hematoma with transtentorial herniation, secondary compression of the oculomotor nerve. Urgent surgery is mandatory.
- Shearing forces may injure the intraparenchymatous part of the nerve; other brainstem structures can be involved (Weber and Benedikt syndrome).
- With stretching or avulsion at the pedunculopontine junction, normal consciousness is regained, but cranial nerve III deficit remains complete [11].
- Associated oculomotor nerve lesions point to lesions in the cavernous sinus or superior orbital fissure; skull base fractures can also be found. Ocular pulsations and a bruit over the

eyeball suggest a carotid–cavernous fistula. Sometimes surgery is necessary.

- In orbital trauma with bony wall fractures, extraocular muscles can be injured.

In compressive lesions, removal of the causative factor ameliorates nerve function [5]. Nerve recovery is often slow and incomplete. Regeneration may be aberrant (lid elevation or pupillo-constriction with eye adduction) [12]. In complete lesions, extraocular muscle surgery is an option, aiming for binocular vision in a primary eye position [13].

Cranial Nerve IV

Trochlear palsy is the most common cause of vertical diplopia [14]. The nerve is vulnerable in blows to the head, with sudden deceleration causing compression by the brainstem against the tentorium cerebelli. Its thinness and the length of its passage after exiting the midbrain up to the cavernous sinus make it vulnerable in head trauma, with an incidence of approximately 2% [15, 16]. It is usually injured together with other oculomotor nerves. A recent study has shown that the etiology was traumatic in 14.2% of isolated trochlear nerve palsies. Bilateral trochlear nerve palsy is caused by craniocerebral trauma in about 50% of cases [17].

Diagnosis requires a cooperating patient with diplopia compensated by head tilt (Bielschowsky's sign). Diplopia is accentuated when reading or walking downstairs.

Cranial Nerve VI

Head trauma is responsible for 3–15% of abducens nerve lesions [18]. It can be injured together with other ocular motor nerves in the cavernous sinus. The fixed position between the petroclinoid ligament and the cavernous sinus makes it susceptible to stretching and tearing. It is vulnerable in skull base fractures.

Abducens palsies have favorable outcomes with recovery in a few months. Isolated abducens nerve lesions have better prognosis than cases with multiple cranial nerve lesions. In persistent, significant deficits, surgery can help.

Cranial Nerve V

Head trauma can injure branches of the trigeminal nerve. The supraorbital and supratrochlear nerves are injured in trauma of the forehead and orbit. Lesion of the infraorbital nerve is seen in maxillofacial trauma. Mandible fractures can cause lesions of the mandibular branch of the trigeminal nerve. In skull base fractures involving the cavernous sinus, injury of the ophthalmic branch is associated with ocular motor nerve lesions. The clinical picture is similar in injuries at the superior orbital fissure after orbital fractures. Skull base fractures of the middle cerebral fossa can extend into the foramen rotundum and foramen ovale, injuring the maxillary and mandibular divisions, respectively. Injuries of branches of the trigeminal nerve cause sensory disturbances in their cutaneous distribution. Usually, hypoesthesia is dominant, but sometimes hyperpathia may occur [19].

Management depends on the clinical situation. In trigeminal neuralgia, carbamazepine or gabapentin is used. In refractory cases, root section or radiofrequency ablation can be done. When possible, surgical treatment is considered. Microsurgical approaches with end-to-end anastomosis or nerve grafting have favorable outcomes [20]. Early repair is ideal.

Cranial Nerve VII

Head trauma is the second most common lesion cause after Bell's palsy. Injuries can occur intracranially or extracranially. Head trauma can act as a deceleration force, with nerve injury at its tethering at the geniculate ganglion. Shearing forces result, with intraneural contusion, edema and hemorrhage, and even nerve transection. Temporal bone fractures (Figs. 32.1 and 32.2) are classified into longitudinal and transverse, depending on the orientation of the fracture line

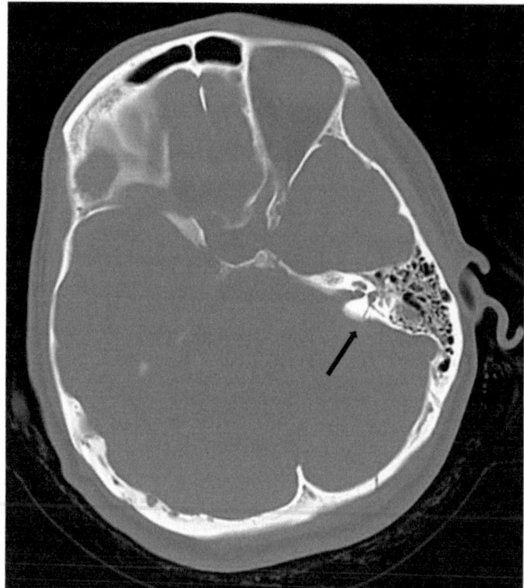

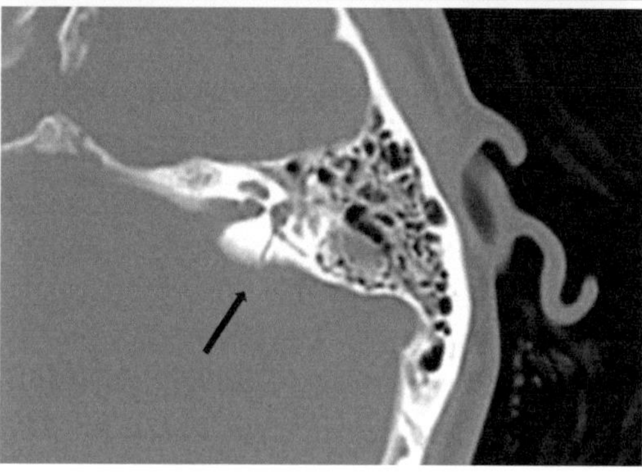

Fig. 32.1 Transverse temporal bone fracture (arrows)

Neurophysiology and imaging are useful for establishing a therapeutic plan. Electromyography and conduction studies (EMG) evaluate nerve continuity and the degree of injury. A motor response amplitude reduction to less than 10% compared to the healthy side is seen in severe lesions and decompressive surgery is considered. Voluntary activity recorded with needle electrodes from facial muscles carries a good prognosis for recovery.

In delayed facial nerve palsy, nerve integrity is assumed; a conservative approach is indicated with a good recovery in most of the cases. In immediate, complete paralysis, the question is whether nerve continuity is preserved or not (axonotmesis vs. neurotmesis). Electrodiagnosis is helpful and, together with the clinical progression, guides the therapeutic pathway towards either a conservative approach or surgical nerve decompression. Recent studies show a better outcome with early decompression, mainly in patients with severe denervation 6 days from the onset.

Corticosteroids can be used either alone or before surgery, especially in incomplete or delayed facial nerve palsies, and act by reducing nerve edema within the bony facial canal. Although their efficacy is debated, there are studies that show they might hasten recovery [23–25].

In nerve transections, end-to-end nerve anastomosis is the best option, provided that the connection is tension-free. Alternatively, interpositional nerve grafting (sural or greater auricular nerves) is considered.

In extratemporal traumatic lesions, surgical repair of the nerve is urgent. The zygomatic and buccal branches have priority, being essential for eye closure and facial expression.

With incomplete eye closure, lubricating substances are applied. During sleep a tape keeps the eyelids closed. A temporary tarsorrhaphy can be performed. Later, placement of a gold weight, permanent tarsorrhaphy, or shortening of the lids is considered [18].

with regard to the long axis of the petrous bone [21]. Longitudinal fractures are more frequent (75%), but associate with fewer facial nerve injuries. They are caused by edema and inflammation, secondary to compression within the inextensible bony canal. Although rare, transverse fractures more often (in 50% of cases) cause severe nerve injuries (transections) [21, 22]. Extracranially, the nerve is injured in traumatic penetrating lesions that intercept it after exiting the stylomastoid foramen. After head trauma, facial palsy can occur immediately, or later, up to 24 h. Delayed paralysis has a better prognosis, being caused by edema within the epineurium or an expanding hematoma.

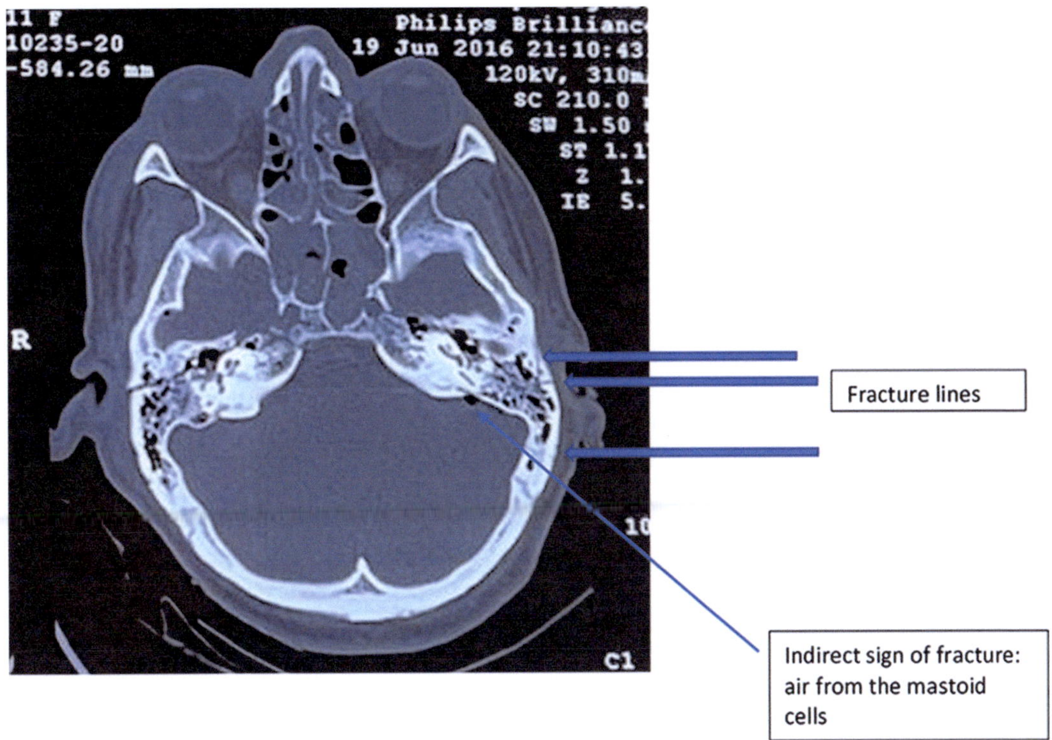

Fig. 32.2 Skull base fracture extending to the mastoid

Cranial Nerve VIII

The vestibulocochlear nerve is vulnerable within the auditory canal in petrous bone fractures. Injury of the vestibule and the cochlea can be associated. Another potential lesion site is at the internal acoustic meatus. In severe craniocerebral trauma with bleeding from the ear or a Battle sign, there is high suspicion of injury of cranial nerve VIII. Otoscopy can show hemotympanum or liquor tympanum. Facial nerve trauma is often associated.

Specific diagnostic tests are useful. Audiograms differentiate sensorineural from conductive hearing loss. Electrocochleography and auditory brainstem responses can identify the affected structure (end organ, nerve, central structures). In blast injuries caused by explosions, hearing loss and tinnitus are often seen [26].

Sometimes posttraumatic vertigo can be very disabling. With injury of the labyrinthine end organ, the loss of balance is very severe. MRI shows hemorrhage in a semicircular canal. Conservative treatment is applied. If this approach fails, labyrinthectomy (hearing sacrificing) or selective vestibular nerve section (hearing preserving) is considered. Disconnection from the injured vestibular end organ is expected to promote central nervous system plasticity, with compensation from the contralateral healthy side as well as from vision and proprioception [27].

Cranial Nerves IX, X, and XI

The glossopharyngeal, vagus, and accessory nerves share a common pathway after exiting the jugular foramen. They can be injured in traumatic lesions of the posterior skull base, in fractures of the petrous bone that extend to the jugular foramen, and in penetrating injuries to the ear or neck (e.g., gunshot, stabbing). The glossopharyngeal nerve is rarely injured alone in trauma [28, 29].

Lesions of the vagus nerve can cause severe dysfunction of the larynx and the pharynx. In acute unilateral recurrent laryngeal nerve lesions, surgical repair is not required. Recording voluntary activity in laryngeal EMG carries a good prognosis but needs special expertise. With persistent absence of voluntary activity in laryngeal muscles, complete nerve degeneration is assumed and surgery is indicated. Another approach is early surgical exploration of the lesion along with nerve reconstruction. Various techniques are used (e.g., end-to-end anastomosis, free nerve graft), with reasonably positive outcomes.

Stridor is an alarming symptom of airway obstruction in bilateral recurrent laryngeal nerve lesions. Tracheotomy must be performed urgently.

Cranial Nerve XI

The accessory nerve can be injured either proximally near the skull base and the jugular foramen (together with cranial nerves IX and X) or distally in the posterior triangle of the neck (more common). Distal palsies are caused by blows to the shoulder in motor vehicle accidents, shoulder dislocation with nerve traction, or more rarely bites to the neck or attempted hanging and strangulation.

In blunt trauma and traction injuries, physical therapy is recommended initially. With no clinical and EMG signs of recovery, surgery is indicated within a few months. Neurolysis, neurorrhaphy, or nerve grafting can be done, usually with a favorable outcome. In penetrating injuries with nerve transection, either primary repair or tagging the terminal ends can be performed [30].

Cranial Nerve XII

Cranial nerve XII is rarely injured in head trauma [31, 32]. Delayed onset of a hypoglossal nerve palsy after a hyperextension neck injury, usually from a traffic accident, should alert to an internal carotid artery dissection. Prompt ther-

apy can prevent a potentially devastating stroke. Imaging studies are essential, with MRI to assess lesions close to the medulla, magnetic resonance angiography for internal carotid artery dissection, and CT scan for bony lesions. In acute nerve injuries, surgical repair should be performed immediately. A tension-free repair is essential, either by end-to-end anastomosis or interposition grafts [33].

Multiple CN Lesions in Trauma

In about two-thirds of traumatic injury cases there are isolated cranial nerve injuries, while in one-third there are multiple cranial nerves involved [15]. The involvement of multiple cranial nerves can occur due to either a lesion in regions where more cranial nerves have a common trajectory or after an intense traumatic impact with extended bony lesions, i.e., fracture of the skull base that extends to the clivus or that intercepts the foramen jugulare.

Skull base fractures are often seen in severe craniocerebral trauma. The fracture lines often extend to other neighboring structures and can involve the olfactory, oculomotor, trigeminal, glossopharyngeal, vagus, and accessory nerves.

Some cranial nerve injuries are almost always associated with specific skull lesions, e.g., optic nerve lesions are almost always associated with orbital fracture. Similarly, nuclear and infranuclear facial and vestibulocochlear nerve palsies are associated with temporal bone fractures in almost all cases.

Imaging

Imaging studies in patients with head trauma and cranial nerve injuries show important findings in approximately two-thirds of cases, most frequently skull fracture, epidural hematomas, and brain contusions. Significant data are obtained by MRI for nerve integrity and CT scan for bone lesions (e.g., fractures, bony fragments).

Electrophysiology

Neurophysiological investigations are used in cases in which functional data were important in the diagnostic evaluation. Visual evoked potentials have been shown to reliably evaluate the function of the optic nerves and can be used even in comatose patients. In facial nerve lesions, nerve conduction velocity and EMG are used to evaluate the extent of the lesion, the prognosis, and thus the indication for surgery. Surgical results can be monitored.

Multidisciplinary Approach

Traumatic cranial nerve lesions are not isolated; they are seen in complex patients that have been exposed to severe traumatic events that may have involved other organs and body parts. Specialists in emergency medicine stabilize the vital functions in severe cases. These patients may suffer important bone lesions, sometimes including the spine, that must be dealt with by orthopedic surgeons. A detailed neurological examination is very important. Neurosurgery is frequently mandatory in such cases. Depending on the associated lesions, ophthalmology and ENT specialists are needed. Plastic and reconstructive surgery is necessary in nerve repair procedures.

Discussion

Recognizing cranial nerve lesions in traumatic injuries is important for two reasons. First, they may represent an important clue to recognizing potentially life-threatening conditions. Second, with the proper and prompt therapeutic management, some of the nerve lesions can be treated (Table 32.1).

Any cranial nerve can be injured in head trauma. In one-third of cases, more than one cranial nerve is affected. Frequently involved are the olfactory, facial, trochlear, and optic nerves.

Table 32.1 Positive and negative prognostic factors in cranial nerve trauma

	Positive prognosis	Negative prognosis
Olfactory nerve	Temporary compression by edema or a hematoma	Imaging: lesions of lamina cribrosa
Optic nerve	Preserved (even if) diminished visual acuity No significant bone lesions (CT), present visual evoked potentials Decompressive surgery	Orbital fracture Absent visual acuity Absent visual evoked potentials Declining visual acuity
Oculomotor nerves	Removal of the causative factor in compressive lesions, incomplete nerve lesion No CT lesion	Skull base fracture
Trigeminal nerve	Incomplete nerve lesion	Skull base fracture involving cavernous sinus, foramen ovale, or foramen rotundum
Facial nerve	Intact nerve, incomplete facial palsy, delayed onset Preserved nerve conduction, voluntary EMG activity	Transverse temporal bone fracture (transection) Absent nerve conduction Absent voluntary EMG activity
Vestibulocochlear nerve	Conductive hearing loss Tinnitus	Transverse temporal bone fracture (nerve transection) Complete deafness
Glossopharyngeal, vagus, accessory	Accessory elongation	Skull base fracture with foramen jugulare syndrome Crush injuries
Hypoglossal nerve	Neck stretch/hyperextension injuries with secondary carotid artery dissections and tongue paresis	Penetrating wounds

Clinical evaluation must be followed by imaging studies, e.g., CT scan and MRI. Although cranial nerves may be injured in minor head trauma, evidence of fractures of the skull base, temporal bones, or orbit is associated with an increased probability of severe cranial nerve injuries, with low chances for a significant recovery. When bony fragments compress a nerve, urgent surgery can have a positive outcome.

Neurophysiology (visual evoked potentials, EMG) may help in the assessment of optic and facial nerve functional status. Complete lesions of cranial nerves are followed by important disabilities: anosmia, blindness, or deafness. Some of the lesions can benefit from plastic surgery nerve repair procedures.

Recommendations

- A thorough evaluation, including knowledge regarding the traumatic circumstances, a clinical examination, and imaging and neurophysiological data, shapes the therapeutic approach.
- In cases with incomplete nerve lesions with preserved function and rapid improvement, the outcome is good with a conservative approach.
- In cases with important cranial nerve dysfunction, early surgery is essential for preservation of nerve viability and functional recovery.

References

1. Keane JR, Baloh RW. Post-traumatic cranial neuropathies. In: Evans RW, editor. The neurology of trauma. Philadelphia: Saunders; 1992. p. 849–68.
2. Huckhagel T, Riedel C, Rohde V. Cranial nerve injuries in patients with moderate to severe head trauma—analysis of 91196 patients from Trauma Register DGUÒ between 2008 and 2017. Clin Neurol Neurosurg. 2022;212:107089.
3. Coello AF, Canals AG, Gonzalez JM. Cranial nerve injury after minor head trauma. J Neurosurg. 2010;113:547–55.
4. Tay A, Zuniga G. Clinical characteristics of trigeminal nerve injury referrals to a university center. Int J Oral Maxillofac Surg. 2007;36:922–7.
5. Bhatoe HS. Trauma to the cranial nerves. Indian J Neurotrauma. 2007;4(2):89–100.
6. Jin H, Wang S, Hou L, Pan C, Li B, Wang H. Clinical treatment of traumatic brain injury complicated by cranial nerve injury. Injury. 2010;41:918–23.
7. Dubal PM, Svider PF, Gupta A, Eloy JA. Injuries of the cranial nerves. In: Nerves and nerve injuries, vol. 2. Elsevier Ltd.; 2015. p. 459–60.
8. Gross CE, DeKock JR, Panje WR. Evidence for orbital deformity that may contribute to monocular blindness following minor frontal head trauma. J Neurosurg. 1981;55:963–6.
9. Mahapatra AK, Tandon DA. A prospective study of 250 patients with optic nerve injury. In: Samii M, editor. Skull base: anatomy, radiology and management. Basel: S Karger; 1994. p. 305–9.
10. Murari G, Duraipandi K. Cranial nerve injuries in adult faciomaxillary trauma: prospective study in a tertiary referral centre. Int J Otorhinolaryngol Head Neck Surg. 2019;5(5):1264–9.
11. Memon MY, Paine KWE. Direct injury of the oculomotor nerve in craniocerebral trauma. J Neurosurg. 1971;35:461–4.
12. Walsh FB. Third nerve regeneration. Br J Ophthalmol. 1957;41:577–98.
13. Arias MJ. Bilateral traumatic abducens nerve palsy without skull fracture and with cervical spine fracture: case report and review of literature. Neurosurgery. 1985;16:232–4.
14. Kline LB, Demeter JL, Tavakoli M. Disorders of the fourth cranial nerve. J Neuro-Oncol. 2021;41(2):176–93.
15. Patel P, Kalyanaraman S, Reginal J. Post-traumatic cranial nerve injury. Indian J Neurotrauma. 2005;2(1):27–32.
16. Sydnor CF, Seaber JH, Buckley E. Traumatic superior oblique palsies. Ophthalmology. 1982;89:134–8.
17. Kim HJ, Kim H, Choi JY. Etiologic distribution of isolated trochlear palsy: analysis of 1020 patients and literature review. Eur J Neurol. 2022;29(12):3658–65.
18. Roofe SB, Kolb CM, Seibert J. Cranial nerve injuries (Chap 18). In: Brennan JA, Holt GR, Thomas RW, editors. Otorlaryngology/head and neck surgery combat casualty care in operation Iraqi freedom and operation enduring freedom. Fort Sam Houston, TX: Borden Institute; 2015. p. 214–7.
19. Becker M, Kohler R, Delavelle J. Pathology of the trigeminal nerve. Neuroimaging Clin N Am. 2008;18:283–307.
20. Bagheri SC, Meyer RA, Khan HA. Microsurgical repair of peripheral trigeminal nerve injuries from maxillofacial trauma. J Oral Maxillofac Surg. 2009;67:1791–9.
21. Hasso AN, Ledington JA. Traumatic injuries of the temporal bone. Otolaryngol Clin N Am. 1988;21:295–316.
22. Coker NJ, Kendall KA, Jenkins HA. Traumatic intratemporal facial nerve injury: management rationale for preservation of function. Otolaryngol Head Neck Surg. 1987;97:262–9.
23. Kim J, Moon IS, Lee W-S. Effect of delayed decompression after early steroid treatment on facial func-

tion of patients with facial paralysis. Acta Otolaryngol (Stockh). 2010;130(1):179–84.

24. Lee PH, Liang CC, Huang SF, Liao HT. The outcome analysis of traumatic facial nerve palsy treated with systemic steroid therapy. J Craniofac Surg. 2018;29(7):1842–7.

25. Siang PG, Ying XT, Dayang Suhana AM, Ing PT. Surgical outcomes of transmastoid facial nerve decompression: preliminary data from a Malaysian tertiary hospital from 2013–2018. Med J Malaysia. 2020;75(3):281–5.

26. Lew HL, Jerger JF, Guillory SB, Henry JA. Auditory dysfunction in traumatic brain injury. J Rehab Res Dev. 2007;44(7):921–8.

27. Aziz KM, Alexander KY, Douglas C, Raymond FS. Chapter 204: Management of cranial nerve injuries. In: Schmidek & Sweet operative neurosurgical techniques—indications, methods, and results. 6th ed. Elsevier/Saunders; 2012. p. 2329–38.

28. Eibling DE, Boyd EM. Rehabilitation of lower cranial nerve deficits. Otolaryngol Clin N Am. 1997;30(5):865–75.

29. Legros B, Fournier P, Chiaroni P. Basal fracture of the skull and lower cranial nerves palsy: four case reports including two fractures of the occipital condyle—a literature review. J Trauma. 2000;48(2):342–8.

30. Kim DH, Cho YJ, Tiel RL, et al. Surgical outcomes of 111 spinal accessory nerve injuries. Neurosurgery. 2003;53(5):1106–12.

31. Delamont RS, Boyle RS. Traumatic hypoglossal nerve palsy. Clin Exp Neurol. 1989;26:239–41.

32. Keane JR. Twelfth-nerve palsy. Analysis of 100 cases. Arch Neurol. 1996;53:561–6.

33. Avitia S, Osborne RF. Surgical management of iatrogenic hypoglossal nerve injury. Ear Nose Throat J. 2008;87:672–6.

Bullet Points

- Autoimmune myasthenia gravis is the most frequent cause of fluctuating ocular symptoms. Several tests exist to diagnose ocular myasthenia clinically.
- Botulism is a rare cause of diplopia and usually associated with ptosis and mydriasis, which are typically preceded by gastrointestinal and autonomic symptoms.
- Neurovascular compression is the most frequent cause of the other rare forms of paroxysmal cranial nerve disorders: superior oblique myokymia, primary facial hemispasm, vestibular paroxysmia, and hemilingual spasm.

Neuromuscular Transmission Disorders

Myasthenia Gravis

Myasthenia gravis (MG) has a prevalence of 15–35/100,000 and an annual incidence of 0.8–2.9/100,000 [1, 2] and is caused by an immune-mediated postsynaptic defect of neuromuscular transmission. Approximately 15% of patients have pure ocular symptoms, and some display only bulbar symptoms, while the remainder have more generalized weakness. However, ocular symptoms are frequently the presenting symptom, and generalized weakness develops in the course of the disease.

The typical feature of MG is use-dependent weakness: symptoms emerge or get worse with repeated use and as the day progresses. Typical ocular symptoms are ptosis and diplopia. Ptosis is frequently asymmetric, and diplopia varies in severity and muscles involved. Involvement of bulbar muscles results in slurred dysarthric speech, impaired swallowing, or neck extensor weakness, which can in severe cases cause a dropped head syndrome.

A number of clinical signs and tests can aid the diagnosis of ocular or bulbar MG:

- *Cogan's lid twitch sign*: Patients with ptosis are asked to gaze downwards for 15 s and then return to primary gaze. The sign is present when the affected eye lid briefly "twitches" upward on returning to primary gaze.
- *Curtain sign*: Performed in patients with asymmetric ptosis; when the examiner lifts the eyelid of the more affected eye, ptosis in the less affected eye increases.
- *Rest test*: Performed in patients with ptosis; following 2 min of rest with eyes closed, there is an improvement in ptosis.
- *Ice pack test*: Performed in patients with ptosis; an ice pack is placed over the ptotic eyelid

---

Author of this chapter: Wolfgang N. Löscher.

for up to 2 min. An improvement of ptosis is considered as positive.

- *Simson test*: Worsening of ptosis during 1–2 min of upwards gaze.
- *Edrophonium (tensilon) test*: Intravenous injection of up to 10 mg of edrophonium results in sudden improvement of ptosis, diplopia, or dysarthria, which lasts for a few minutes only. Asthma and bradyarrhythmias are contraindications.

Of these, the ice pack tests and the edrophonium test have has the highest sensitivity and specificity, especially in the evaluation of ptosis [3, 4].

A neuromuscular transmission defect can also be ascertained using repetitive low-frequency 3-Hz nerve stimulation or single-fiber electromyography (EMG). Repetitive nerve stimulation is easily performed, but its sensitivity in ocular MG is low (<50%). Single-fiber EMG has a high sensitivity of 90%; however, it is not widely available.

Another cornerstone in the diagnosis of MG is testing for specific antibodies directed against postsynaptic structures at the neuromuscular junction [1, 2]. Antibodies against the acetylcholine receptor (AChR-Ab) are the most frequent antibodies detected but are only present in up to 50% of MG patients with ocular myasthenia. Antibodies against muscle-specific kinase (MuSK) are typically found in middle-aged females with bulbar symptoms, although ocular symptoms can be the presenting complaints. LDL receptor-related protein 4 (LRP4)/agrin are the least frequent antibodies. In 10–15% of MG patients, none of these antibodies can be detected. AchR-Ab-positive MG can be a paraneoplastic disorder, and therefore, imaging studies to exclude a thymoma are mandatory in these patients.

Treatment of ocular MG is usually started with the acetylcholinesterase inhibitor pyridostigmine at 60 mg three to four times daily. If patients are still symptomatic despite pyridostigmine, prednisolone is started at a dose of 5–10 mg/day and increased slowly until clinical remission is achieved [5–7]. For patients who do not respond to pyridostigmine and steroids, several escalating immunosuppressive treatment regimens have been recommended [5–8].

Lambert Eaton Myasthenic Syndrome

Lambert–Eaton myasthenic syndrome (LEMS) is a rare disease with a prevalence of 2.3–2.5/1,000,000 and an incidence of 0.17–0.4/1,000,000 [1]. It is caused by antibodies against presynaptic P/Q-type voltage-gated calcium channels (VGCC) in the majority of cases. In contrast to MG, isolated ocular symptoms are rare and show fewer fluctuations in LEMS, but eye muscle weakness can develop in 30% over the course of the disease [1]. A small-cell lung cancer is found in 50–60% of cases with LEMS; however, the clinical symptoms usually occur before the diagnosis of small-cell lung cancer is made. While paraneoplastic LEMS affects mainly men at a median age of 60, nontumorous affects mostly young females [9, 10].

The presynaptic neuromuscular transmission defect can be demonstrated in repetitive nerve stimulation studies. Low-frequency 3-Hz repetitive nerve stimulation shows a decremental response similar to MG, but high-frequency 30-Hz repetitive nerve stimulation reveals a dramatic increment of more than 60%.

Serum antibodies against P/Q-type VGCC are detected in paraneoplastic and autoimmune cases, but SRY-box transcription factor 1 (SOX1) antibodies are only found in paraneoplastic LEMS. In any case, repeated and intensive screening for small-cell lung cancer is mandatory.

The treatment of choice is amifampridine (3,4-diaminopyridin) and cancer treatment in paraneoplastic cases. If the treatment response is incomplete, pyridostigmin, intravenous immunoglobulins, steroids, azathioprine, and rituximab can be tried [1, 10, 11].

Botulism

Foodborne botulism is an extremely rare but potentially life-threatening illness cause by botulinum neurotoxins (BoNTs). Between 2001 and 2017, 326 laboratory confirmed cases were reported in the USA [12]. BoNTs are produced by *Clostridium botulinum*, an anaerobe and spore-forming bacterium, and seven types of toxin (A–G) exist. Foodborne botulism is the most frequent form, with the others being infantile and adult intestinal, wound, iatrogenic, and inhalation botulism. Foodborne botulism typically results from the consumption of preformed toxins in home-canned food or traditional local food [13].

The BoNTs impair the calcium-associated presynaptic release of acetylcholine at the neuromuscular endplate and at cholinergic synapses within the autonomic nervous system. Symptoms typically occur within 12–48 h after ingestion of contaminated food. Gastrointestinal symptoms, pain, nausea, vomiting, and diarrhea are usually transient and observed in approximately 70% of cases. Autonomic symptoms, such as dry mouth and postural hypotension, typically precede other neurological symptoms, which cause an afebrile descending flaccid paralysis. Initial symptoms are dysarthria, dysphonia, and dysphagia. Typically, patients develop ptosis, mydriasis, blurred vision, and weakness of extraocular muscles (Fig. 33.1). Sensation is normal. In severe cases, diaphragmatic weakness and respiratory failure develops, necessitating ventilatory support. In these cases, recovery is frequently incomplete. In a large series of wound and food-borne botulism cases, 46% of patients required mechanical ventilation with a median duration of 26.5 days. In general, recovery originates from reinnervation of paralyzed muscles and therefore can be slow, depending on the severity of the disease [13–15].

The diagnostic gold standard to diagnose botulism is the in vivo mouse lethality bioassay, which involves intraperitoneal injection of mice with patient serum. However, this test is not readily available and takes up to 4 days to provide conclusive results. Other options include the detection of BoTNs in serum, stool, and food and the isolation of BoTN-producing clostridia in stool samples.

Treatment of foodborne botulism consists of gastrointestinal decontamination, administration of antitoxin, and supportive measures including mechanical ventilation when necessary. Gastrointestinal decontamination is performed to remove bacteria and toxins. It can be challenging due to toxin-induced autonomic failure resulting in gastroparesis. An antidote should be given as early as possible to neutralize circulating BoTNs, as this seems to reduce the need for mechanical ventilation [13].

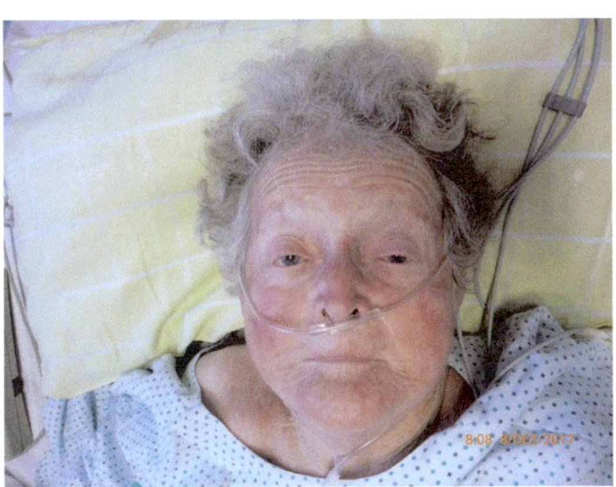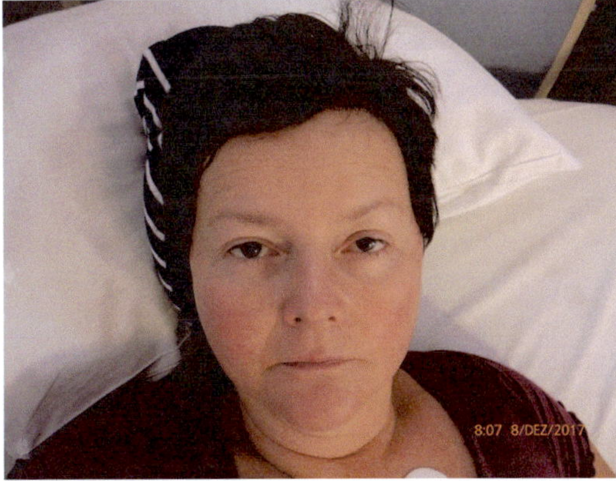

Fig. 33.1 Mother (left) and her daughter (right) with food-borne botulism after ingestion of expired bore spread. Note ptosis and mydriasis; extraocular muscle weakness was also present

Paroxysmal CN Disorders

CN III, IV, VI: Ocular Neuromyotonia

Ocular neuromyotonia results in intermitted diplopia due to spasms in eye muscles innervated by a single oculomotor CN, mostly the oculomotor and more rarely the trochlear or abducens nerve [16, 17]. It may be triggered by ocular movement in the direction of the involved muscle or occur spontaneously. When involving the superior oblique muscle, it can be differentiated from superior oblique myokymia by the absence of oscillopsia in ocular neuromyotonia. Most cases were reported after radiation therapy of the skull base, and ephaptic transmission is assumed to be the underlying mechanism. Treatment with cellular membrane stabilizing medications, e.g., carbamazepine, lacosamid, phenytoin, and gabapentin, usually is effective in suppressing ocular neuromyotonia.

CN IV: Superior Oblique Myokymia

Superior oblique myokymia, a rare disorder of CN IV, is experienced as monocular oscillopsia due to paroxysmal high-frequency contractions of the musculus obliquus superior [17]. These low-amplitude, high-frequency torsional eye movements last for a few seconds to minutes and may occur several times a day, but may then remit for even months to years. The presumed causes are ephaptic transmission within CN IV or a compression of the nerve by the superior cerebellar artery. Rare cases due to posterior fossa astrocytoma and dural arteriovenous fistula have been reported [17]. The condition usually is benign and does not necessitate treatment. Pharmacological treatment options, including topical beta-blocker eye drops, systemic beta blockers, carbamazepine, and gabapentin, have successfully been used. Eye muscle surgery and neurosurgical interventions are reserved for severe and refractory cases.

CN V: Trigeminal Neuralgia and Auriculotemporal Neuralgia

See Chap. 34.

CN VII: Facial Hemispasm

Primary hemifacial spasm is a rare disorder with a prevalence of 9.8–11/100,000 that affects women more frequently than men (2:1). Age of onset usually is after the age of 40 years, and familial cases are the exception [18].

Symptoms typically start with brief repetitive contractions of the orbicularis oculi muscle, resulting in short involuntary twitches around the eye. Over time, these involuntary contractions spread to other facial muscles but remain unilateral in most cases. The "other Babinski sign" (or Babinski-2 sign) can be observed: with eyelid closure there is rise of the eyebrow [18, 19]. Paroxysmal clicking sounds in the ear of the affected side may occur due to contractions of the stapedius muscle. Hearing loss and mild facial palsy are extremely rare. The involuntary contractions persist during sleep.

Primary and secondary hemifacial spasms are distinguished. Primary hemifacial spasm is caused by vascular compression of the nerve at its root entry zone by the superior cerebellar, anterior inferior cerebellar, or vertebral artery. Other aberrant vessels, including veins, have also been observed. Secondary hemifacial spasm can be found with posterior fossa tumors and cysts, brainstem lesions, facial nerve lesions, and vascular malformations. The pathophysiology is considered to be due to focal demyelination and ephaptic transmission in most cases [18].

The clinical presentation suggests the diagnosis. Additional investigations, such as electrophysiological and imaging studies, are primarily performed to rule out secondary forms. High-resolution MRI with special sequences, such as CISS (constructive interference in steady-state) sequences and 3D time-of-flight MRI angiography, are necessary to demonstrate vascular compression in primary hemifacial spasm. Electrophysiological studies show spread of the blink reflex to muscles other than the orbicularis oculi muscle in response to stimulation of the supraorbital nerve.

Treatment of secondary hemifacial spasms aims to remove the underlying cause. For primary hemifacial spasms, several treatment options exist. Drugs, such as carbamazepine or gabapentin, can be tried but their use is limited by side effects or poor efficacy. Botulinum toxin is the treatment of choice. It is injected into the most severe affected muscles, and the first effects can be overserved after 3–6 days and usually last for 2–3 months. Side effects, such as mild facial weakness or ptosis, are transient and usually mild and depend on the site of injection. When these treatments fail, microvascular decompression of the facial nerve can be performed. The reported success rates are 85–90%; however, the risk for serious complications, such as hearing loss, permanent facial palsy, CSF leakage, and disease recurrence, is relatively high [18, 19].

CN VII: Geniculate Neuralgia

See Chap. 34.

CN VIII: Vestibular Paroxysmia

Vestibular paroxysmia is characterized by brief attacks or positional or rotatory vertigo and instability of posture and gait, which are triggered by head movements, a particular head position, and hyperventilation. These attacks last for seconds to a minute and occur in series of 30 or more attacks, and hypoacusis and tinnitus can also occur [20]. In a series of 17,718 patients at a specialized clinic, 3.7% were diagnosed with vestibular paroxysmia [20]. The pathophysiology in the majority of cases is a compression of the vestibular nerve at its root entry zone by an either aberrant or ateriosclerotic elongated artery. This

compression results in focal demyelination, which causes ephaptic discharges or conduction block. Neuroimaging is mandatory to exclude rear secondary causes, such as arteriovenous malformations, arachnoid cysts, brainstem lesions, or plaques or cerebellopontine angle tumors. Neurovascular compression can be visualized by MRI with CISS sequences and 3D time-of-flight MRI angiography. However, in a series of 32 patients with vestibular paroxysmia, a neurovascular contact was present bilaterally in 42% [21], which makes it difficult to decide which side is affected.

The treatment of choice is medical. Most patients respond to low doses of carbamazepine (200–600 mg/day) or oxcarbazepine (300–900 mg/day). Lamotrigine, topiramate, baclofen, and gabapentin have also been used in selected cases. Surgical treatment for microvascular decompression is reserved for patients refractory to medical treatment [20, 21].

CN IX: Glossopharyngeal Neuralgia

See Chap. 34.

CN X: Superior Laryngeal Neuralgia

See Chap. 34.

CN XII: Hemilingual Spasm

In 2002, De Ridder et al. described a patient with paroxysmal spasms of the right side of the tongue and proposed the term hemilingual spasm [22]. In this patient, a premedullary arachnoid cyst was seen in imaging studies, and the spasms resolved immediately after resection of the cyst. A couple of additional cases have been reported due to vascular compression of the hypoglossal nerve [23, 24]. In all cases, neurovascular decompression led to an immediate termination of the spasms.

References

1. Punga AR, Maddison P, Heckmann JM, et al. Epidemiology, diagnostics, and biomarkers of autoimmune neuromuscular junction disorders. Lancet Neurol. 2022;21:176–88. https://doi.org/10.1016/s1474-4422(21)00297-0.
2. Gilhus NE, Tzartos S, Evoli A, et al. Myasthenia gravis. Nat Rev Dis Primers. 2019;5:30–19. https://doi.org/10.1038/s41572-019-0079-y.
3. Giannoccaro MP, Paolucci M, Zenesini C, et al. Comparison of ice-pack test and single fiber EMG diagnostic accuracy in patients referred for myasthenic ptosis. Neurology. 2020;95:e1800. https://doi.org/10.1212/wnl.0000000000010619.
4. Benatar M. A systematic review of diagnostic studies in myasthenia gravis. Neuromuscul Disord. 2006;16:459–67. https://doi.org/10.1016/j.nmd.2006.05.006.
5. Sussman J, Farrugia ME, Maddison P, et al. Myasthenia gravis: Association of British Neurologists' management guidelines. Pract Neurol. 2015;15:199–206. https://doi.org/10.1136/practneurol-2015-001126.
6. Narayanaswami P, Sanders DB, Wolfe G, et al. International consensus guidance for management of myasthenia gravis. Neurology. 2021;96:114–22. https://doi.org/10.1212/wnl.0000000000011124.
7. Narayanaswami P, Sanders DB, Wolfe G, et al. International consensus guidance for management of myasthenia gravis: 2020 update. Neurology. 2020;96:114–22. https://doi.org/10.1212/wnl.0000000000011124.
8. Gronseth GS, Barohn R, Narayanaswami P. Practice advisory: thymectomy for myasthenia gravis (practice parameter update). Neurology. 2020;94:705. https://doi.org/10.1212/wnl.0000000000009294.
9. Titulaer MJ, Maddison P, Sont JK, et al. Clinical Dutch-English Lambert-Eaton myasthenic syndrome (LEMS) tumor association prediction score accurately predicts small-cell lung cancer in the LEMS. J Clin Oncol. 2011;29:902–8. https://doi.org/10.1200/jco.2010.32.0440.
10. Titulaer MJ, Lang B, Verschuuren JJ. Lambert-Eaton myasthenic syndrome: from clinical characteristics to therapeutic strategies. Lancet Neurol. 2011;10:1098–107. https://doi.org/10.1016/s1474-4422(11)70245-9.
11. Wirtz PW, Verschuuren JJ, van Dijk JG, et al. Efficacy of 3,4-diaminopyridine and pyridostigmine in the treatment of Lambert-Eaton myasthenic syndrome: a randomized, double-blind, placebo-controlled, crossover study. Nature. 2009;86:44–8. https://doi.org/10.1038/clpt.2009.35.
12. Lúquez C, Edwards L, Griffin C, et al. Foodborne botulism outbreaks in the United States, 2001–2017. Front Microbiol. 2021;12:713101. https://doi.org/10.3389/fmicb.2021.713101.
13. Lonati D, Schicchi A, Crevani M, et al. Foodborne botulism: clinical diagnosis and medical treatment. Toxins. 2020;12:509. https://doi.org/10.3390/toxins12080509.
14. Gable K, Massey J. Presynaptic disorders: Lambert-Eaton myasthenic syndrome and botulism. Semin Neurol. 2015;35:340–6. https://doi.org/10.1055/s-0035-1558976.
15. Chatham-Stephens K, Fleck-Derderian S, Johnson SD, et al. Clinical features of foodborne and wound botulism: a systematic review of the literature, 1932–2015. Clin Infect Dis. 2017;66:S11–6. https://doi.org/10.1093/cid/cix811.
16. Tabba S, Kini A, Othman BA, et al. Shared features of the Heimann–Bielshowsky phenomenon and ocular neuromyotonia. Neuro-Ophthalmology. 2019;44:1–3. https://doi.org/10.1080/01658107.2019.1648520.
17. Kline LB, Demer JL, Vaphiades MS, et al. Disorders of the fourth cranial nerve. J Neuroophthalmol. 2021;41:176–93. https://doi.org/10.1097/wno.0000000000001261.
18. Chaudhry N, Srivastava A, Joshi L. Hemifacial spasm: the past, present and future. J Neurol Sci. 2015;356:27–31. https://doi.org/10.1016/j.jns.2015.06.032.
19. Baldauf J, Rosenstengel C, Schroeder HWS. Nerve compression syndromes in the posterior cranial fossa. Deutsches Ärzteblatt Int. 2019;116:54–60. https://doi.org/10.3238/arztebl.2019.0054.
20. Brandt T, Strupp M, Dieterich M. Vestibular paroxysmia: a treatable neurovascular cross-compression syndrome. J Neurol. 2016;263:90–6. https://doi.org/10.1007/s00415-015-7973-3.
21. Hufner K, Barresi D, Glaser M, et al. Vestibular paroxysmia: diagnostic features and medical treatment. Neurology. 2008;71:1006–14. https://doi.org/10.1212/01.wnl.0000326594.91291.f8.
22. Ridder DD, Alessi G, Lemmerling M, et al. Hemilingual spasm: a new neurosurgical entity? Case report. J Neurosurg. 2002;97:205–7. https://doi.org/10.3171/jns.2002.97.1.0205.
23. Heckmann JG, Marthol H, Bickel A, et al. Hemilingual spasm associated with tortuosity of the extracranial internal carotid artery. Cerebrovasc Dis. 2005;20:208–10. https://doi.org/10.1159/000087329.
24. Osburn LL, Møller AR, Bhatt JR, et al. Hemilingual spasm: defining a new entity, its electrophysiological correlates and surgical treatment through microvascular decompression. Neurosurgery. 2010;67:192–6. https://doi.org/10.1227/01.neu.0000370596.78384.2b.

Bullet Points

- Trigeminal neuralgia frequently responds to carbamazepine and is often caused by compression of the trigeminal nerve root by an artery (classical trigeminal neuralgia). High-resolution three-dimensional T2-weighted MR imaging with thin-slice sequences through the pontocerebellar angle together with 3D *time-of-flight* magnetic resonance *angiography must be done to rule* out relevant neurovascular conflict.
- Secondary causes of trigeminal neuralgia should be ruled out by neuroimaging.
- In refractory trigeminal neuralgia surgical procedures such as neurovascular decompression should be considered.
- Trigeminal neuropathy is caused by nerve injury related to trauma or infection and is associated with sensory dysfunction.
- Glossopharyngeal neuralgia is treated in analogy to trigeminal neuralgia.

Authors of this chapter: Franz Riederer, Stefan Leis, and Johannes Herta.

Introduction

Cranial nerve pain syndromes can be subdivided into cranial neuralgias with minor damage or irritation of the still functional nerve and cranial neuropathies where nerve lesions cause sensory loss. Cranial neuralgias are classified according to MRI findings into the following: (1) classical, if significant nerve–vessel conflict that causes morphological changes is present; (2) idiopathic, if this is not the case; or (3) secondary, if other causes such as multiple sclerosis or tumoral lesions are present. Neuropathies of cranial nerves are associated with nerve dysfunction and can be attributed to specific causes, such as viral agents (e.g., varicella zoster virus [VZV]) and inflammation, but may also be idiopathic. It has to be mentioned that diseases of cranial nerves, like oculomotor nerve palsy or optic neuritis, may be associated with pain [1], but these will not be discussed in the present chapter that focuses on diseases where pain is the main symptom.

Trigeminal Neuralgia

Clinical Presentation and Diagnosis

Trigeminal neuralgia (TN) is an extremely painful disorder characterized by unilateral, short-lasting, electric shock-like pain paroxysms in the distribution of one or more branches of the trigeminal nerve, with the second and third branches being most frequently affected. It is frequently triggered by innocuous stimuli, such as touching or chewing, and may be characterized by a refractory period, with less sensitivity to mechanical stimuli. Pain may also occur spontaneously without triggers. Pain paroxysms may be accompanied by jerky movement of the facial muscles, which has traditionally been termed as "tic douloureux." TN can critically affect adequate food and fluid intake and may be associated with depression. TN may be purely paroxysmal, but continuous concomitant pain between the attacks can also exist [1]. Sensation is usually normal in the affected nerve territories, although subtle hypoesthesia has been found with quantitative sensory testing [2]. In most cases, TN is unilateral and affects the third or second division of the trigeminal nerve alone or, most commonly, in combination [3]. The ophthalmic branch is rarely affected in less than 10% of cases and may be accompanied by trigemino-autonomic symptoms, such as ciliary injection and tearing. In this case, the differential diagnosis to SUNCT syndrome (short-lasting unilateral neuralgiform headache attacks with conjunctival injection and tearing) may be challenging. This very rare unilateral headache syndrome with very frequent unilateral shooting or stabbing pain paroxysms belongs to the trigemino-autonomic cephalalgias, which also include cluster headache, paroxysmal hemicrania, and hemicrania continua. Discriminatory symptoms between TN and SUNCT are mechanical triggers and a refractory period which are typically seen in TN, although SUNCT can also be triggered. However, as in TN, nerve–vessel contacts between the trigeminal nerve and surrounding vessels have also been described in SUNCT syndrome [4], suggesting a continuum between the two disorders [5].

The lifetime prevalence of trigeminal neuralgia is 0.3%, with an incidence of up to 27 new cases per 100,000, with women being affected more frequently (in 60% of cases) [6, 7]. It usually manifests between the sixth and seventh

decades [8]. Manifestation in younger ages is associated with symptomatic TN, caused, for instance, by multiple sclerosis. Familial forms of TN have been described [7].

According to the current classification [1], primary TN comprises the terms classical trigeminal neuralgia and idiopathic TN. Classical trigeminal neuralgia is caused by a neurovascular conflict with nerve compression (Fig. 34.1), while such a contact is absent in idiopathic trigeminal neuralgia. It must be emphasized that a mere contact between a vessel (frequently the superior cerebellar artery) and the trigeminal nerve is not a sufficient cause. Rather, nerve compression, dislocation, or atrophy has to be demonstrated with adequate MRI sequences, such as CISS (constructive interface in steady state) [9]. According to current guidelines, a combination of three high-resolution sequences—3D T2-weighted, 3D TOF-MRA, and 3D T1-gadolinium—should be used [10]. It has been suggested that the neuroradiologist should be blinded to the site of pain [10], as insignificant nerve–vessel contact is frequently observed on the healthy side and also in healthy individuals.

Secondary TN may be attributable to multiple sclerosis, space-occupying lesions such as vascular malformations, neurinomas, and other tumors, or other causes like ischemic brainstem lesions. About 15% of TN cases are secondary [6]. Younger age at onset, prominent sensory deficits and bilateral manifestation could point towards secondary TN.

The International Headache Society [1] and the International Association for the Study of Pain (IASP) [11] have defined the diagnostic criteria outlined in Table 34.1.

According to current guidelines, testing trigeminal brainstem reflexes, such as masseter or blink reflex, and trigeminal somatosensory evoked potentials can be helpful to distinguish primary from secondary TN if MRI is not possible [10]. In this case, CT with contrast agent should be performed to detect space-occupying lesions.

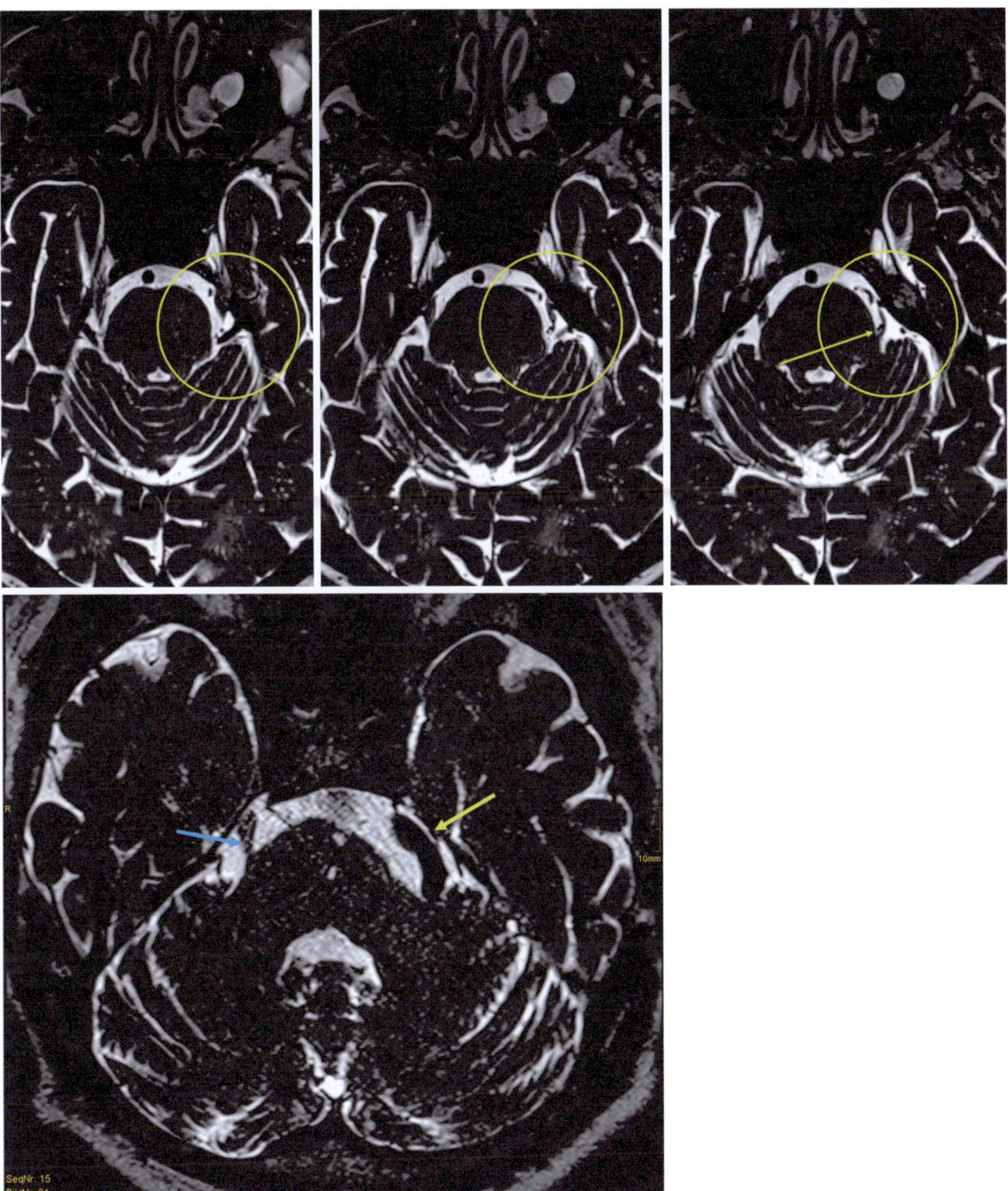

Fig. 34.1 Upper panel: neurovascular conflict between trigeminal nerve and superior cerebellar artery (yellow circle). Lower panel: compression of trigeminal root by megadolicobasilar artery (yellow arrow). The healthy side is indicated by a blue arrow

Table 34.1 Diagnostic criteria of trigeminal neuralgia

A. Recurrent paroxysms of unilateral facial pain in the distribution(s) of one or more divisions of the trigeminal nerve, with no radiation beyond and fulfilling criteria B and C
B. Pain has all of the following characteristics: 1. Lasting from a fraction of a second to 2 min 2. Severe intensity 3. Electric shock-like, shooting, stabbing, or sharp in quality
C. Precipitated by innocuous stimuli within the affected trigeminal distribution
D. Not better accounted for by another ICHD-3 diagnosis

Pathophysiology

The trigeminal nerve seems to be vulnerable to compression by vessels or lesions near the root entry zone, where myelinization changes from peripheral Schwann cells to central oligodendroglia cells. In this region, demyelination and dysmyelination of nerve fibers by compression may allow ephaptic impulses to "jump" from sensory to nociceptive nerve fibers or trigger the generation of spontaneous impulses from ectopic pacemaker sites [8]. Advanced MRI techniques, such as diffusion tensor imaging (DTI), have shown changes in the affected trigeminal nerve, such as alterations in relative fractional anisotropy values, as a result of nerve compression [12]. Central mechanisms, such as sensitization [13] or gain-of-function mutations of voltage-gated sodium channels, are being discussed in the pathophysiology of TN [6]. Also, pontine multiple sclerosis plaques affecting presynaptic afferents can cause TN. About 2–6% of multiple sclerosis patients suffer from TN [7]. In this case, TN manifests in younger ages and is more often bilateral. Frequently, plaques between the root entry zone and trigeminal nuclei affecting afferent pathways have been described [14].

Treatment of Trigeminal Neuralgia

The natural course of trigeminal neuralgia is fluctuating in terms of intensity and frequency of pain attacks; thus, increasing and decreasing of dosages for treatment may be appropriate. First-line treatment of TN is carbamazepine 200–1200 mg/day or oxcarbazepine 300–1800 mg/day [10], both of which are sodium channel blockers. Doses should be gradually increased. Carbamazepine can be started with a daily dose of 300 mg, increasing the dose by 100 mg every 3 days. Further drugs that can be used alone or in combination are lamotrigine (up to 400 mg), gabapentin (up to 3600 mg), pregabalin (up to 600 mg), or baclofen (up to 100 mg) [6]. Gabapentin and pregabalin target $\alpha2\delta$ auxiliary subunit of the voltage-gated calcium channel [15]. Some of the drugs, such as lamotrigine, require slow dose titration to avoid potentially serious adverse events such as rash. Acute intervention with intravenous fosphenytoin or lidocaine, which also act as sodium channel blockers, under cardiac monitoring has been suggested as a transitional approach for exacerbations of trigeminal neuralgia as a weak recommendation in current treatment guidelines [10] and is supported by data from a small prospective series [16]. According to a recent retrospective series, the sodium channel blocker lacosamide may be similarly efficacious and better tolerated than phenytoin [17]. Another treatment option is botulinum toxin type A injections into the pain area and trigger points [18] with different techniques (intradermally, in submucosa, subcutaneously) using a dose from 25 to 100 U [10]. A presumed mechanism of botulinum toxin A in neuropathic pain is beyond muscle relaxation and probably involves an interaction with synaptic vesicle proteins so that the release of various pain modulatory neurotransmitters, like glutamate or calcitonin gene-related peptide (CGRP), are impaired [15]. Carbamazepine and oxcarbazepine may cause dizziness or sedation and are enzyme inducers, which may be relevant in elderly patients suffering from various comorbidities and osteoporosis. Considering these side effects, there is a need for the development of new drugs for TN. Currently, the sodium channel blocker vixotrigine is being investigated for the treatment of TN [19].

Based on expert opinion, it has been suggested that combinations of carbamazepine or oxcarbazepine with gabapentin, pregabalin, or lamotrigine should be tried before referral to surgery [6]. In general, if pain cannot be sufficiently controlled in terms of efficacy and side effects by medical treatment in adequate doses with appropriate monitoring, surgical options should be offered [10]. Microvascular decompression, also known by its describer as the *Jannetta* procedure, is a surgical procedure where compressing vessels at the trigeminal nerve root entry zone are repositioned and isolated from the nerve [20]. During surgery, the cerebellopontine cistern is entered over a retrosigmoid approach and a Teflon padding or other agents in combination with fibrin glue are used to isolate the offending vessel [6]. If possible, microvascular decompression surgery should be given priority over other surgical interventions as it is potentially curative, nondestructive to the trigeminal system, and associated with low morbidity. According to a pooled analysis which included 5149 patients, microvascular decompression was shown to be effective, with pain-free rates ranging from 62% to 89% at follow-up from 3 to 11 years [6]. Microvascular decompression is a major surgical procedure that can have complications, such as cranial nerve palsy (4%), CSF leak (1.5%), ipsilateral hearing loss (1.8%), stroke (0.6%), or meningitis (0.4%), with an overall mortality of about 0.3% [10, 20]. Patients should be referred to high-volume centers, as the morbidity rate decreases significantly. In eligible patients with classical TN, microvascular decompression has been suggested as the first-choice option for a surgical procedure. A shorter disease duration as well as type 1 Burchiel classification (typical paroxysmal facial pain) have shown to be predictors of pain freedom in a meta-analysis [21]. Therefore, if there is a poor response to drug therapy or if side effects are intolerable, the patient should be informed about the possibility of surgery at an early stage. However, patients with idiopathic TN are good candidates for surgery, as even with more sophisticated MRI sequences a neurovascular conflict cannot be detected in more than 45% [22]. This can be explained by the complex 3D structure of the trigeminal nerve, but also by, for example, arachnoid adhesions that are not visible in the MRI (Fig. 34.2). Even in rare cases of multiple sclerosis and assumed secondary TN, microvascular decompression surgery may be indicated [23]. Here, however, the indication must be checked carefully: the clinical picture of a typical triggerable TN must exist, and in MRI there should be no evidence of multiple sclerosis plaques in the area of the trigeminal nuclei with a simultaneous clear vessel–nerve contact.

Neuroablative therapies are generally less invasive but destructive procedures involving controlled lesions of the trigeminal ganglion or root. They involve penetration of the foramen ovale with a cannula to provide a thermal (radiofrequency thermocoagulation), mechanical (balloon compression), or

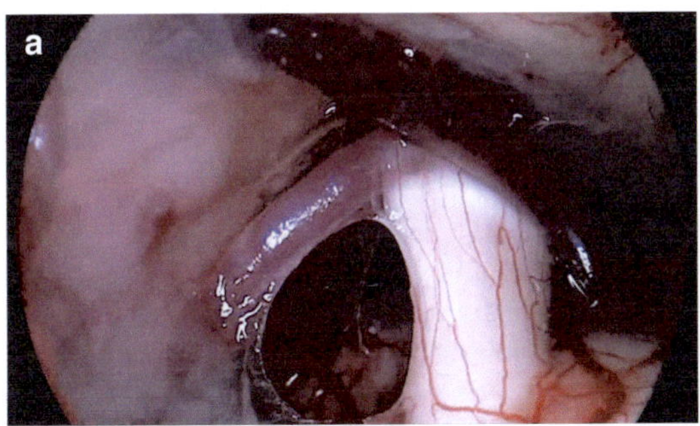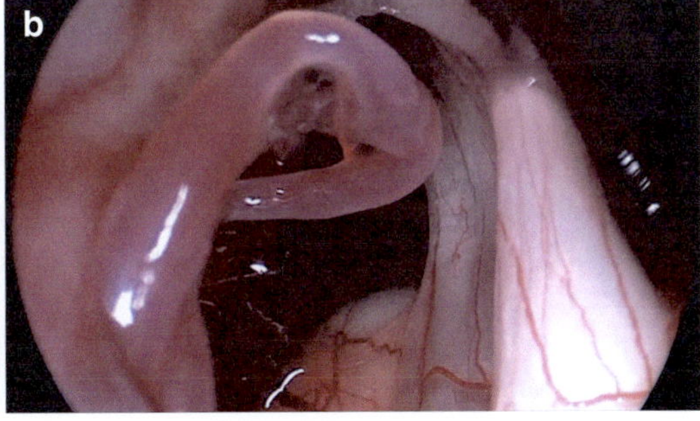

Fig. 34.2 The patient was diagnosed with idiopathic trigeminal neuralgia as MRI showed a neurovascular contact without morphological changes to the nerve root. During surgery, the continuity of the nerve without displacement, which could also be seen in the preoperative MRI, is initially evident (**a**). Only after closer observation, loosening of adhesions, and decompression of the nerve root, the arterial loop appears clearly that presses into the nerve root and deforms it (**b**)

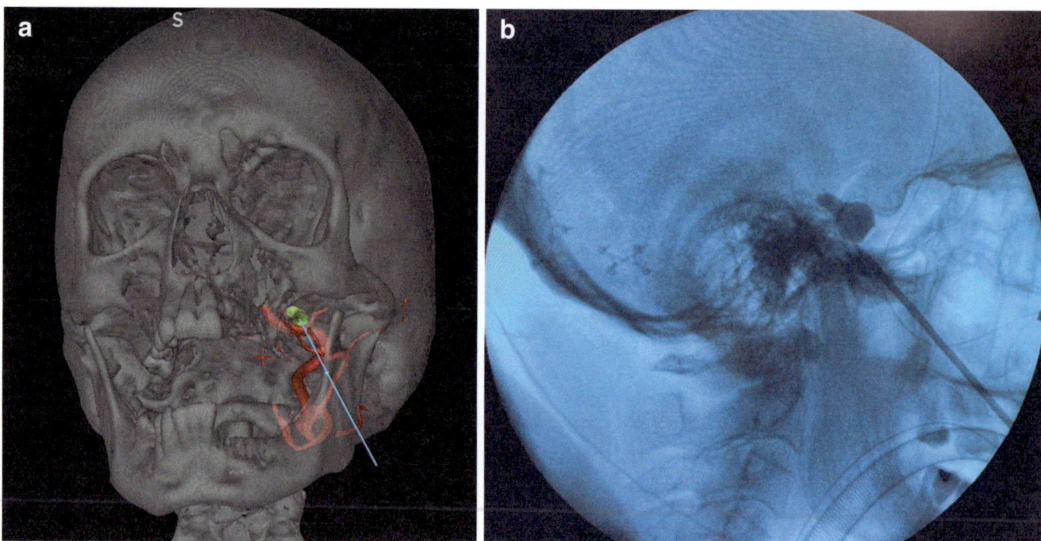

Fig. 34.3 (**a**) Shows the typical trajectory for a percutaneous approach to the trigeminal ganglion (green). During balloon compression, (**b**) the bear-shaped form of the inflated balloon indicates adequate placement in Meckel's cave

chemical (glycerol) lesion [6]. Ablative techniques are recommended in patients with classical and idiopathic TN if patients are not eligible for microvascular decompression surgery, decide against an open neurosurgical treatment, or if previous surgery was unsuccessful. Additionally, patients with secondary TN, such as in multiple sclerosis, benefit from an ablative procedure (Fig. 34.3). In general, the recurrence rate after ablative therapies is higher, but most procedures, such as balloon compression and radiofrequency thermocoagulation, may be repeated. Pooled analyses reported pain-free rates of 55–80% in TN patients after balloon compression, 26–82% after radiofrequency thermocoagulation, and 19–58% after glycerol injection (follow-up 4–11 years) [10]. Stereotactic radiosurgery (Gamma Knife) is also an ablative method focusing on the root entry zone of the trigeminal nerve. While the onset of effect may be delayed, it has the clear advantage that patients do not need to be anesthetized or sedated. A systematic review showed pain-free rates between 30% and 45% at 10 years [24]. The most common side effect of neurodestructive methods is facial hypoesthesia (19%) that usually improves in the months after the procedure but can occasionally remain permanent. Other common side effects include corneal hypoesthesia (5%) that occurs most frequently after radiofrequency ther-

mocoagulation and trigeminal motor weakness (5%), while anesthesia dolorosa is rare (0.5%) [10].

During ganglionic local opioid analgesia (GLOA), a diluted buprenorphine solution is injected transorally near the superior cervical ganglion as part of the autonomic nervous system. The technique is used for TN as well as for neuropathic facial pain syndromes [25]. The prognostic value of the sympathetic blockade on the long-term course of the pain, however, remains unclear since no high-quality studies exist to date.

In clinical practice, patients should be informed about the various procedures with regard to efficacy and potential side effects.

Auriculotemporal Neuralgia

The auriculotemporal nerve originates from the mandibular division of the trigeminal nerve. Auriculotemporal neuralgia manifests in periods of pain lasting from seconds to 30 min, and mild continuous pain may be present in some cases. The throbbing and stabbing pain is unilateral, located around the temple, temporomandibular joint, ear, and preauricular and parotid area. Paresthesias in the painful areas may occur [26].

Auriculotemporal neuralgia can be caused by compression of the auriculotemporal nerve by its passage through the lateral pterygoid muscle or by other structures, such as cysts or aneurysms. Disorders of the temporomandibular joint must be ruled out. A single local anesthetic nerve block can result in pain relief for up to 1–2 years. Carbamazepine and gabapentin may also be effective [26, 27].

Painful Trigeminal Neuropathy

Clinical Description and Diagnosis

Lesions in the peripheral trigeminal branches (neuropathy), the trigeminal ganglion (ganglionopathy), or the central trigeminal pathways can cause neuropathic pain. Lesion of the trigeminal pathway can occur by mechanical, thermal, or chemical trauma or by radiation [28]. Trauma, such as dental extraction or surgery, are the most common etiologies [28]. The pain follows the dermatome and has the typical neuropathic features, with positive (hyperalgesia, allodynia) or negative (hypoesthesia, hypoalgesia) signs of nerve dysfunction. It may mimic TN, with either spontaneous or triggered pain paroxysms superimposed on a dull burning background pain, usually without a refractory period, but these paroxysms are not the predominant type of pain. A possible associated symptom of trigeminal neuropathy is masticatory weakness. The clinical exam should include sensory testing of trigeminal regions, including intraoral sensation and trigeminal reflexes such as jaw jerk reflex and corneal reflex [28]. Neuroimaging such as MRI with contrast is mandatory. Possible causes are dental implants, tooth extractions, root canal therapy, and local anesthesia [28]. Prognosis is rather poor, with only one-third of patients reporting improvement.

Other possible etiologies include neoplastic disease, autoimmune diseases such as Sjogren's syndrome, progressive systemic sclerosis, and infectious agents such as herpes zoster, herpes simplex, *Borrelia burgdorferi*, syphilis, or leprosis.

Treatment of Trigeminal Neuropathy

Treatment of painful trigeminal neuropathy should include a multidisciplinary setting. Medical treatment follows recommendations for neuropathic pain [29], such as tricyclic antidepressants, SNRIs, gabapentin, or pregabalin. Topical therapies, such as lidocaine plasters, intraoral botulinum toxin, or topical capsaicin, as well as neuromodulation have been proposed [28].

Herpes Zoster Neuropathy

Herpes zoster manifestation is associated with acute painful neuropathy and postherpetic neuropathy in 10% of cases [7], which can become a chronic potentially disabling condition. Traditionally, it has been termed post-herpetic neuralgia, although it is a neuropathy as described in current classifications [1, 11]. The incidence of post-herpetic trigeminal neuropathy is 3.3/100,000 [7]. It affects the first branch in 10–15% of cases and can cause acute and persistent neuropathic pain. Risk factors for the development of post-herpetic neuropathy are prodromal pain, severe acute pain, severe rash, ophthalmic involvement, and older age [30]. It can be prevented by vaccination.

Allodynia and pain can precede herpes zoster efflorescence for some days (Fig. 34.4). Gabapentin, pregabalin, tricyclic antidepressants, or opioids can be used for the treatment of post-herpetic neuralgia [31]. Further treatment options may include carbamazepine or oxcarbazepine, topical capsaicin, or lidocaine [28].

Differential Diagnoses of Trigeminal Neuropathy

An important differential diagnosis for painful cranial nerve diseases is persistent idiopathic facial pain. In this pain condition, pain can be poorly localized and does not follow peripheral nerve distribution. The neurological examination is normal, which precludes gross sensory abnormalities. This difficult to treat primary pain syn-

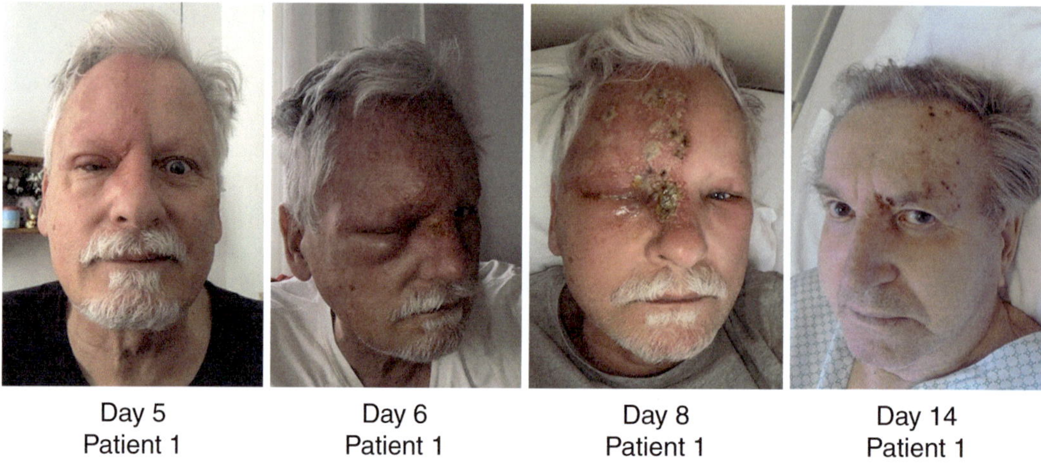

Fig. 34.4 Temporal evolution of zoster ophthalmicus in two patients (64 and 80 years old) with acute painful trigeminal neuropathy. Patient 1 (left 3 images) had shooting pain and allodynia in V1 distributions 3 days before the rash

drome requires extensive diagnostic workup, including dentists and neuroimaging, and remains a diagnosis of exclusion. A continuum with trigeminal neuropathy has been discussed.

Note that facial pain can be a symptom of primary headaches, such as orofacial migraine or cluster headache. Therefore, particular focus should be given to accompanying symptoms, such as nausea, vomiting, or sensoriphobia, which point towards migraine. Accompanying trigemino-autonomic symptoms, such as tearing, lacrimation, or rhinorrhea, point towards a trigemino-autonomic cephalalgia, even in patients with pain only in the face. Another prominent feature of trigeminal autonomic cephalalgias is restlessness (frequently observed as "pacing around") and sometimes even aggressive behavior. Temporomandibular joint dysfunction (TMD) is another important differential diagnosis for facial pain.

Glossopharyngeal Neuralgia

Clinical Description and Diagnosis

Glossopharyngeal neuralgia (GN) is characterized by unilateral excruciating paroxysms of pain in the distribution of the sensory branches of the glossopharyngeal and vagus nerves, such as ear, base of the tongue, tonsillar fossa, pharynx, and beneath the angle of the jaw, that may be triggered by swallowing, talking, yawning, or coughing [1, 32]. Swallowing and yawning are typical triggers for GN, while other triggers are less specific. Further triggers which may overlap with other cranial neuralgias include turning the head to the painful side, chewing, sneezing, clearing the throat, sneezing, or laughing. GN occurs mostly unilateral, although side alternating or bilateral cases have been described [32]. It occurs mostly during daytime, but can eventually wake up the patient during the night [32]. Like TN, severe GN can affect adequate nutrition intake. GN can also occur spontaneously without triggers. GN may be accompanied by autonomic symptoms, such as coughing, bradycardia, or syncope, in up to 10% of cases [32]. The symptomatology can be derived from nerve function. The glossopharyngeal nerve provides sensory supply to the eustachian tube, middle ear, base of the tongue, tonsillar fossa, and pharynx [33]. Together with the vagus nerve, it provides motor supply to the pharynx and it innervates the stylopharyngeal muscle, which is involved in swallowing. The nerve also conducts impulses from the sinus and chemoreceptors of the carotid body [33], which explains possible accompanying autonomic symptoms such as bradycardia or syncope. Intervals between pain paroxysms last from a few minutes to a few hours. Similar to TN, GN can

Table 34.2 Diagnostic criteria of glossopharyngeal neuralgia

A. Recurring paroxysmal attacks of unilateral pain in the distribution of the glossopharyngeal nerve and fulfilling criterion B
B. Pain has all of the following characteristics: 1. Lasting from a few seconds to 2 min   2. Severe intensity   3. Electric shock-like, shooting, stabbing, or sharp in quality   4. Precipitated by swallowing, coughing, talking, or yawning
C. Not better accounted for by another ICHD-3 diagnosis

follow a relapsing–remitting period, with remission from weeks to months.

Glossopharyngeal neuralgia is a very rare disorder, accounting for 0.2–1.3% of facial pain syndromes [32]. Like TN, it has a female preponderance [32]. The incidence is 0.8 per 100,000 [7]. Concurrence of GN and TN have been described [32]. GN seems to concur rarely with multiple sclerosis [14].

Diagnostic criteria of GN are given in Table 34.2.

Following the same taxonomy as TN, classical GN is caused by a significant nerve–vessel conflict, whereas such a conflict or other pathologies are absent in idiopathic GN. In a Chinese series, posterior inferior cerebellar artery was most frequently found as the culprit, followed by veins, anterior inferior cerebellar artery, and vertebral artery [34].

Secondary GN is caused by lesions other than significant nerve–vessel conflict [1]. Diagnostic workup should include an MRI of the brain, with particular focus on brain stem and cranial nerves including the base of the skull, and an evaluation by an ear–nose–throat (ENT) specialist to rule out oropharyngeal tumors [35]. Further secondary causes include cerebellopontine angle or skull-base tumors. Like TN, GN can rarely be caused by multiple sclerosis [14]. Another rare syndrome, Eagle's syndrome, which is caused by an elongated styloid process of more than 4 cm (the normal length being 2.5–3 cm) [35] may have overlapping symptoms with GN, such as pain localization in the angle of the jaw or ear presenting as otalgia. Pain can also be located in the anterior part of the neck. Trigger factors include yawning, chewing, and turning the neck. Symptoms may include dysphagia and foreign body sensation [35]. Eagle's syndrome may be overdiagnosed since a prolonged styloid process is not always related to pain.

Primary GN can have overlapping symptoms with TN or superior laryngeal neuralgia (the respective nerve is a branch of the vagus nerve), which can cause throat pain or nervus intermedius neuralgia which causes otalgia [35]. Laryngeal topical anesthesia or blockade can help to establish the diagnosis of superior laryngeal neuralgia. For differential symptoms, vasovagal symptoms and throat pain are typical for GN, as is swallowing as a trigger.

Treatment of Glossopharyngeal Neuralgia

Treatment of GN is similar to the treatment of TN, although evidence is generally far less robust than for TN. Medical treatment options include oxcarbazepine, carbamazepine, lamotrigine, phenytoin, gabapentin, pregabalin, and baclofen [32]. Nerve blocks of the glossopharyngeal nerve are possible treatment options [32]. Ultrasound-guided block of the glossopharyngeal nerve via the styloid process has been proposed as a repeatable, less invasive procedure [36]. Microvascular decompression is a surgical treatment option in refractory cases with compression of the glossopharyngeal nerve by an artery or vein, with a pain-free response rate of 89.7% at 1 year and 66.3% after 10 years [34]. Patients with venous compressions had a higher recurrence rate. Complications include cranial nerve paresis associated with dysphagia, hoarseness, facial paresis, or hearing loss, which were transient in most cases [32]. As with TN, microsurgical, endoscopic, endoscopic-assisted, and exoscopic techniques have been described for microvascular decompression [37, 38] with good response rates.

Surgical treatment options for cases without a nerve–vessel conflict include rhizotomy of the glossopharyngeal and vagus nerves and Gamma Knife surgery of the root entry zone [32, 39].

Nervus Intermedius Neuralgia (Geniculate Neuralgia)

Clinical Description and Diagnosis

Nervus intermedius neuralgia (NIN) is a very rare form of neuralgic otalgia that was previously termed geniculate neuralgia. The pain location is deep in the auditory canal, with possible radiation to the mastoid, temporal regions, or angle of the jaw. Pain characteristics with shock-like, shooting, sharp, or stabbing pain paroxysms are similar to other neuralgias. Frequently, constant pain was reported in NIN [40]. NIN can be triggered in the posterior wall of the auditory canal and/or the periauricular region, but triggers may be absent [40]. As the nerve carries parasympathetic fibers, pain paroxysms in NIN may be associated with auto-nomic symptoms, such as lacrimation and hypersalivation, or by taste changes, although this is not required in the diagnostic criteria [40]. Neuralgic otalgia necessitates an extensive diagnostic workup, including neuroimaging and ENT consultation. Innervation of the ear involves the trigeminal nerve (auriculotemporal nerve), nervus intermedius, glossopharyngeal, and vagus nerves, as well as occipital nerves with greater auricular nerve [40]. Thus, attribution of neuralgias to a single nerve may not be easy in this body region (Fig. 34.5) [1].

Thus, the differential diagnosis of neuralgic otalgia is broad and may include TN, GN, NIN, occipital neuralgia, cervicogenic headache, trigemino-autonomic cephalalgia, temporomandibular disorder, or red ear syndrome (if the ear becomes red during pain paroxysms) [41]. Diagnostic criteria for NIN are given in Table 34.3.

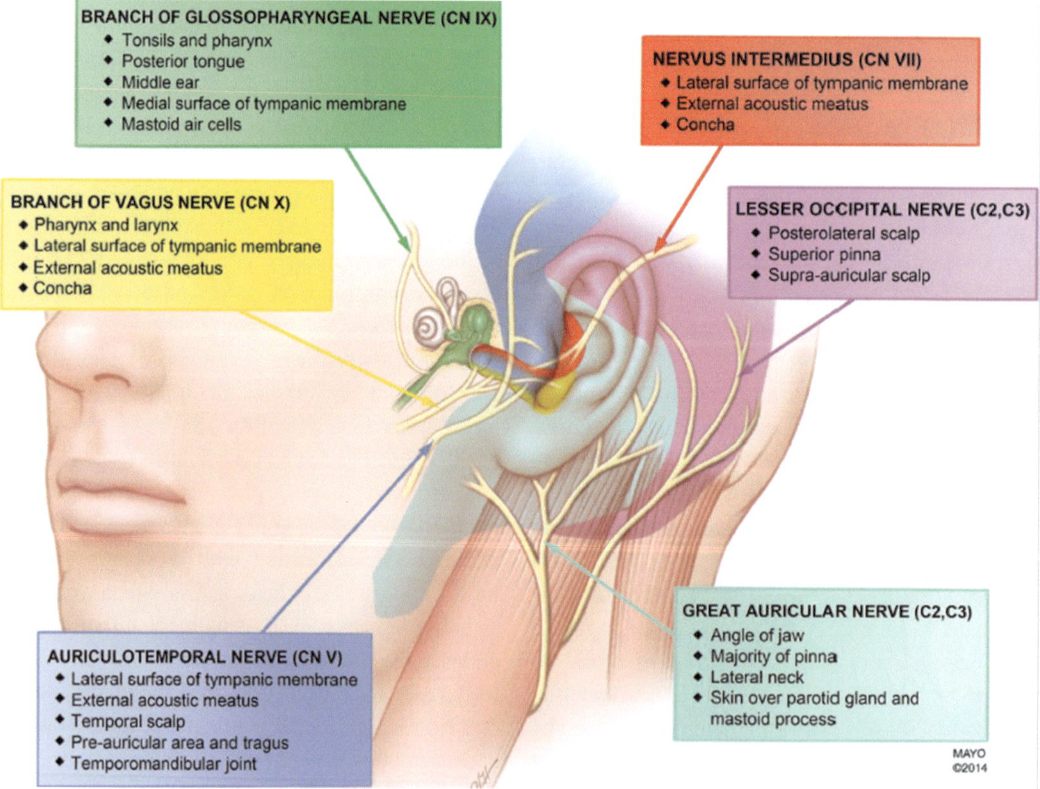

Fig. 34.5 Overlapping innervation of the ear. (Reproduced with kind permission by Mayo Foundation for Medical Education and Research)

Table 34.3 Diagnostic criteria of nervus intermedius neuralgia

A. Paroxysmal attacks of unilateral pain in the distribution of the nervus intermedius[a] and fulfilling criterion B
B. Pain has all of the following characteristics: 1. Lasting from a few seconds to minutes 2. Severe intensity 3. Shooting, stabbing or sharp in quality 4. Precipitated by stimulation of a trigger area in the posterior wall of the auditory canal and/or periauricular region
C. Not better accounted for by another ICHD-3 diagnosis

[a] Pain is located in the auditory canal, auricle, in the region of the mastoid process, and occasionally the soft palate, and may sometimes radiate to the temporal region or the angle of the mandible

Treatment of Nervus Intermedius Neuralgia

Evidence for treatment strategies is generally limited and mostly based on retrospective case series. Treatment strategies for NIN are analogous to TN and GN, with medications against neuropathic pain as a first-line option, nerve block, microvascular decompression in cases of significant nerve compression, or neuroablative strategies or rhizotomy [40].

Following the classification scheme for cranial neuralgias, NIN can be classified into classical (with nerve–vessel conflict), secondary, and idiopathic cases [1].

Nervus Intermedius Neuropathy

Painful neuropathy after herpes zoster reactivation has been described [40]. In zoster oticus, the varicella zoster virus persists in the geniculate ganglion, which contains neurons for cutaneous sensory fibers and taste fibers of the nervus intermedius [33, 40]. The clinical picture of zoster efflorescence in the ear with peripheral facial palsy, which may also involve the vestibulocochlear nerve, has been termed Ramsay Hunt syndrome [42]. Spreading of varicella zoster virus to the glossopharyngeal and vagus nerves thus (multiple cranial neuropathy) has been described in Ramsay Hunt syndrome [43], with multiple mechanisms of viral spreading being discussed. Please note that the term "Ramsay Hunt syndrome" has also been used for progressive myoclonus epilepsy, which may be misleading.

Occipital Neuralgia

Clinical Description and Diagnosis

Occipital neuralgia (ON) is characterized by usually unilateral pain paroxysms in the distribution of the greater, lesser, and/or third occipital nerves [44]. Pain paroxysms last seconds to minutes. The pain is perceived as severe with shooting, stabbing, or sharp quality. The pain is frequently associated with positive symptoms, such as dysesthesia or allodynia, and tenderness over the affected nerve branches. Pain is temporarily eased by blockade of the affected nerve branches with a local anesthetic. In most cases (90%), the greater occipital nerve is affected and in 10% the lesser occipital nerve [44]. The greater and lesser occipital nerve may also be affected together.

Possible causes include anatomic, traumatic, and iatrogenic etiologies. Posterior head trauma, including fractures or whiplash injury, has been implicated in occipital neuralgia. Nerve compression by the occipital artery has been described [44], and nerve entrapment by muscles is another possible cause. ON may occur as a secondary headache related to schwannoma of the occipital nerve [45].

MRI of the head and the neck is considered the imaging modality of choice, but diagnostic procedures may include X-rays of the cervical spine to diagnose C2 facet joint arthritis or CT to identify osseous pathologies such as osteoma. Sonography of the occipital nerve may be an emerging diagnostic strategy (Table 34.4).

Differential diagnoses include cervicogenic headache and migraine. Pain characteristics with pain paroxysms from seconds to minutes as well as occipital trigger zones are typical for ON and not for cervicogenic headache or migraine, although occipital tenderness and allodynia may also be seen in migraine. Unilateral pain is typi-

Table 34.4 Diagnostic criteria for occipital neuralgia

A. Unilateral or bilateral pain in the distribution(s) of the greater, lesser, and/or third occipital nerves and fulfilling criteria B–D
B. Pain has at least two of the following three characteristics: 1. Recurring in paroxysmal attacks lasting from a few seconds to minutes 2. Severe in intensity 3. Shooting, stabbing, or sharp in quality
C. Pain is associated with both of the following 1. Dysesthesia and/or allodynia apparent during innocuous stimulation of the scalp and/or hair 2. Either or both of the following: (a) Tenderness over the affected nerve branches (b) Trigger points at the emergence of the greater occipital nerve or in the distribution of C2
D. Pain is eased temporarily by local anesthetic block of the affected nerve(s)
E. Not better accounted for by another ICHD-3 diagnosis

cal for ON and cervicogenic headache, while migraine may also be bilateral. Neck stiffness and decreased cervical range of motion are typical for cervicogenic headache, although this may also be observed in migraine. Even though response to greater occipital nerve (GON) infiltration is a diagnostic criterion for ON, this is not specific for ON since other headache disorders, such as cervicogenic headache, cluster headache, or even chronic migraine, may also respond [46].

Treatment of Occipital Neuralgia

ON is at least temporarily eased by nerve block, as mentioned above. A combination of local anesthetics and steroids can be used. Ultrasound-guided techniques have been proposed [47]. In our experience, GON infiltration based on anatomical landmarks as has been done in cluster headache [48] is also useful. Physical therapy and massage can be tried as additional treatment [44]. Treatment of ON includes medications against neuropathic pain, such as carbamazepine, oxcarbazepine, amitriptyline, gabapentin, pregabalin, or baclofen. In refractory cases, botulinum toxin applied to occipital cervical regions may also be useful according to a small case series [49]. Further, more invasive treatment options,

which should only be performed in experienced centers, include pulsed radiofrequency stimulation of the occipital nerve [49, 50], occipital nerve stimulation [51], or radiofrequency ablation of the C2 dorsal root ganglion or third occipital nerve [52].

Superior Laryngeal Neuralgia

This rare disorder features attacks of severe pain which radiate to the lateral aspect of the anterior neck and lasts seconds to minutes. Hoarseness and cough can also occur. Attacks are triggered by palpation of the superior laryngeal nerve when it enters the larynx and also by swallowing, talking, coughing, or yawning. Superior laryngeal neuralgia is caused by inflammation, upper respiratory infection, trauma, or surgery. Imaging of the neck region is mandatory to exclude serious disorders, such as pharyngeal carcinoma. Carbamazepine, gabapentin, amitriptyline, and nerve blocks with lidocaine are reported to be effective [26, 27].

References

1. Headache Classification Committee of the International Headache Society (IHS) the International Classification of Headache Disorders, 3rd edition. Cephalalgia. 2018;38(1):1–211.
2. Younis S, Maarbjerg S, Reimer M, Wolfram F, Olesen J, Baron R, et al. Quantitative sensory testing in classical trigeminal neuralgia-a blinded study in patients with and without concomitant persistent pain. Pain. 2016;157(7):1407–14.
3. Rozen TD, Capobianco DJ, Dalessio DJ. Cranial neuralgia and atypical facial pain. In: Silberstein SD, Lipton RB, Dalessio D, editors. Woff's headache. Oxford: Oxford University Press; 2001. p. 509–24.
4. Lambru G, Rantell K, O'Connor E, Levy A, Davagnanam I, Zrinzo L, et al. Trigeminal neurovascular contact in SUNCT and SUNA: a cross-sectional magnetic resonance study. Brain. 2020;143(12):3619–28.
5. Lambru G, Matharu MS. SUNCT, SUNA and trigeminal neuralgia: different disorders or variants of the same disorder? Curr Opin Neurol. 2014;27(3):325–31.
6. Bendtsen L, Zakrzewska JM, Heinskou TB, Hodaie M, Leal PRL, Nurmikko T, et al. Advances in diagnosis, classification, pathophysiology, and man-

agement of trigeminal neuralgia. Lancet Neurol. 2020;19(9):784–96.

7. Manzoni GC, Torelli P. Epidemiology of typical and atypical craniofacial neuralgias. Neurol Sci. 2005;26(Suppl 2):s65–7.

8. Maarbjerg S, Di Stefano G, Bendtsen L, Cruccu G. Trigeminal neuralgia—diagnosis and treatment. Cephalalgia. 2017;37(7):648–57.

9. Maarbjerg S, Wolfram F, Gozalov A, Olesen J, Bendtsen L. Significance of neurovascular contact in classical trigeminal neuralgia. Brain. 2015;138(Pt 2):311–9.

10. Bendtsen L, Zakrzewska JM, Abbott J, Braschinsky M, Di Stefano G, Donnet A, et al. European Academy of Neurology guideline on trigeminal neuralgia. Eur J Neurol. 2019;26(6):831–49.

11. International Classification of Orofacial Pain, 1st edition (ICOP). Cephalalgia. 2020;40(2):129–221.

12. Fujiwara S, Sasaki M, Wada T, Kudo K, Hirooka R, Ishigaki D, et al. High-resolution diffusion tensor imaging for the detection of diffusion abnormalities in the trigeminal nerves of patients with trigeminal neuralgia caused by neurovascular compression. J Neuroimaging. 2011;21(2):e102–8.

13. Obermann M, Rodriguez-Raecke R, Naegel S, Holle D, Mueller D, Yoon MS, et al. Gray matter volume reduction reflects chronic pain in trigeminal neuralgia. NeuroImage. 2013;74:352–8.

14. Nick ST, Roberts C, Billiodeaux S, Davis DE, Zamanifekri B, Sahraian MA, et al. Multiple sclerosis and pain. Neurol Res. 2012;34(9):829–41.

15. Gambeta E, Chichorro JG, Zamponi GW. Trigeminal neuralgia: an overview from pathophysiology to pharmacological treatments. Mol Pain. 2020;16:1744806920901890.

16. Andersen ASS, Heinskou TB, Asghar MS, Rossen B, Noory N, Smilkov EA, et al. Intravenous fosphenytoin as treatment for acute exacerbation of trigeminal neuralgia: a prospective systematic study of 15 patients. Cephalalgia. 2022;42:1138.

17. Munoz-Vendrell A, Teixidor S, Sala-Padro J, Campoy S, Huerta-Villanueva M. Intravenous lacosamide and phenytoin for the treatment of acute exacerbations of trigeminal neuralgia: a retrospective analysis of 144 cases. Cephalalgia. 2022;42:1031.

18. Morra ME, Elgebaly A, Elmaraezy A, Khalil AM, Altibi AM, Vu TL, et al. Therapeutic efficacy and safety of botulinum toxin A therapy in trigeminal neuralgia: a systematic review and meta-analysis of randomized controlled trials. J Headache Pain. 2016;17(1):63.

19. Kotecha M, Cheshire WP, Finnigan H, Giblin K, Naik H, Palmer J, et al. Design of phase 3 studies evaluating vixotrigine for treatment of trigeminal neuralgia. J Pain Res. 2020;13:1601–9.

20. Barker FG 2nd, Jannetta PJ, Bissonette DJ, Larkins MV, Jho HD. The long-term outcome of microvascular decompression for trigeminal neuralgia. N Engl J Med. 1996;334(17):1077–83.

21. Holste K, Chan AY, Rolston JD, Englot DJ. Pain outcomes following microvascular decompression for drug-resistant trigeminal neuralgia: a systematic review and meta-analysis. Neurosurgery. 2020;86(2):182–90.

22. Brinzeu A, Drogba L, Sindou M. Reliability of MRI for predicting characteristics of neurovascular conflicts in trigeminal neuralgia: implications for surgical decision making. J Neurosurg. 2018;1-11:1.

23. Sandell T, Eide PK. The effect of microvascular decompression in patients with multiple sclerosis and trigeminal neuralgia. Neurosurgery. 2010;67(3):749–53; discussion 53–4.

24. Tuleasca C, Regis J, Sahgal A, De Salles A, Hayashi M, Ma L, et al. Stereotactic radiosurgery for trigeminal neuralgia: a systematic review. J Neurosurg. 2018;130(3):733–57.

25. Spacek A, Bohm D, Kress HG. Ganglionic local opioid analgesia for refractory trigeminal neuralgia. Lancet. 1997;349(9064):1521.

26. O'Neill F, Nurmikko T, Sommer C. Other facial neuralgias. Cephalalgia. 2017;37(7):658–69.

27. Wilhour D, Nahas SJ. The neuralgias. Curr Neurol Neurosci Rep. 2018;18(10):69.

28. Smith JH, Cutrer FM. Numbness matters: a clinical review of trigeminal neuropathy. Cephalalgia. 2011;31(10):1131–44.

29. Attal N, Bouhassira D. Advances in the treatment of neuropathic pain. Curr Opin Neurol. 2021;34(5):631–7.

30. Forbes HJ, Thomas SL, Smeeth L, Clayton T, Farmer R, Bhaskaran K, et al. A systematic review and meta-analysis of risk factors for postherpetic neuralgia. Pain. 2016;157(1):30–54.

31. Hadley GR, Gayle JA, Ripoll J, Jones MR, Argoff CE, Kaye RJ, et al. Post-herpetic neuralgia: a review. Curr Pain Headache Rep. 2016;20(3):17.

32. Blumenfeld A, Nikolskaya G. Glossopharyngeal neuralgia. Curr Pain Headache Rep. 2013;17(7):343.

33. Kahle W, Leonhardt H, Platzer W. Brain stem and cranial nerves. In: Kahle W, editor. Color atlas and textbook of human anatomy, Nervous system and sensory organs, G. Thieme; 1976. p. 110–1. ISBN 10: 0815149662ISBN 13: 9780815149668.

34. Zheng W, Zhao P, Song H, Liu B, Zhou J, Fan C, et al. Prognostic factors for long-term outcomes of microvascular decompression in the treatment of glossopharyngeal neuralgia: a retrospective analysis of 97 patients. J Neurosurg. 2021:1–8. https://doi.org/10.3171/2021.9.JNS21877.

35. Badhey A, Jategaonkar A, Kovacs AJA, et al. Eagle syndrome: A comprehensive review. Clinical Neurology and Neurosurgery. 2017: 159:34–38.

36. Liu Q, Zhong Q, Tang G, He G. Ultrasound-guided glossopharyngeal nerve block via the styloid process for glossopharyngeal neuralgia: a retrospective study. J Pain Res. 2019;12:2503–10.

37. Kabil MS, Eby JB, Shahinian HK. Endoscopic vascular decompression versus microvascular decom-

pression of the trigeminal nerve. Minim Invasive Neurosurg. 2005;48(4):207–12.

38. Li Y, Mao F, Cheng F, Peng C, Guo D, Wang B. A meta-analysis of endoscopic microvascular decompression versus microscopic microvascular decompression for the treatment for cranial nerve syndrome caused by vascular compression. World Neurosurg. 2019;126:647–655.e7.

39. Lara-Almunia M, Moreno NEM, Sarraga JG, Alvarez RM. Gamma knife radiosurgery and refractory glossopharyngeal neuralgia: a single-center series with long-term follow-up. Neurosurg Rev. 2022;45(1):525–31.

40. Robblee J. A pain in the ear: two case reports of nervus intermedius neuralgia and narrative review. Headache. 2021;61(3):414–21.

41. Patel I, Desai D, Desai S. Red ear syndrome: case series and review of a less recognized headache disorder. Ann Indian Acad Neurol. 2020;23(5):715–8.

42. Hunt JR. On herpetic inflammations of the geniculate ganglion. A new syndrome and its complications. Arch Neurol. 1968;18(5):584–9.

43. Ananthapadmanabhan S, Soodin D, Sritharan N, Sivapathasingam V. Ramsay Hunt syndrome with multiple cranial neuropathy: a literature review. Eur Arch Otorhinolaryngol. 2022;279(5):2239–44.

44. Pan W, Peng J, Elmofty D. Occipital neuralgia. Curr Pain Headache Rep. 2021;25(9):61.

45. Ballesteros-Del Rio B, Ares-Luque A, Tejada-Garcia J, Muela-Molinero A. Occipital (Arnold) neuralgia secondary to greater occipital nerve schwannoma. Headache. 2003;43(7):804–7.

46. Gomez R, Frenandez R, Guttierez J, Perez J, Verduras MJ, Sanchez P, et al. [Use of microporous-expanded polytetrafluoroethylene (PTFE) in systemic-pulmonary shunts in infants]. Ann Chir. 1983;37(2):169–74.

47. Pingree MJ, Sole JS, O'Brien TG, Eldrige JS, Moeschler SM. Clinical efficacy of an ultrasound-guided greater occipital nerve block at the level of C2. Reg Anesth Pain Med. 2017;42(1):99–104.

48. Gantenbein AR, Lutz NJ, Riederer F, Sandor PS. Efficacy and safety of 121 injections of the greater occipital nerve in episodic and chronic cluster headache. Cephalalgia. 2012;32(8):630–4.

49. Wamsley CE, Chung M, Amirlak B. Occipital neuralgia: advances in the operative management. Neurol India. 2021;69(Suppl):S219–S27.

50. Orhurhu V, Huang L, Quispe RC, Khan F, Karri J, Urits I, et al. Use of radiofrequency ablation for the management of headache: a systematic review. Pain Physician. 2021;24(7):E973–E87.

51. Keifer OP Jr, Diaz A, Campbell M, Bezchlibnyk YB, Boulis NM. Occipital nerve stimulation for the treatment of refractory occipital neuralgia: a case series. World Neurosurg. 2017;105:599–604.

52. Hamer JF, Purath TA. Response of cervicogenic headaches and occipital neuralgia to radiofrequency ablation of the C2 dorsal root ganglion and/or third occipital nerve. Headache. 2014;54(3):500–10.

Bullet Points
- Hallucinations occur in the general population as well as in patients with psychiatric disorders. When examining patients with auditory, visual, gustatory, or olfactory hallucinations, it might be challenging for the clinician to discern those two.
- Because the said modalities of sensual hallucinations concern the areas (imitate the function?) of some cranial nerves, it is important to know what defines a functional (neurological) and a psychiatric disorder.
- This chapter aims to give an overview regarding occurrence, characteristics, and differential diagnoses of hallucinations corresponding to cranial nerves.

Introduction

Hallucinations are a sensory experience without an external stimulus and can occur in the modalities of all five senses. Auditory, visual, olfactory, gustatory, tactile (haptic), and cenesthetic (visceral) hallucinations are described, with auditory being the most common [1]. The DSM-IV criteria describe hallucination as "sensory perception that has the compelling sense of reality of a true perception but that occurs without external stimulation of the relevant sensory organ" [2].

There are ongoing debates about the origin of the word hallucination. It might derive from the Latin verb *(h)allucinere*, meaning "to wander in mind," the term first being used by the English physician Thomas Brown in 1642 [2]. In the nineteenth century, the understanding of this sensual phenomenon changed due to a new understanding of nature and natural processes and the catTegorization of phenomena in different scientific areas. Hallucinations were no longer loaded with religious beliefs and ascribed transcendental functions, but were considered a disorder of perception. The class of these now medicalized and pathological phenomena was termed hallucinations and seen as an entity itself [3]. The French psychiatrist Jean-Étienne Dominique Esquirol (1772–1840) stated that a hallucination is a "form of delirium that makes patients believe they have a perception" and tried to explain the phenomenon within an intellectual misleading of the mind. According to another French psychiatrist Jean-Pierre Falret (1794–1870), "the hallucination is a perception without object, as has been often repeated." The German psychiatrist Wilhelm Griesinger (1817–1868) explained hallucinations as the external projection of internal images, which then seem to exist in reality [4]. In the

Author of this chapter: Simon Grisold.

twentieth century, other models of explanation were developed. Hallucinations were regarded as a form of delusion, and thus perception disturbance, caused by unconscious processes or anatomical and biochemical changes.

The phenomenon of hallucinations continues to be puzzling and hard to pin down, because it is not possible to describe them in an objective manner due to the subjective experience and reports of hallucinating people.

Prevalence

In general, the most common hallucinations are auditory followed by visual, olfactory, and gustatory. Data regarding the prevalence of hallucinations vary greatly. "Hearing voices" is described to be the most common both in patient and general population. It is estimated that up to 85% of healthy individuals have experienced persecutory hallucinations and 15% have heard voices throughout their lifetime [5]. Others suggest that the prevalence is up to 28% in the general population.

Hearing voices or auditory verbal hallucinations (AVH) are very common in psychiatric patients with schizophrenia (75%), bipolar disorder (20–50%), major depression (10%), and posttraumatic stress disorder (PTSD) (up to 40%). The prevalence ranges from 5% to 16% [6] in children and adolescents.

So-called pseudo-hallucinations occur in people without mental illness with a lifetime prevalence of about 10% in men and 15% in women [2]. They occur in times of psychological distress and emotional crisis in otherwise healthy individuals and seem to have a functional quality. In contrast to hallucinations with schizophrenia, they are experienced as internal and part of the person. Some patients afflicted by psychiatric diseases, such as PTSD or borderline personality disorder, are more likely to experience pseudo-hallucinations [7]. It is argued that the term pseudo-hallucinations might be misleading, meaning "false–false perception" and thus being illogical. The term might imply that the patients' complaints about hearing voices are not real or the patients might be lying [8].

In this chapter, characteristics, such as frequency, appearance, quality, possible causes, and association with organic diseases of hallucinations, will be discussed.

Auditory Hallucinations

Auditory hallucinations are the most common hallucinations and appear in the patient as well as the general population. The average prevalence of "hearing voices" might be around 13%, ranging widely from 0.6% to 84% in the general population [9]. It is thus important to emphasize that auditory hallucinations are not necessarily linked with psychiatric disorders. However, the association in mental diseases, such as schizophrenia, bipolar disorder, or major depression, is strong. Up to 74% of patients with schizophrenia report about hearing voices in their medical history [2].

As AVH appear in the patient as well as the general population, it is important to look at differences regarding appearance and quality. The most significant factor in discerning the voices is the negative content of the verbal hallucinations and the psychic stress associated with them. AVH in a healthy population are referred to as neutral or even pleasant in quality and positive in content [9]. Alternatively, the content of AVH in patients with schizophrenia is described as threatening and menacing, derogatory, or persecutory. Patients are hearing accusations, threats, commands, or personal comments on their actions or themselves. Naturally, this leads to negative emotions and distress, arouses anger, anxiety, and frustration and impedes social functioning and everyday life [5]. The voices are said to be intrusive, unwanted, and uncontrollable and are localized outside the head [10]. A key feature of AVH in patients is the negative value and the emotional distress they cause. The most common kind of auditory hallucinations is hearing voices followed by unintelligible sounds, such as whispering and murmuring or distant footsteps.

Performing the clinical examination, some information could be helpful to differentiate between clinical psychotic and nonclinical AVH. Voices speaking in third person are twofold higher in the patient than in the non-patient group, whereas the latter can control the voices up to 87% of the time compared to a maximum of 20% in patients. The duration in the healthy population is about 2–3 min, which is much shorter compared with 40 min in affected patients. As mentioned, the types of voices are demeaning and commenting to a higher degree (up to 72%) in patients, leading to a massive disturbance of daily functioning. The emotional valence of the AVH in patients is unpleasant and distressing, causing anxiety and anger, whereas in population with nonclinical AVH between 4% and 53% do have negative content. Characteristically, voices have a strong effect on patients and can be frightening and trigger depression, anger, or anxiety and strong emotional responses [11].

Organic diseases could also be a reason for auditory hallucinations. For example, *Toxoplasmosis gondii* may cause auditory hallucinations or other symptoms of psychosis. It is estimated that about 15,000 cases of new psychosis in the USA are caused by an infection with toxoplasmosis, the symptoms besides auditory hallucinations being mostly affective disorders [12]. Other possible organic causes of auditory hallucinations to be considered include anti-NMDA-R encephalitis, leucine-rich glioma-inactivated 1 (LGI1) encephalitis, or neuropsychiatric systemic lupus erythematosus (NPSLE) [13].

Visual Hallucinations

Visual hallucinations often are related to organic causes. Organic disorders may include neurodegenerative diseases, such as Alzheimer's disease, intoxication with drugs, alcohol, or other toxic agents, structural brain lesions (e.g., due to a cerebral tumor), delirium tremens, or other systemic diseases, such as infections or hormonal changes [5].

Visual hallucinations occur with schizophrenia in up to 72% of patients and may be an indicator for a more severe state of disease or psychosis [14]. Vivid scenes with relatives, friends, or animals (usually normally sized) are typical. On the contrary, in delirium, figures and persons are also seen, but they are described as much smaller than the patient and seem to be busily working (Lilliputian hallucination) [15]. Other visual hallucinations could include parts of people (faces, heads), streaks of light or color, shadows, and distortions of the world [5].

Various neurological diseases might at some time be associated with characteristic visual hallucinations. In delirium, they occur in up to 27% and show unpleasant hallucinations, like crawling insects (zoopsia), or neutral or pleasant ones, like Lilliputian distortion [16]. They are an index for the severity of delirium, and the probability is much higher if a somatic diagnosis exists or some substance abuse is recorded [14]. The hallucinations usually appear within 3 days after the last alcohol consummation [17]. Around 20% of patients with dementia with Lewy bodies (DLB) hallucinate complex scenarios, including vivid scenes of people, animals, and inanimate objects, which might be an important clue for the clinician, while up to 50% of patients with Parkinson's disease might also visualize delicately shaped figures, animals, or objects [14].

Visual hallucinations in combination with epileptic seizures are well known and described. Their quality is that of color–light phenomena and often described as spots, indistinct shapes, or shadows [14]. The visual hallucinations in focal epilepsy are described as "brief, stereotyped and fragmentary" [18].

Another example for a genuine neurological disease with visual hallucinations or visual symptoms is migraine. Here, a prodromal aura might appear as blurring of the vision, photophobia, the sensation of falling snow, zigzag lines, flashes of light, or difficulties in face recognition which may be a kind of prosopagnosia [18–20].

The Heidenhain variant of Creutzfeldt–Jakob disease (CJD) is associated with a wide range of visual symptoms, such as changes in perception of color, visual impairment, distortion of proportions, and vivid visual hallucinations [14, 21]. It might look similar to Charles Bonnet syndrome, with visual impairment and images of living figures; however, patients with Bonnet syndrome are aware of reality and no other psychopathology can be described [5].

Drugs or toxic agents might also be a cause for visual hallucinations. This was first described for digitalis in 1901 [22, 23], but could also be caused by different drugs, such as rasagiline, zolpidem, methylphenidat, baclofen, ertapenem, or valacyclovir [24].

Olfactory Hallucinations

Olfactory hallucinations are olfactory perceptions without a chemical stimulus (phantosmia). It is described to occur in the Norwegian general population in around 4–54% in combination with hallucinations in other modalities [25].

Olfactory hallucinations are strongly associated with psychiatric conditions, such as schizophrenia (11–83%) or major depressive disorder (19–33%). About 25% of patients with major depressive disorder describe the so-called olfactory reference syndrome, i.e., they perceive a foul odor emanating from parts of their body or the skin [26]. Other sensations might be the smell of rotting meat, garbage, or feces, often occurring in combination [5].

In general, olfactory hallucinations seem to be associated with different kinds of psychological distress, with or without a concomitant psychiatric disease. The hallucinations of patients with an uncinated epileptic fit are brief and accompanied by other symptoms of a seizure. They are also described as stereotypical, meaning the perceived odor is always the same [27]. Brief olfactory sensations may also occur as an aura shortly before the seizure and are often accompanied with sensations in other modalities (visual, gustatory, and autonomic). Other neurological conditions with olfactory hallucinations include traumatic brain injury, multiple sclerosis, or Parkinson's disease.

Gustatory Hallucinations

Gustatory hallucinations are the least frequent after auditory, visual, and olfactory hallucinations. They might occur in the general population or in the patient population in combination with psychiatric disorders. Gustatory hallucinations can be divided into ageusia which is the inability to experience tastes, hypogeusia which is the reduced ability to experience tastes, and dysgeusia which is a different perception of tastes. Data about the incidence is scarce and ranges from 0.5% to 4% in the general population and between 11% and 38% in patients with schizoaffective disorder [28]. Gustatory hallucinations might occur in healthy people or as secondary symptoms related to organic diseases, such as brain tumors or temporal lobe epilepsy, misuse of substances and drugs, or in psychotic conditions. Tactile, olfactory, and gustatory hallucination (TOGH) seems to be associated with male gender, severe mental illness like schizophrenia, and black ethnicity [28].

Rare Diseases

There are rare syndromes with hallucinations in psychiatry and neurology which do not fit into classical diagnostic schemes. Relevant for this chapter are the Charles Bonnet syndrome, musical hallucinosis, or olfactory reference syndrome [29].

Charles Bonnet Syndrome

First described by Charles Bonnet in 1860, this syndrome with visual hallucinations can be noticed in elderly patients with ocular pathology and visual impairment. Cognitive functions are not impaired, and the patients recognize the visual hallucinations as unreal and located in external space [30]. It is important to notice that there is no underlying organic, neurological, or psychiatric cause to explain these phenomena. The mean age of onset is 81 years, with male gender being affected more frequently. The hallucinations may occur suddenly in full intensity or develop slowly from simple forms to elaborate scenes. The visual hallucinations include human figures, animals, or flowers and they might be colorful or monochromatic.

Musical Hallucinations

Musical hallucinations can appear in various forms, from whole songs to single musical instruments. Female gender, left-sided hearing impairment, and age over 60 years increase the probability. The hallucinations seem to be associated with depression, anxiety, or bipolar disorder and thus might be interesting for psychiatry [30]. There might also be organic causes, like neurodegenerative disorders, seizures, and encephalitis. With dementia, they most frequently occur in Lewy body dementia followed by Parkinson's dementia. Psychiatric diseases, like depression or psychosis, could also be associated with musical hallucinations.

Olfactory Reference Syndrome

In 1971, Pryse-Phillips described a condition where patients believed that a smell or foul odor emanates from their skin and bodies [30]. In reaction, they take actions against it, such as excessive showering or washing or changing their clothes very frequently. In olfactory reference syndrome, no neurological or psychiatric condition can explain the phenomenon. The belief that one emanates an unpleasant and offending smell leads from social awkwardness to impairments in daily life and finally to social withdrawal, all causing strong emotional distress. The afflicted live in constant fear of social rejection, are sure to lose their social standing, and constantly are afraid of being judged by others. The age of onset is around 20 years, with males being afflicted more frequently. The smell is most frequently perceived as coming from the mouth, armpits, or genitals and is either described as unspecific, such as foul and bad, or quite distinct, such as garbage gases, burning fish, or cigarettes. Olfactory reference syndrome is associated with low mood and anxiety. The risk for suicide is increased because of the massive impairment, problems in social functioning, social withdrawal, and social avoidance.

Conclusion

In summary, the occurrence of hallucinations might be challenging for general physicians, neurologists, or even psychiatrists. It is important to know that they occur in the general healthy population as well as in patients with psychiatric or organic disorders. Exploring the medical and psychiatric history, conducting a thorough examination, and assessing the present psychopathological state are crucial for differentiating between organic and psychiatric causes.

When exploring hallucinations, it is also crucial to assess their quality and concomitant affective states and reactions. Patients tend to react to the hallucinations, especially because they often seem to have a frightening quality. Conversations with hallucinations or verbal reactions, like yelling or shouting, can be tell-tale signs for an organic hallucinosis. Patients with schizophrenia hearing voices often try to pinpoint the source of the voices, sometimes also mumbling or muttering. The assumed cause for the voices or other auditory hallucinations is typically external.

Visual hallucinations are mostly associated with organic cerebral dysfunction (e.g., Alzheimer's disease, Lewy body dementia, intoxication). The hallucinations occur in combination with other pathognomonic symptoms of dementia or organic cerebral dysfunction.

Auditory or visual hallucinations in schizophrenia are associated with strong emotional responses, like fear, anger, or agitation, and do not occur isolated. Auditory hallucinations might also occur in affective disorders, such as schizoaffective, bipolar, or depressive disorder. It is important to check the anamnesis of family history, previous psychotic episodes, and former psychiatric treatment.

Olfactory and gustatory occur quite rarely, and rare diseases, such as Charles Bonnet syndrome or olfactory reference syndrome, should be considered.

References

1. Linszen MMJ, de Boer JN, Schutte MJL, Begemann MJH, de Vries J, Koops S, Blom RE, Bohlken MM, Heringa SM, Blom JD, Sommer IEC. Occurrence and phenomenology of hallucinations in the general population: a large online survey. Schizophrenia (Heidelb). 2022;8(1):41.
2. Choong C, Hunter MD, Woodruff PW. Auditory hallucinations in those populations that do not suffer from schizophrenia. Curr Psychiatry Rep. 2007;9(3):206–12.
3. Berrios GE. On the fantastic apparitions of vision by Johannes Müller. Hist Psychiatry. 2005;16(2):229–46.
4. Telles-Correia D, Moreira AL, Gonçalves JS. Hallucinations and related concepts—their conceptual background. Front Psychol. 2015;6:991.
5. Kaplan HI, Sadock BJ, editors. Kaplan & Sadock's comprehensive textbook of psychiatry, vol. 1. 10th ed. Wolters Kluwer; 2017.
6. Thakur T, Gupta V. Auditory hallucinations. In: StatPearls. Treasure Island, FL: StatPearls Publishing; 2022.
7. Mustafa FA. Pseudohallucinations as functional cognitive disorders. Lancet Psychiatry. 2020;7(3):230.
8. Poole R, Higgo R. Psychiatric interviewing and assessment. 2nd ed. Cambridge: Cambridge University Press; 2017.
9. Johns LC, Kompus K, Connell M, Humpston C, Lincoln TM, Longden E, Preti A, Alderson-Day B, Badcock JC, Cella M, Fernyhough C, McCarthy-Jones S, Peters E, Raballo A, Scott J, Siddi S, Sommer IE, Larøi F. Auditory verbal hallucinations in persons with and without a need for care. Schizophr Bull. 2014;40(Suppl 4):S255–64.
10. Hugdahl K. Auditory hallucinations: a review of the ERC "VOICE" project. World J Psychiatry. 2015;5(2):193–209.
11. De Leede-Smith S, Barkus E. A comprehensive review of auditory verbal hallucinations: lifetime prevalence, correlates and mechanisms in healthy and clinical individuals. Front Hum Neurosci. 2013;16(7):367.
12. Fuller Torrey E. Parasites, pussycats and psychosis: the unknown dangers of human toxoplasmosis. Springer; 2022.
13. Khandaker G, Harrison N, Dantzer R, editors. Textbook of immunopsychiatry. University of Texas, MD Anderson Cancer Center, Cambridge University Press; 2021.
14. Teeple RC, Caplan JP, Stern TA. Visual hallucinations: differential diagnosis and treatment. Prim Care Companion J Clin Psychiatry. 2009;11(1):26–32.
15. Semple D, Smyth R. Oxford handbook of psychiatry. Oxford University Press; 2019.
16. Ffytche DH. Visual hallucinatory syndromes: past, present, and future. Dialogues Clin Neurosci. 2007;9(2):173–89.
17. Brust JCM. Handbook of clinical neurology. Elsevier; 2014.
18. Gillig PM, Sanders RD. Cranial nerve II: vision. Psychiatry (Edgmont). 2009;6(9):32–7.
19. van Dongen RM, Haan J: Symptoms related to the visual system in migraine. F1000Res. 2019;8. https://doi.org/10.12688/f1000research.18768.1
20. Yetkin-Ozden S, Ekizoglu E, Baykan B. Face recognition in patients with migraine. Pain Pract. 2015;15(4):319–22.
21. Miranda GP, Bolaños AA. A case of Heidenhain variant of Creutzfeldt-Jakob disease mimicking a Charles Bonnet syndrome. J Geriatr Med Gerontol. 2021;7:120.
22. Closson RG. Visual hallucinations as the earliest symptom of digoxin intoxication. Arch Neurol. 1983;40(6):386.
23. Volpe BT, Soave R. Formed visual hallucinations as digitalis toxicity. Ann Intern Med. 1979;91(6):865–6.
24. Abou Taam M, de Boissieu P, Abou Taam R, Breton A, Trenque T. Drug-induced hallucination: a case/non case study in the French Pharmacovigilance Database. Eur J Psychiat. 2015;29(1):21–31.
25. Wehling E, Bless JJ, Hirnstein M, Kråkvik B, Vedul-Kjelsås E, Hugdahl K, Kalhovde AM, Larøi F. Olfactory hallucinations in a population-based sample. Psychiatry Res. 2021;304:114117.
26. Henkin RI, Potolicchio SJ, Levy LM. Olfactory hallucinations without clinical motor activity: a comparison of unirhinal with birhinal phantosmia. Brain Sci. 2013;3(4):1483–553.
27. Moini J, Piran P, editors. Functional and clinical neuroanatomy: limbic, olfactory, and gustatory systems. Elsevier; 2019. p. 467–495 (Chapter 15).
28. Birnie KI, Stewart R, Kolliakou A. Recorded atypical hallucinations in psychotic and affective disorders and associations with non-benzodiazepine hypnotic use: the South London and Maudsley Case Register. BMJ Open. 2018;8(9):e025216.
29. Oyebode F. Psychopathology of rare and unusual syndromes. RCPsych Publications; 2021.
30. Pang L. Hallucinations experienced by visually impaired: Charles Bonnet syndrome. Optom Vis Sci. 2016;93(12):1466–78.

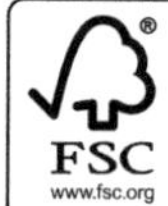

If you have any concerns about our products,
you can contact us on
ProductSafety@springernature.com

In case Publisher is established outside the EU,
the EU authorized representative is:
Springer Nature Customer Service Center GmbH
Europaplatz 3, 69115 Heidelberg, Germany

Printed by Libri Plureos GmbH
in Hamburg, Germany